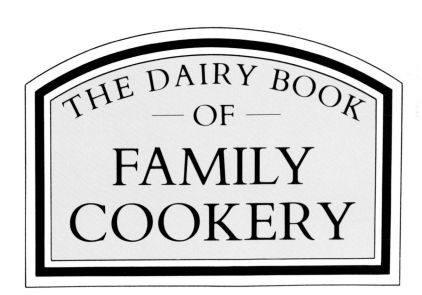

THE DAIRY BOOK
— OF —
FAMILY
COOKERY

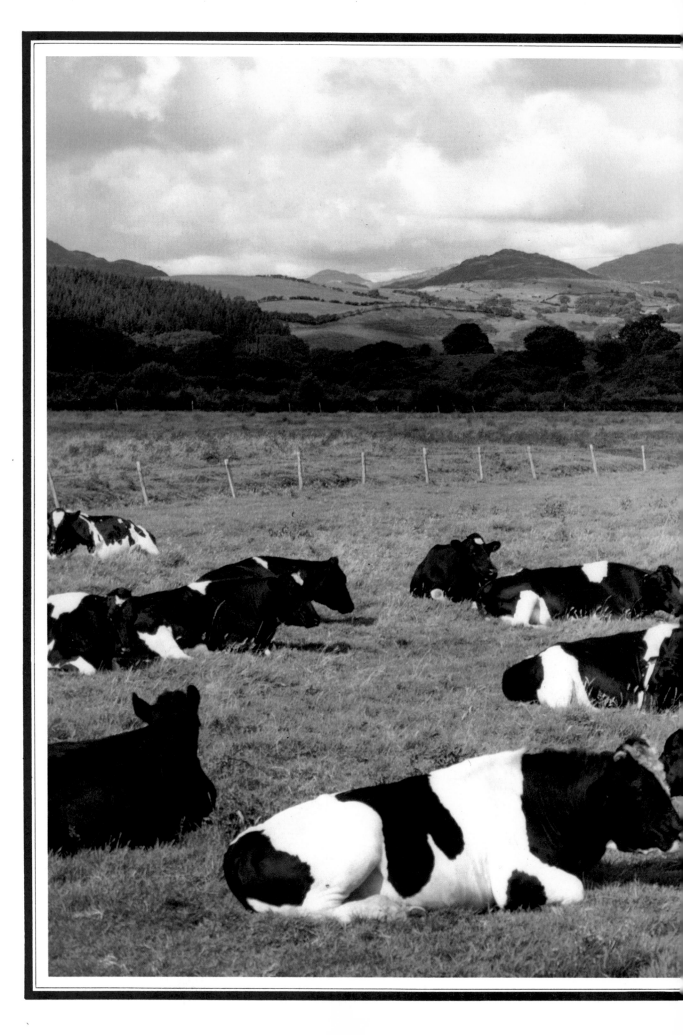

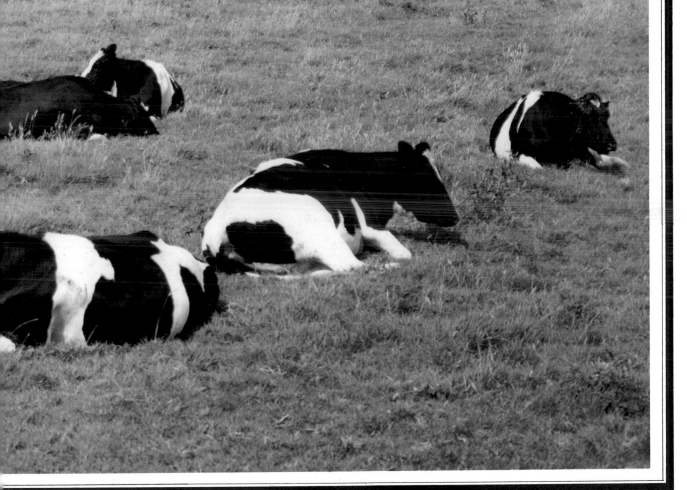

THE DAIRY BOOK
— OF —
FAMILY
COOKERY

OVER 700 RECIPES FOR EVERY OCCASION

THIS EDITION PUBLISHED BY DOLPHIN PUBLICATIONS
PUBLISHED BY ARRANGEMENT WITH EBURY PRESS
AN IMPRINT OF RANDOM HOUSE UK
20 VAUXHALL BRIDGE ROAD, LONDON SW1V 2SA
ON BEHALF OF THE MILK MARKETING BOARD

ISBN 0 09 177811 5

EDITOR: ALEXANDRA ARTLEY
CHIEF HOME ECONOMIST: SUSANNA TEE
DESIGNERS: BOB HOOK AND IVOR CLAYDON
FOOD PHOTOGRAPHY: MELVIN GREY, PAUL KEMP (INCLUDING COVER),
AND PAUL WILLIAMS
STEP-BY-STEP ILLUSTRATIONS: RAY BURROWS

HISTORICAL AND TECHNICAL DATA: JACQUI HURST; THE MUSEUM OF RURAL
LIFE; UNIVERSITY OF READING; FINE ART PHOTOGRAPHS; THE MARY EVANS
PICTURE LIBRARY; RICHARD GREEN GALLERIES, LONDON; FOTOBANK
INTERNATIONAL COLOUR LIBRARY; BRIDGEMAN ART LIBRARY; FOTOMAS INDEX;
THE MANSELL COLLECTION

THE PUBLISHERS WOULD ALSO LIKE TO THANK THE DAIRY PRODUCE ADVISORY
SERVICE, MILK MARKETING BOARD FOR THEIR HELP IN COMPILING RECIPES AND
ALSO COVENT GARDEN KITCHEN SUPPLIES, DIVERTIMENTI AND DAVID MELLOR
FOR THEIR HELP IN PROVIDING ACCESSORIES FOR PHOTOGRAPHY

FILMSET, PRINTED AND BOUND BY JARROLD PRINTING, NORWICH

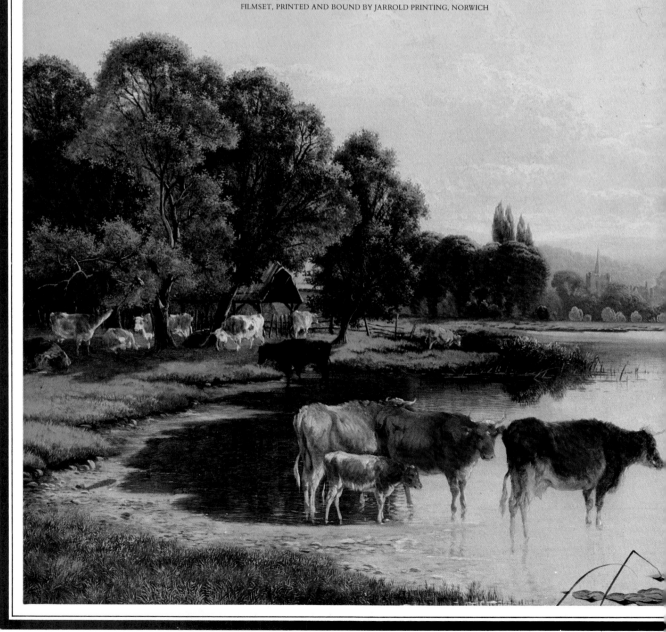

—CONTENTS—

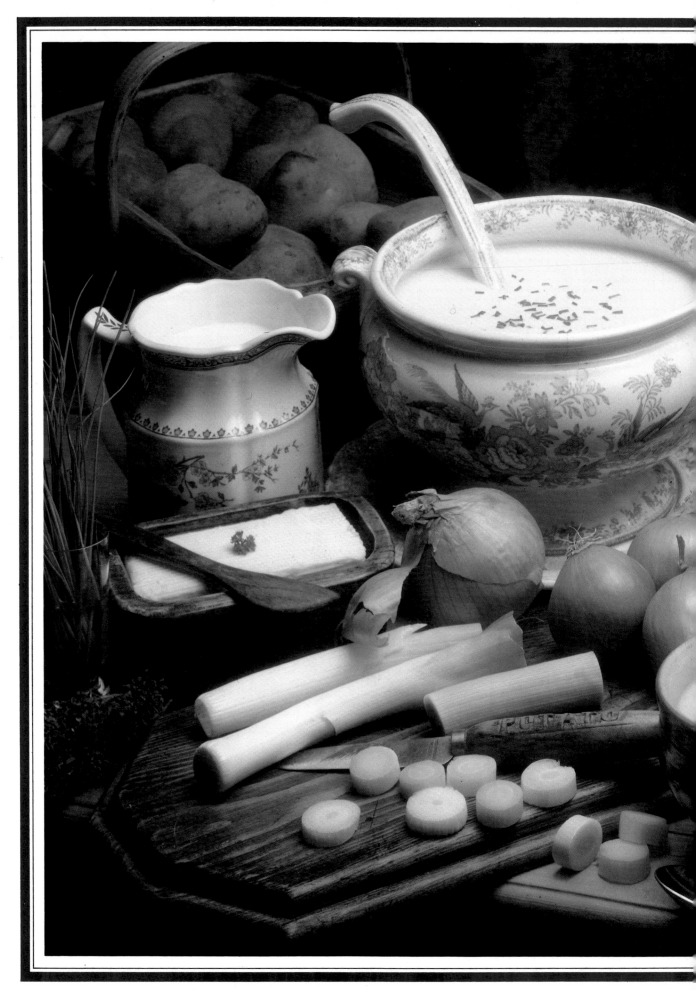

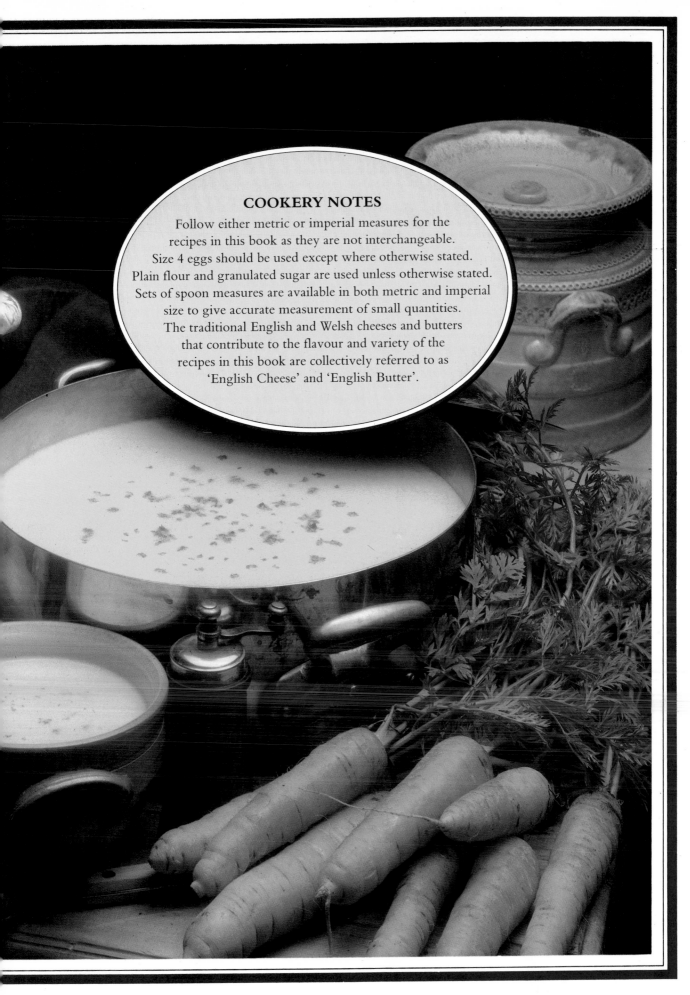

COOKERY NOTES

Follow either metric or imperial measures for the
recipes in this book as they are not interchangeable.
Size 4 eggs should be used except where otherwise stated.
Plain flour and granulated sugar are used unless otherwise stated.
Sets of spoon measures are available in both metric and imperial
size to give accurate measurement of small quantities.
The traditional English and Welsh cheeses and butters
that contribute to the flavour and variety of the
recipes in this book are collectively referred to as
'English Cheese' and 'English Butter'.

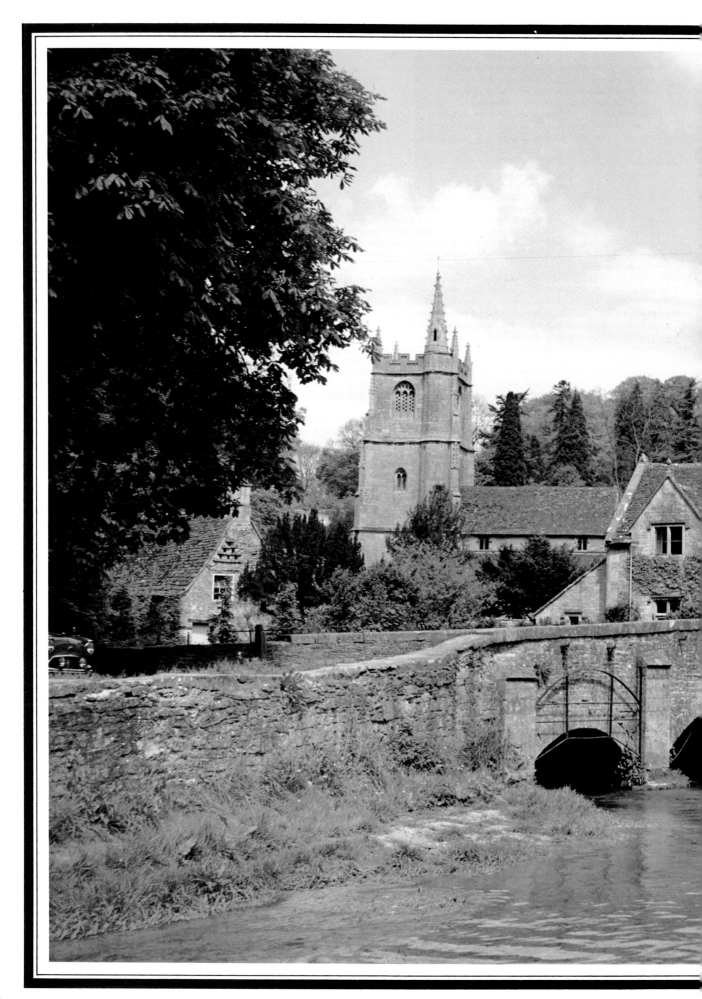

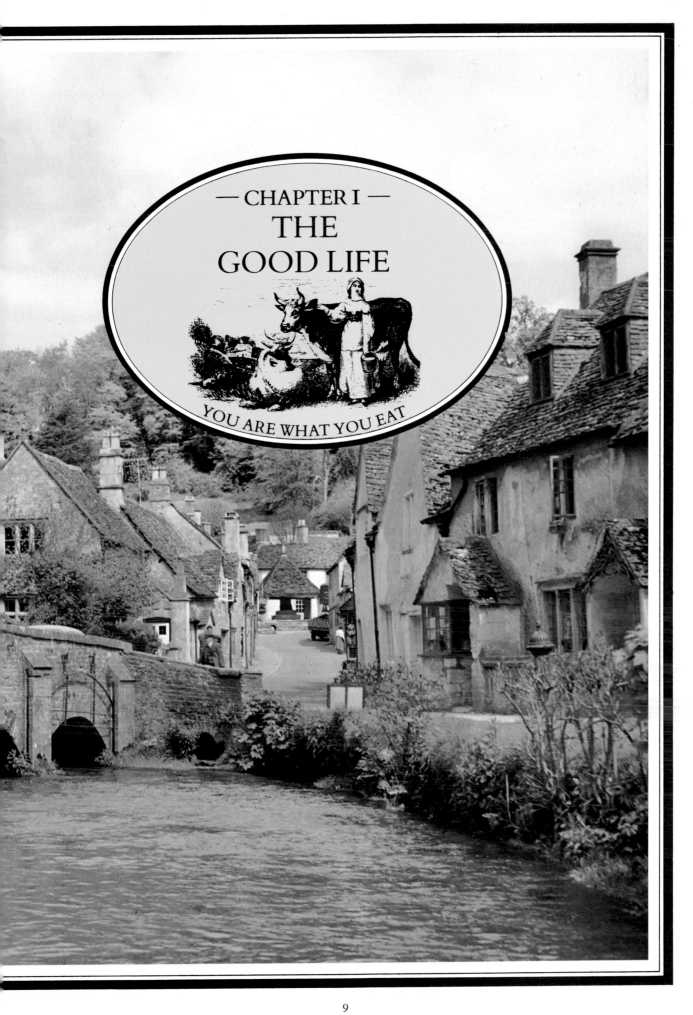

— CHAPTER I —
THE
GOOD LIFE

YOU ARE WHAT YOU EAT

It is often said you are what you eat. This makes sense because your body depends on a regular supply of food to grow and keep healthy.

When it comes to choosing a healthy diet and enjoying food, variety really is the spice of life. Eat mainly sweet or fried foods and you're likely to overload your system with sugar, fat or salt. Fail to eat plenty of cereal based foods, fresh fruit and vegetables, you'll go short on fibre and some vitamins too.

Luckily, good nutrition is not as complicated as it may sound. The *Wheel of Food* below has been designed to take the hard work out of choosing a healthy diet. It groups foods according to their nutritional value. Simply choose *different* foods from *each* group every day. Quantity is important too, so use the size of the segments in the Wheel to guide you. Reading the sections that follow will tell you more about the nutrients we need, their role and the foods that provide them.

Eating healthily does not mean any food has to be avoided, although you may find you need to eat some of your 'favourites' less often or in smaller portions. It certainly shouldn't lead to a boring diet.

EAT WISELY, EAT WELL

Most foods contain a range of nutrients, in varying amounts; so when, for example, we talk of 'protein' foods, we don't mean they contain nothing but

THE WHEEL OF FOOD AND GOOD HEALTH

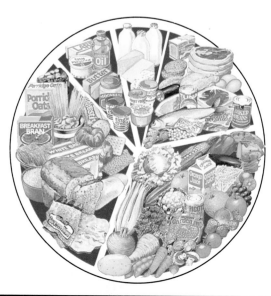

protein, rather that of all the nutrients they contain, protein is present in a significant amount. Below we list the nutrients found in the food and drink available today.

Protein must be first digested and then it can be used to form the frame-work of our bodies – muscle and bone, hormones such as insulin and the many enzymes that keep our bodies working efficiently. Protein is rarely lacking in the British diet and in fact most of us eat more than enough. Milk, cheese, meat, poultry, eggs and fish are the best known sources, but it is also found in yogurt, bread and cereal foods, pulses such as baked beans and lentils, and nuts, which can all be used to bring interest to the daily round of meals.

Fat is a concentrated source of energy present in varying amounts in most foods except fruit and vegetables. It adds flavour and texture to food. Fat can be 'hidden' as in lean meat, pâté and processed meats, cheese and chocolate, or 'visible' as in spreading and cooking fats, oils, streaky bacon or fat around meat.

Carbohydrate is another source of energy. In bread, potatoes and pulses it is found as starch and is accompanied by important nutrients. As sugar itself, or in foods and drinks with a predominantly sweet taste, it rarely brings many nutrients with it.

Alcohol is not really a nutrient but is an often forgotten source of energy. A pint of lager or a couple of gin and tonics is fast approaching 200 calories.

Fibre isn't really a nutrient either, but it does play an important role in keeping the digestive system functioning properly. Fibre is found in bread and cereals, particularly wholegrain, pulses, fresh fruits and vegetables.

Calcium along with Vitamin D is essential for all age groups for the development and maintenance of strong teeth and bones. Major sources in the UK diet are milk, cheese, yogurt and white bread.

Iron prevents anaemia and ensures healthy blood. It is important that children, adolescents and women of child-bearing age get enough iron. Meat, liver and kidneys are excellent sources. Iron is also present in eggs, bread, pulses, leafy vegetables and cocoa. The body absorbs the iron in these more readily if a food rich in Vitamin C is eaten at the same meal.

Vitamin A and **Carotene** promote healthy skin and eyes. They can be found in carrots, liver, milk, hard cheese, butter and fortified spreading fats, leafy vegetables and tomatoes.

Vitamin B complex is important for general good health. The most well known B vitamins are – thiamin (B_1), riboflavin (B_2), nicotinic acid, folic acid and B_{12}. This range of vitamins is found in milk, cheese, yogurt, meat, offal and cereals.

Vitamin C is essential for growth and rapid healing. No one is really sure if it helps to prevent or cure colds. It is found in citrus fruits, fresh and canned soft fruits, potatoes, cauliflower, swede and leafy vegetables. It should be remembered that overcooking destroys Vitamin C, as does contact with the air on cut surfaces, so prepare your vegetables just before cooking, do not soak them, always add them to boiling water and cook them in the minimum of water for the shortest length of time. Finally, serve cooked vegetables as soon as they're done. That way, they'll not only do you more good, they'll taste better too.

Vitamin D is important for the formation of strong bones and teeth and is found in oily fish, liver and fortified spreading fats. It is also formed in the body by the action of summer sun on the skin.

Using the Wheel of Food it *is* possible to plan a balanced diet easily and to ensure that all your family will benefit. You can also see how valuable milk, butter, cheese and yogurt can be in that diet. It is worth taking a closer look at exactly what makes milk so nutritious, before we tell you how every member of the family, from babies, toddlers and schoolchildren, to hardworking adults and older members of the family, can benefit from a daily ration of milk products.

MILK – UNIQUELY NUTRITIOUS

Milk is one of our most complete foods, containing some of virtually every nutrient on our list. It is an important source of Vitamin A (especially in summer) and certain B group vitamins, the minerals – calcium and phosphorus – and valuable protein. And, of course, cheese and yogurt, which all began as milk, have many of the same nutritional characteristics.

A lot has been said recently about a possible link between the consumption of fat and coronary heart disease, but there is no conclusive evidence either way. As Professor John Yudkin, Emeritus Professor of Nutrition at the University of London has said: 'Butter fat has been very much discussed in the past 25 years, since it has been claimed to be an important cause of coronary heart disease. This claim has been strongly supported by many serious and respected research workers, but rejected by many others equally serious and respected.' You all have to make up your own mind of course, but there's really no reason to cut milk products out of your diet. Remember, *balance* is the key to healthy eating – a little of a lot of foods.

Milk has yet another benefit which we haven't mentioned – it is very easy to digest. Milk is always useful when someone in the family is unwell or needs building up. A milk pudding or milkshake slips down easily and won't upset a delicate stomach.

HOW MILK COMPARES WITH OTHER FOODS

Milk is one of the most complete foods and, of course, it is also one of the most versatile protein sources. But exactly

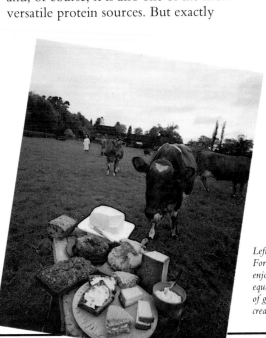

Above:
Eating habits are picked up when we are very young and often become ingrained, so affecting our food choice throughout our adult life. To give their child a healthy start in life, parents should try to establish sensible eating habits at this impressionable age, for lasting results.

Left:
For cooking, baking and enjoyment there is nothing to equal the pure wholesome taste of good English butter and fresh cream.

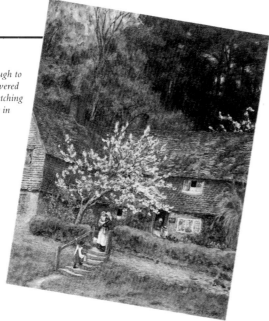

Right:
Before we were lucky enough to have fresh, pure milk delivered straight to our doorstep, fetching the milk was a daily chore in town and country alike.

how well does it line up against some of the other things we eat regularly?

Let's compare 100-calories worth of milk with the same amount of pork sausages. The meat would do better than the milk on iron and nicotinic acid. There would be roughly the same amount of protein, but the milk would be streets ahead on calcium and B_2. And, on top of that, the milk has Vitamin A, which is not in sausages at all.

Compare 100-calories worth of milk with the same amount of biscuits and the contrast is even more impressive. True, you would get *some* protein, calcium, Vitamin B_1 and nicotinic acid from the biscuits. But you'd get much, much more from the milk. They're just not in the same class.

So there we have it – milk, cheese and yogurt are extremely nourishing and relatively inexpensive. Of course, everyone needs food for slightly different reasons, so below we take a close look at every age group and explain their special needs.

THE DIET OF A LIFETIME

A good diet is vitally important even before you're pregnant. You want to be fit and healthy to prepare your body for the demands of pregnancy as, of course, a baby is formed from the nutrients absorbed by your body from foods you eat. Eating well during pregnancy is important for successful breast-feeding, too. To make sure you get a good helping of all the important nutrients you and your baby need, try to eat

Right:
Milk has long been recognised as one of our most complete foods and is a particularly good source of protein, calcium and some vitamins.

When a baby is born, the best food is its mother's milk. A mother who is breast-feeding her baby has extra demands for protein and calcium and so she should make sure there is enough milk, cheese and yogurt in her own diet. Once a baby is six months old, fresh milk can be given just as a drink or in recipes such as soups, sauces and milk puddings. If you buy untreated (green top) milk, it should be boiled and cooled before being given to infants.

some of these foods every day and remember you shouldn't be eating *quantities* for two!

Milk – at least one pint. The calcium, protein and vitamins will help build strong, healthy bones and tissues for your baby. Drink the milk ice cold, or add it to cereals, drinks, puddings or custards. For a change, you can have yogurt – one small carton of natural yogurt equals about $\frac{1}{3}$ pint of milk.

Cheese can be eaten alone as a snack, or used in savoury dishes. One ounce of hard cheese equals about $\frac{1}{3}$ pint of milk.

Meat, fish, eggs, cheese, beans and lentils are good sources of protein and you should aim to feature one of these in your diet at least twice each day. Try to include liver or kidney once a week as they are concentrated sources of many nutrients. Oily fish like kippers, herrings and sardines are often cheap and contain lots of Vitamin D.

Fruit and vegetables – at least four servings a day. It sounds like a lot, but raw fresh fruit counts and so do fresh fruit juices and salads. Include all types – green and root vegetables – and cook them with care to preserve the most vitamins.

Bread and cereals – try wholemeal or wholegrain varieties, particularly if you have a problem with constipation. Pasta and rice fall into this group, too.

Fats and oils – don't be too extravagant with these, particularly if you are gaining weight too quickly.

A diet based on these foods should provide you with all you need for a healthy pregnancy, although, if you are

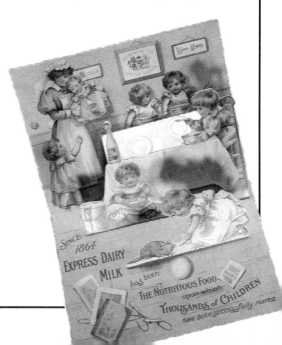

given vitamin or iron supplements at the ante-natal clinic you should take these as well. If in any doubt, ask at your clinic.

Keep an eye on your weight gain during pregnancy but serious slimming diets should not be contemplated while pregnant or breastfeeding.

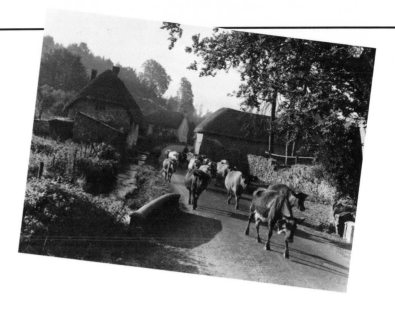

WHEN THE BABY ARRIVES

Breast-feeding is the most natural and convenient way to feed your baby and you should carry on paying attention to a very healthy diet for yourself while you are feeding. Follow a similar diet to the one given above. If you have gained more weight than you hoped, watch spreading fats, fried foods, sweets, cakes and biscuits. Don't embark on any serious slimming campaigns while you're breast-feeding. Producing $1-1\frac{1}{2}$ pints of nutrient-rich breast milk each day places considerable demands on your body, so be patient – you could find the extra flab disappears of its own accord over the first few months.

Once again, take vitamin supplements if advised by your health visitor or doctor. Make sure you drink enough, but avoid fizzy drinks and squashes, which are often high in sugar. Some foods which you enjoy, such as garlic and spices, may upset your baby's stomach slightly, so simply steer clear of them while you're still breast-feeding.

Don't worry too much about getting into a routine straight away. Once the milk supply is established, after the early weeks, you and your baby will find your own routine. Just make sure you get plenty of rest and try to stay relaxed about the whole procedure.

TAKING TO THE BOTTLE

If you cannot breast-feed for some reason, or you decide not to, there is no need to worry. Feed your baby on one of the specially marketed baby milks – your health visitor or midwife can advise you. Make up the feeds according to the instructions on the packet and also give the baby cooled, boiled water or unsweetened natural fruit juices to drink between feeds, especially in hot weather. You still need to keep an eye on your own diet – make sure it is

balanced, and if weight has crept on, don't have large portions of food, and limit fatty foods, sugary foods and drinks. Aim to get back to your ideal weight gradually.

Above:
Milking time: an idyllic country scene as the cows amble home through an unspoilt West Country village.

STARTING ON SOLIDS

Between 4–6 months, babies begin to need solids and these should be introduced bit by bit. Don't encourage a sweet tooth by offering too many sugary things, and don't add salt to the food either. Carry on with milk feeds, decreasing them gradually as the baby takes more solids. Weaning is a process which takes place over weeks or even months. Let your baby set the pace and if you are breast-feeding carry on for as long as you both want to.

When the baby is six months old, or more, she or he will be able to cope with the higher protein and mineral content of doorstep milk. There is no need to dilute the milk or boil it, unless it is untreated or has been standing on a warm doorstep or in the kitchen for some time. Choose silver top and make sure you keep it cool, clean – preferably in its original container – and covered.

If the milk has to be boiled, bring it *quickly* to the boil, then cool it *quickly* by standing the covered pan in cold water.

Your baby will probably enjoy cheese and yogurt. Start off with yogurt and cottage cheese at 5–6 months and work up to finely grated Cheddar at around eight months. Try natural yogurt and flavour it yourself with fresh fruit juice or pieces of fruit. Your clinic and health visitor can give much more

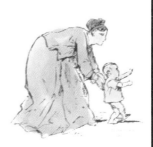

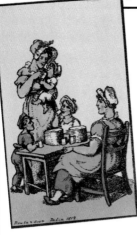

Above:
The years from one to five are very important – not only because the child is growing and developing fast, but because its eating habits are being formed. One pint of milk each day provides nearly half of the child's protein and all his calcium requirements at this stage.

detailed help with feeding, so be guided by them, and remember that even at this early age, a balanced diet is vitally important.

TEMPTING A TODDLER

Every parent knows about the 'terrible twos' – the age children start to assert independence and go to great lengths to get their own way. If your toddler turns up its nose at all the foods you know are good for it, try tempting it with different tastes and textures. Imaginative presentation of food may be more time-consuming for you, but it can certainly pay dividends. Try, for example, cheesy mashed potato hedgehog, with sliced sausage and carrot spines. Toddlers like handling their food, so savoury cookies they can hold are a good idea. The important thing is to ensure that the child gets all the nutrients it needs. If it refuses meat, try fish and eggs. Milk doesn't have to be served as a drink: try savoury sauces, pancakes, custard, milk puddings, cheese or yogurt. Or try a simple trick – flavour milk with fruit syrup or add some dairy ice cream to make a frothy milkshake. But don't give in to your toddler's demands for sweets and ice cream too often. Between meals foods like these cause tooth decay, so give fresh fruit, savoury biscuits, a finger of cheese, a glass of milk or unsweetened fruit juice instead of sweet, sticky things. If you are around to supervise, dried fruit and nuts can be enjoyed, too. Go for milk, cheese, yogurt, fruit and vegetables and you can save your child some unpleasant sessions with the dentist later on.

THE BEST YEARS OF THEIR LIVES

Growing children need proportionally more protein, calcium and other nutrients than adults. Milk is such a balanced food that it obviously makes good sense to encourage children to drink it. It is a sad fact that once children start school and can be easily influenced by friends, they will tend to go for 'tuck shop type foods' whenever they get the chance. There is not much parents can do to discourage this except to make sure that when children eat at home they get a healthy all-round diet.

Tooth decay is a common problem among school children. Being overweight can also make a school child's life a misery. Milk can help guard against both of these problems. When children choose milk, instead of sweet or fatty foods like biscuit bars or chips, they get a sugar-free balanced food that in many cases provides fewer calories. Milk has other bonuses, too, where dental care is concerned – it does not encourage acid to develop in the mouth whereas sugary foods and drinks do. Acid production is the cause of tooth decay.

With younger children it is relatively easy for parents to keep an eye on what they eat, but as they get older, the task gets harder. All you can do with stroppy teenagers is try gentle persuasion. If they are just plain picky, you might be able to lure them into eating nutritious foods by serving up small portions of healthy dishes you know they enjoy. Once they have had enough to get the juices flowing, they might just ask for seconds. This is a good tactic to try on faddy eaters of any age. If it doesn't work, you will just have to resort to making sure that what they *do* eat is as good for them as possible, and remember that many of us probably eat far more nutrients than we need.

If there is a teenage athlete in the family, he or she will need to think especially about what food to choose. There is no need to put them on to a regime of fillet steak to build up their strength! Once again, balance is the key, but children who lead a very active life need plenty of energy-giving foods. Milk, cheese and yogurt can all help, without breaking the bank.

SLIMMING SENSIBLY

Most teenagers are totally preoccupied with their appearance and suspicion of overweight is greeted with horror – whether the problem is imaginary or not. If a teenager or anyone else in the family has a weight worry, sensible eating can cure it over a period of time, without letting general health suffer. There is absolutely no need to indulge in crazy crash diets, followed by periods of bingeing to control weight. The best,

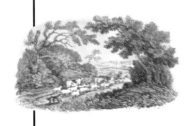

and least painless way to lose those extra pounds is to eat only when you feel hungry, stop as soon as you've had enough and take a lively interest in food values. Once you realise that calories consumed in the form of sweets, biscuits, chips and fizzy drinks, are not likely to satisfy you for as long as those you get from meat, fish, cheese or milk, it becomes easier to choose the right foods to help you slim and keep well.

There is no need for any slimmer to become fanatical about food – a cream cake every now and then won't hurt anyone. With an intelligent and informed approach to eating, everyone can control his or her own weight without ever thinking about it. And, of course, there are low-fat dairy foods such as natural yogurt and cottage cheese which all help in keeping the daily calorie count down. The recipes on pages 125–139 are specially good for slimmers, and you will find lots of others throughout this book.

COOKING FOR ONE

Not everyone has the demands of a large family to think of at every meal. Plenty of people live alone and, if anything, they need to take more positive care over their diet than people who have to cook a balanced meal for others every single day. When you are catering for one, the temptation is often to nibble rather than eat regular meals. Whatever your age – pensioner, student or somewhere in between – living alone is no reason for eating badly.

There are several simple ways to make easy meals more fun to prepare and better for you:

★ Invest in a few single-portion dishes and pans – you will find them much easier to use than large ones for small quantities.

★ Take the time to garnish food. A lemon or cucumber twist, a slice or two of tomato, a couple of sprigs of parsley or a sprinkling chopped fresh herbs can all help to cheer up what might otherwise be a plain dish.

★ Puddings for one are easy – fresh fruit, cheese or yogurt should fit the bill most days.

★ If you eat by yourself during the day and cook for the family in the evening, you can save fuel by preparing food in advance for the main meal and putting your lunch along with it in the oven. Something simple, like a cheesy jacket potato or a little liver casserole would be nice and easy.

★ If you often use packet meals or soups, enrich them by using all or part milk instead of water to make them up. The finished result will be much creamier. Or sprinkle a little grated cheese on top of soups to add flavour, texture and protein.

★ You can cook several vegetables together in the same pan if you wrap each one in a small foil parcel before adding it to the water. You can bake them like this, too – top each one with a knob of butter before you seal the package.

MILK: THE VERSATILE FOOD

Now you've seen how valuable milk can be – and how important a balanced diet is, not just to babies, or children or older people, but to the whole family – you'll want to try some new ways of using milk, cheese and yogurt in your cooking. In Chapters 4–12 you will find mouthwatering recipes for all sorts of different dishes. Read on and start enjoying the good life!

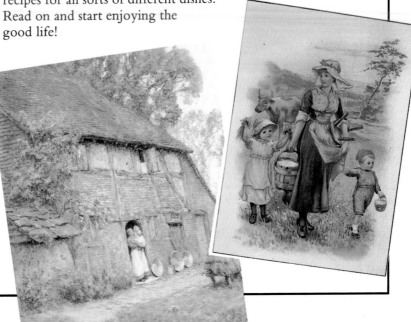

Below:
The good life: a balanced diet will help your child to enjoy working and playing hard and will keep him or her healthy. But taking care of the food needs of the family is a big responsibility and a mother should not forget to feed herself properly. She needs to keep herself in good health as the family depends on her.

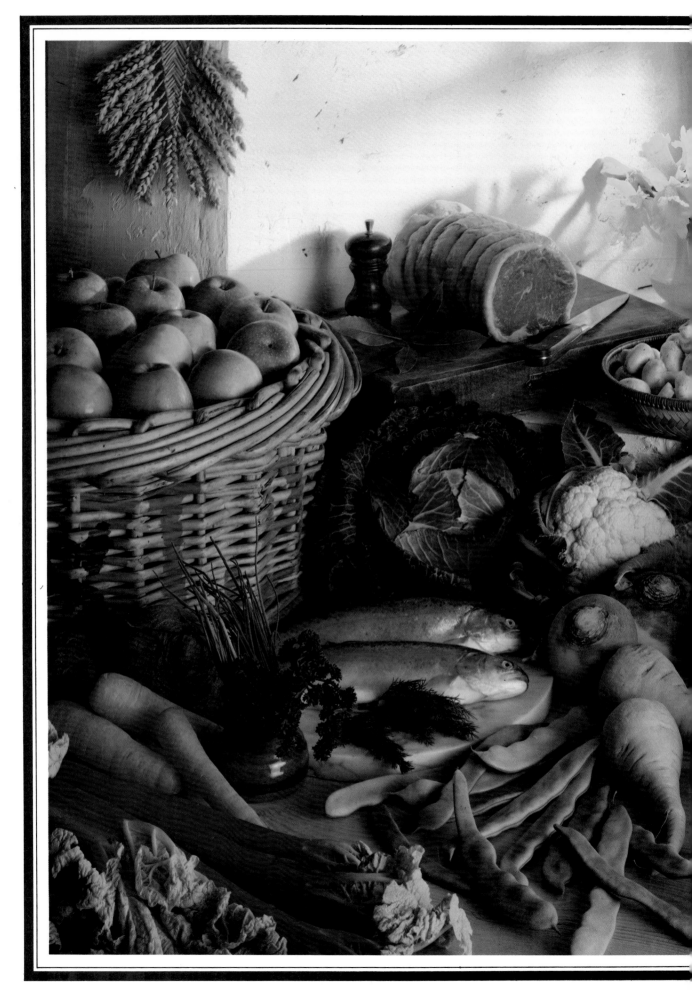

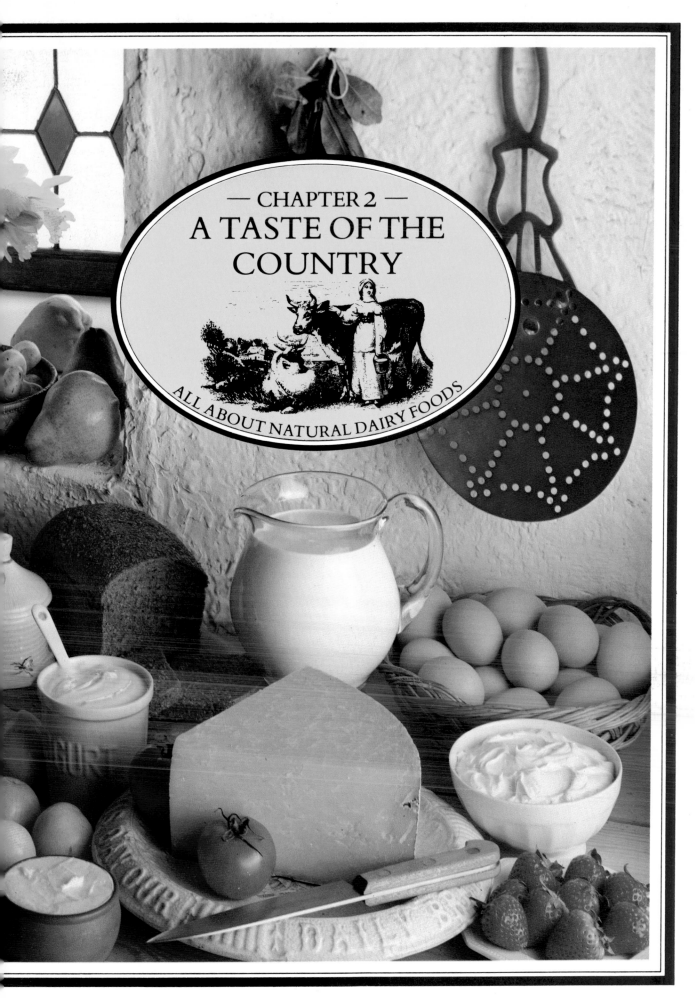

— CHAPTER 2 —

A TASTE OF THE COUNTRY

ALL ABOUT NATURAL DAIRY FOODS

Right:
Until glass bottles came into use, the milkman would push his churns on a 'pram' or drive round the streets with a pony cart.

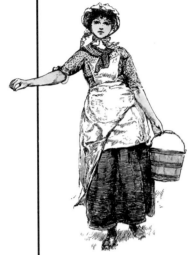

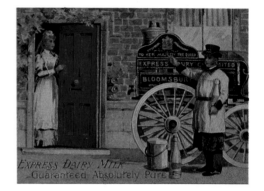

Green pastures and grazing cows are a timeless feature of Britain's rural landscape. Dairying has a long and honourable tradition in British farming and its influence can be clearly seen in our food, from the regional cheeses to the huge range of creamy mouthwatering puddings for which we are famed throughout the world. Centuries ago, most families kept at least one cow and this is reflected in the recipes for puddings to be found in cookery books of bygone days. Sometimes they instructed the cook to milk the cow straight into her pudding mixture so as to create bubbles – hence 'silly bubbles' now called syllabub!

At first, the dairy was not a separate part of the farm or manor house: the farmer's wife or the dairy maid simply made her butter and cheeses in a corner of the kitchen. Gradually, as the need for cool conditions and careful hygiene was recognised, the dairy became a separate building, sited well away from the hot, busy kitchen.

Today we have come a long way from picturesque dairy maids with their yokes and wooden pails selling milk straight from the cow, to hygienic bottles delivered fresh to the doorstep. During the nineteenth century dairying standards gradually improved and with it the health and nutrition of the British family. The development of the railway system in the 1860s meant that milk could be brought to the cities from outlying country areas and from that time milk was available to the urban population. Today over 12,000 million litres of milk are produced in England and Wales each year from cows bred to provide high-yield, top-quality milk. The consumer is offered a choice, from the rich creamy milk of Channel Islands' cows to low-fat milks, both white and flavoured.

GRADES OF MILK IN ENGLAND AND WALES

Milk is graded according to the treatment it receives at the dairy and the grades can be identified by the colour of the bottle cap. With the exception of Channel Islands milk (legal minimum 4% butterfat) whole milk must contain a minimum of 3% butterfat. The average butterfat content of ordinary milk in the UK is 3.8%.

UNTREATED MILK
Ordinary untreated milk is sold in bottles with a green foil cap. Channel Islands milk has a green cap with a gold stripe. All untreated milk must come from brucellosis accredited herds, be bottled on the farm where it was produced and sold by licensed distributors. It must be clearly labelled 'raw unpasteurised milk'.

PASTEURISED MILK
This mild heat treatment destroys any harmful bacteria which may be present and improves the keeping qualities of the milk, while having a negligible effect on its nutritional value. It will keep for 1–2 days in a cool place, or 3–4 days in your refrigerator. There are

Near right:
Interior of a farm dairy in the early nineteenth century. The large shallow pans are called 'setting dishes' and were made of earthenware or tin. Milk for butter-making stood overnight in these to allow the cream to float to the surface, an operation known as 'setting the milk'. Next day, the cream would be skimmed off ready for churning.

Far right:
In early town dairies cows were often kept at the back of a shop and milk was stored in wooden churns from which the dairyman ladled out whatever quantity the customer wanted.

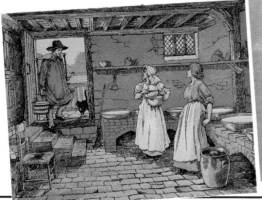

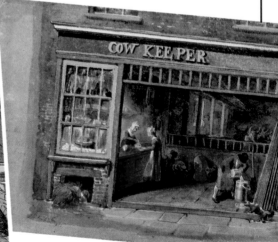

three types of pasteurised milk:

Ordinary The bottles have silver caps. This milk, which has a visible cream line, is ideal for general use, in drinks, in cooking and on cereals.

Homogenised The bottles have red caps. This milk has no cream line because homogenisation distributes the cream evenly through the milk. The milk looks whiter than ordinary pasteurised milk and is ideal on cereals as everyone gets a fair share of the cream!

Channel Islands The bottles have gold caps. This is a rich milk with a definite cream line, produced by Jersey, Guernsey or South Devon cows. Channel Islands is the breed of cow – don't believe the myth that the milk has been shipped daily from Jersey and Guernsey!

UHT MILK

This is sometimes called Long Life, as the milk is homogenised, then given Ultra Heat Treatment, rapidly cooled and aseptically packaged. Unopened, it keeps for up to 6 months out of the refrigerator. Check the date stamp and use before it expires. Once opened, keep as for pasteurised milk. Some Vitamin B_{12} may be lost during storage, but otherwise it is nutritionally similar to pasteurised milk. This milk is ideal for self-catering holidays and to keep as a standby in the store cupboard.

STERILISED MILK

This milk is usually sold in long-necked glass bottles or plastic bottles with a blue foil cap. In some areas it is also available in cartons. Homogenised milk is heated to above boiling point and held for a sufficient length of time to give a sterile milk. Legally, sterilised milk must keep unopened, without refrigeration for at least 7 days, but several weeks is usual for milk in glass bottles. Plastic bottles and cartons are date-stamped with a shelf-life of several months. Keep opened containers in a refrigerator. Sterilised milk has a characteristic caramel-like flavour which makes it excellent for custards and puddings.

SKIMMED MILK

This has had virtually all the fat removed to produce milk with less than 0.3% fat. It may be pasteurised, sterilised or ultra-heat treated. Care should be taken when heating skimmed milk as it easily burns.

SEMI-SKIMMED MILK

This has been partially skimmed and contains between 1.5 and 1.8% fat. It may be pasteurised or UHT treated. Neither skimmed nor semi-skimmed milks are suitable for newly-weaned babies because of the relatively low energy value.

MILK POWDERS

This type of milk is produced by the evaporation of water from milk by heat to produce solids containing 5% or less moisture. Both skimmed and semi-skimmed milk to which vegetable fat has been added (known as 'filled' milk) are available in powdered form. Milk powders are packed in airtight containers and have a long shelf-life if stored at a moderate temperature. Once you have reconstituted powdered milk with water, it should receive the same care as fresh milk.

EVAPORATED MILK

This type of milk is a concentrated, homogenised milk which does not contain added sugar. It is sterilised in the can and its final concentration is about twice that of the original milk. Evaporated milk is another useful store cupboard food as unopened it will keep almost indefinitely.

CONDENSED MILK

This is made from whole, semi-skimmed or skimmed milk with added cane sugar. After processing, condensed milk has a concentration of at least twice that of original milk and unopened will keep almost indefinitely.

HOW TO STORE MILK

Average keeping times for the different types of milk have been given above, but there are a few points to remember

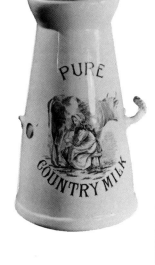

Below:
Milkmaids or dairymaids were important members of the farming community from medieval times onwards. They needed to be strong and healthy as they usually started work at dawn, and after milking the cows they would begin their butter or cheesemaking for the day.

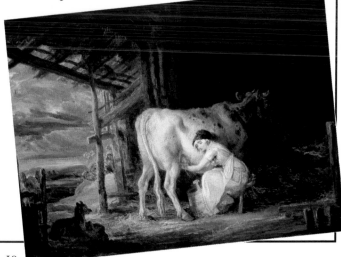

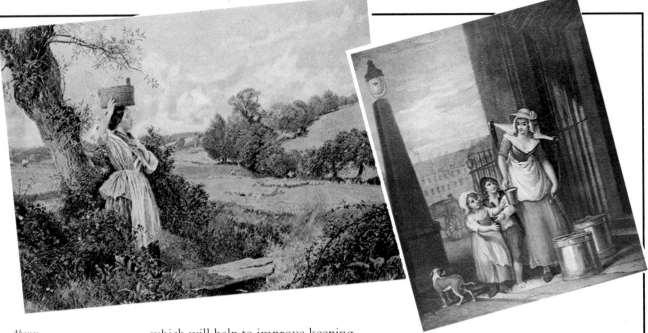

Above:
In the spring, there were many traditional customs connected with milkmaids. At Hornsea and Southorp in the East Riding of Yorkshire, milkmaids collected flowers on Whit Sunday to be made into garlands at the house of the cowherd. Traditionally, he gave them 'possett and white cakes' to eat. On the Monday morning the first milkmaid to reach each pasture received a ribbon and was named the 'queen' or 'lady' of that pasture for the summer.

Above right:
This coloured print, dating from 1798, shows a milkmaid selling milk direct from two pails in the streets of central London. Even in the heart of a busy city, milkmaids held light-hearted celebrations in the spring. The most famous of these was the picturesque frolic held on May Day during which milkmaids and chimney sweeps traditionally danced together through the streets of London.
On 1st May 1667, this dance was described by the great diarist Samuel Pepys, who happened to witness it: 'To Westminster; on the way meeting many milkmaids with their garlands upon their pails, dancing with a fiddler before them.'

which will help to improve keeping quality:

★ Take your milk indoors as soon as it is delivered, as sunlight will affect its vitamin content.

★ Always keep the milk in a cool, dark place – in the refrigerator or a larder.

★ Leave the milk in the bottle it came in if you can, since it is the most hygienic container for milk. Always keep it covered.

★ If using a milk jug, always wash and rinse it carefully. Do not wipe it with a tea-towel. Cover it to keep out dust. Do not add new milk to old before re-washing the jug. Never pour milk back into the milk bottle.

★ Use milk in date order and never mix old with new.

★ Remember that pasteurised milk does not 'sour' in the same way as untreated milk. Don't use it once it has 'gone off' as it will taste nasty. Not suitable for scone-making.

★ Have your milk delivered to the door regularly so you never run short.

★ Be sure to have an extra pint or two in hand or choose UHT or sterilised milk, both of which keep well even without a refrigerator.

★ Red top (homogenised) milk can be frozen in a plastic container for one month, but it is a waste of valuable freezer space.

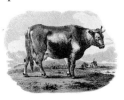

CREAM FROM THE COUNTRYSIDE

Cool, smooth, velvety fresh cream enhances the humblest food. There are so many delicious ways to use it and you certainly don't always need the most expensive ingredients to use with it.

Cream rises to the surface of milk if it is allowed to stand. In the old days the cream was skimmed off by hand, but nowadays it is separated from the milk by centrifugal force in a mechanical separator. Like milk, it is heat-treated to ensure its safety and to improve its keeping qualities. Fresh cream adds a luxurious feel to everyday meals and of course it's great for entertaining. There are many different types to choose from. Here is a guide to help you:

PASTEURISED CREAM
Half cream This cream is rather like the top of the milk and the legal minimum butterfat content is 12%. It is good in coffee, on cereals, in sauces or dressings.
Single cream This type of cream has a legal minimum butterfat content of 18% and is always homogenised. It pours readily and is lovely swirled on to soup or coffee, over fruit, jelly or trifle.
Soured cream This type has the same fat content as single cream. Its refreshing piquant flavour results from incubating cream with a harmless bacterial culture to turn it slightly acid. Soured cream is superb in casseroles, goulash, salad dressings and on cheesecakes.

Double cream This cream has a legal minimum butterfat content of 48%. It is deliciously rich and will float temptingly on soup or coffee. It is ideal for decorating cakes and desserts.

Double cream extra thick This cream needs no whipping. It is homogenised so that it is thick and spoonable and is ideal to dollop on apple pie, strawberries or other fruit.

Whipping cream This cream has a legal minimum butterfat content of 35%. It will at least double in volume if whipped properly (see page 22) so may be used lavishly, piped on to desserts, in cakes or in pastries.

Whipped cream This cream is sold ready whipped and has a legal minimum butterfat content of 35%.

Spoonable cream This cream has been homogenised to make it easily spoonable, but it has the same fat content as whipping cream.

CLOTTED CREAM

This delicious cream is traditionally associated with the West Country. As the surface of clotted cream looks wrinkled and 'folded', the name is thought to come from an old word, 'clout', meaning a wrinkled patch of leather. Traditionally, this cream was made by warming the milk very slowly all day by the fire and then cooling it gradually in shallow pans placed overnight on the cold stone flags of the dairy floor. In the morning a thick layer of cream would have formed on top. These days the process is mechanised, and the resulting cream has a legal minimum butterfat content of 55%. Clotted cream spreads easily and is marvellous with scones and jam for a cream tea.

UHT CREAM

Half cream, single, double and whipping varieties are available. It is ultra heat-treated and aseptically packed in foil-lined containers. Unopened, it will keep for months but check the expiry date stamp. This type of cream is very useful for holidays and in the store cupboard. The whipping cream forms only a soft foam when whipped.

EXTENDED LIFE CREAM

This comes packed in vacuum-sealed bottles and keeps in the refrigerator, unopened for 2–3 weeks. It is spoonable double cream and can be whipped.

STERILISED CREAM

This type of cream keeps unopened for up to 2 years. It comes in cans and has been heat-treated and homogenised. The sterilisation process gives a distinctive caramel flavour and as it is a thick cream it will not whip.

FROZEN CREAM

Double, whipping, and single cream can be bought commercially frozen. It is usually packed in manageable quantities and is a very useful standby.

For home freezing, double and whipping cream freeze particularly well if they are first lightly whipped and then frozen in plastic containers. They will then keep successfully for two months. It is best to add 1 tbsp of milk to each 150 ml (5 fl oz) of double cream before partially whipping. When thawed, finish whipping these creams to the consistency you want. Take care when whipping cream which has been frozen, because it easily overwhips. Clotted cream freezes well for 1 month, then becomes buttery.

If you have some whipped cream left in the piping bag, pipe rosettes on to a non-stick baking tray and open freeze. When frozen, pack the rosettes into a rigid container. Use them while still frozen to decorate cakes and trifles, then allow 45 minutes for them to thaw.

If there is a drop of cream left at the bottom of the carton, tilt the carton

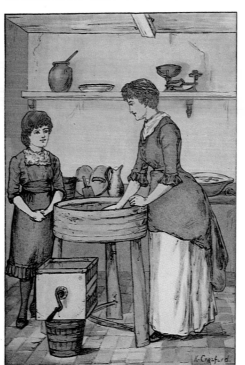

Above:
Judging by the heavy dairy equipment they had to handle, dairy maids and milk girls needed to have good health and physical strength.

Whether they worked in the country or the town, these women had to walk considerable distances over rough ground and literally carrying a weight on their shoulders of about 60 lb. That was the average weight of a wooden yolk with churns, and two heavy buckets full of milk. A milkmaid with a yoke delivered milk to the Burlington Arcade, London until as late as 1907.

Left:
Cleanliness and coolness are still the prime essentials of a dairy building. Traditionally, a dairy had a stone, brick, slate or tiled floor and the shelves were also of slate, if possible. Ideally, the window would face north to keep out the sun and was protected by gauze or louvres.

The dairy was often built in the shade of leafy trees which kept the building cool in summer. Often an elder tree was planted outside a dairy window to keep flies away and also to keep away witches who were thought to be responsible when butter failed to 'come' properly during churning.

WHIPPING AND PIPING CREAM

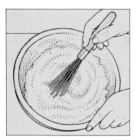

1 Gently tilting the bowl while whipping

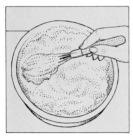

2 Whipping the cream until it holds its shape

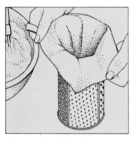

3 Preparing icing bag. Spooning cream into bag

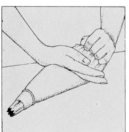

4 Pressing cream towards the nozzle to remove any air pockets

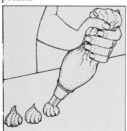

5 Piping quickly and deftly

over a jug of milk to use up the last dregs. For larger amounts freeze it in an ice-cube tray and use it in recipes which need only small amounts. One cube of cream equals about 15 ml (1 tbsp).

STORING FRESH CREAM

When storing any type of fresh cream remember to keep it cool, clean and covered. It should also be kept well away from any strong-flavoured foods which might taint it.

WHIPPING AND PIPING CREAM

Fresh whipped cream makes the perfect decoration for all sorts of desserts, particularly if you pipe it in rosettes, a trellis or some other pretty pattern. Like so many things, it is easy once you know how, and a few simple tips will help.

* Always choose double or whipping cream. To achieve more volume, add 15 ml (1 tbsp) of milk to 150 ml (5 fl oz) double cream, before you whip it.
* Chill the fresh cream and all the utensils thoroughly before you start.
* A spiral whisk gives better results than a rotary or electric one.
* Whip quickly at first until the cream begins to look matt on the surface, then whip a little more slowly until it stands in soft peaks and does not fall off the upturned whisk.
* If you overwhip the cream it will look granular and the flavour will be affected. It is impossible to rescue it if this happens, so carry on whipping and you should end up with butter.
* Fill the cream into a chilled piping bag. This is easier if the bag is held in place over a grater or tall glass while you are filling it with the whipped cream. This helps to prevent you getting covered as well as the cake!
* Remove the bag from the glass and gently force the cream into the end of the bag by twisting the top. Then, holding the bag at the top above the cream, you are ready to pipe.

DELECTABLE DAIRY ICE CREAM

Today we often take dairy ice cream for granted and we assumed it is a thoroughly modern sweet, as much of a twentieth-century invention as the refrigerator. But ice cream has a long history. In Britain it first appeared in the eighteenth century, as a treat reserved strictly for the rich. Before the invention of the freezer, they were the only people who could afford to keep ice cream frozen, and special ice houses were often built in the grounds of large country estates. An ice house was simply a deep brick-lined pit, roofed over and filled with natural ice taken from local lakes and pools in winter. No wonder ice cream was prettily described as 'eating winter with a spoon'.

Today we can buy a vast range of dairy ice creams ready made, but if you want to make something really special, extra creamy and truly delicious, it is really quite simple and you'll find lots of lovely recipes here.

BASIC DAIRY ICE CREAM

568 ml (1 pint) milk
1 vanilla pod
6 egg yolks
175 g (6 oz) sugar
568 ml (1 pint) fresh whipping cream

1. Bring the milk and vanilla pod almost to the boil. Take off the heat and leave for at least 15 minutes.
2. Beat the egg yolks and sugar together, stir in the milk and strain back into the pan. Cook the custard gently over a low heat, stirring until it coats the back of a wooden spoon. Do not boil.
3. Pour into a chilled, shallow freezer container and leave to cool.
4. Freeze for about 2 hours until mushy.
5. Turn into a large, chilled basin and mash with a flat whisk or fork. Lightly whip the fresh cream and fold into the mixture. Freeze again until mushy then mash again.
6. Return to the freezer to become firm.

To freeze Overwrap according to type of container.

Note Do not whip the fresh cream if using a mechanical churn or cream maker. Agitate chilled custard and unwhipped cream together.

Serves 8–10

Variations

Chocolate Break up 175 g (6 oz) plain chocolate, heat with the milk, whisking until smooth.

Coffee Stir 60 ml (4 tbsp) coffee essence into made custard.

Strawberry Purée 350 g (12 oz) strawberries with 25 g (1 oz) icing sugar and 10 ml (2 tsp) lemon juice and stir into made custard.

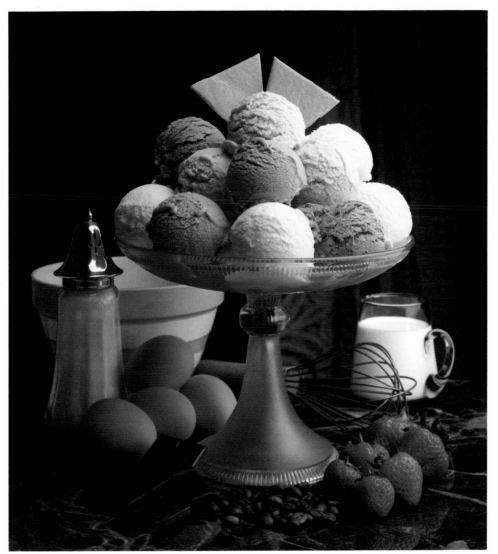

Left:
BASIC VANILLA,
CHOCOLATE, COFFEE
AND STRAWBERRY ICE
CREAM
Nothing can beat the rich fresh taste of real homemade dairy ice cream. Whether you make the creamy vanilla version, or the variations flavoured with luscious strawberry purée, fragrant coffee essence or tempting plain dark chocolate, these delicious treats will be the very best ice cream you have ever tasted.

MAKING DAIRY ICE CREAM

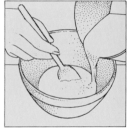

1 Adding the milk to the beaten egg yolks

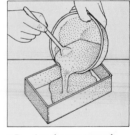

2 Pouring the egg custard into a chilled, shallow freezer container

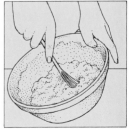

3 Mashing the frozen mixture before folding in the lightly whipped fresh cream and freezing again

FRESH PEACH DAIRY ICE CREAM

350 g (12 oz) fresh ripe peaches

300 ml (½ pint) milk

grated rind and juice of 1 lemon

100 g (4 oz) icing sugar

300 ml (10 fl oz) fresh whipping cream

1. Quarter the peaches and remove the skins, discarding the stones.
2. Roughly slice the peaches into the blender, add the milk, lemon rind and juice, icing sugar and the fresh cream. Blend well until the mixture is quite smooth.
3. Pour out into ice-cube trays or a shallow freezer container, freeze until firm.
4. Allow to soften at room temperature for about 30 minutes before serving. Serve plain or with a chocolate sauce.
To freeze Overwrap according to type of container.

Serves 6

BANANA AND HONEY DAIRY ICE CREAM

450 g (1 lb) bananas

150 ml (5 fl oz) fresh double cream

142 g (5 oz) natural yogurt

juice of 1 large lemon

75 ml (5 level tbsp) thick honey

50 g (2 oz) browned hazelnuts, chopped

2 egg whites

1. Peel and mash the bananas in a large bowl using a fork.
2. Add the unwhipped fresh cream, yogurt, lemon juice, honey and hazelnuts. Beat well to combine.
3. Turn into a rigid container – not too deep. Cover and half freeze to the mushy stage.
4. Whisk the egg whites until stiff; fold into the banana mixture and return to finish freezing.
5. Allow to soften in the refrigerator for 1 hour before serving.
To freeze Overwrap according to type of container.

Serves 8

BLACKCURRANT RIPPLED DAIRY ICE CREAM

400 ml (¾ pint) milk
1 vanilla pod
1 egg, size 2, plus 4 egg yolks
175 g (6 oz) caster sugar
300 ml (10 fl oz) fresh double cream
225 g (8 oz) frozen blackcurrants, thawed
125 g (4 oz) icing sugar

1. Bring the milk and the vanilla pod almost to the boil. Take off the heat and infuse for about 10 minutes.
2. Whisk together the eggs, egg yolks and caster sugar until thick and pale. Strain on the infused milk (wash vanilla pod and dry for re-use). Stir over a low heat without boiling until the mixture thickens a little, cool.
3. Lightly whip the fresh cream and fold into the cooled custard. Pour into a square or oblong rigid freezer container to give a depth of 5 cm (2 inches). Freeze for about 3 hours until mushy. Remove and whisk. Freeze for a further 3–4 hours.
4. Meanwhile in a blender purée together the uncooked blackcurrants and icing sugar. Sieve to remove pips.
5. Take dairy ice cream out of the freezer and whisk again to a spreading consistency. Spoon a layer back into the freezer container. Pour over some of the blackcurrant purée. Continue to layer. Return to freezer.

Below:
BLACKCURRANT RIPPLED DAIRY ICE CREAM
The tempting 'rippled' or 'marbled' effect in this mouthwatering dairy ice cream, is made by freezing alternate layers of blackcurrant purée and rich vanilla custard. Try it for a spectacular summer pudding.

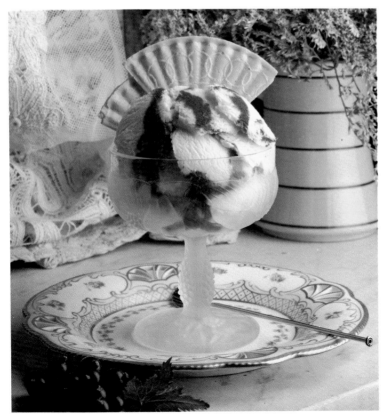

6. To serve, allow to soften in the refrigerator for about 1 hour.
To freeze Overwrap according to type of container.
Serves 8

CHOCOLATE RAISIN DAIRY ICE CREAM

75 g (3 oz) raisins
45 ml (3 tbsp) Irish Cream Liqueur
75 g (3 oz) plain chocolate
300 ml (½ pint) milk
2 eggs
50 g (2 oz) soft brown sugar
150 ml (5 fl oz) fresh double cream

1. Chop the raisins quite finely and place in a medium basin. Pour over the liqueur and leave to stand while preparing the custard.
2. Chop the chocolate and put in a heavy-based pan with 60 ml (4 tbsp) milk. Warm gently until the chocolate melts to a smooth consistency. Whisk in the remaining milk.
3. Beat the eggs and the sugar together until well mixed; add the chocolate milk to this mixture. Return to the pan and cook over a gentle heat until the custard thickens slightly. Strain immediately over the raisins; stir to combine, cool.
4. Lightly whip the fresh cream and stir through the cold custard. Pour into a freezer container and freeze for about 3 hours, or until the ice cream is firm enough to support the weight of the raisins.
5. Stir gently to distribute the raisins evenly, cover and return to the freezer. Freeze for at least 6 hours until firm. Allow to soften in the refrigerator for 1 hour before serving.
To freeze Overwrap according to type of container.
Serves 6–8

PRALINE DAIRY ICE CREAM

50 g (2 oz) whole unblanched almonds
50 g (2 oz) sugar
300 ml (½ pint) milk
1 vanilla pod
1 egg, plus 2 egg yolks
75 g (3 oz) caster sugar
300 ml (10 fl oz) fresh double cream
plain chocolate to decorate

1. Place the almonds and sugar in a heavy-based pan, heat slowly until the sugar caramelises, turning occasionally. Pour on to an oiled baking sheet to cool and harden. Then use a mouli grater to grind to a powder.
2. Bring the milk and vanilla pod to the boil, take off the heat and infuse for 15 minutes.

3. Beat the egg, egg yolks and caster sugar until pale in colour; strain in the milk. Cook slowly until the custard coats the back of the spoon – do not boil. Cool. Lightly whip the fresh cream and fold two-thirds into the custard.

4. Freeze the mixture for about 3 hours until mushy. Beat well then fold in the praline powder.

5. Spoon into a freezer container and freeze for about 6 hours until firm.

6. Transfer to the refrigerator to soften for 30 minutes before serving. Decorate with the remaining fresh cream and coarsely grated chocolate.

To freeze Overwrap according to type of container.

Serves 6

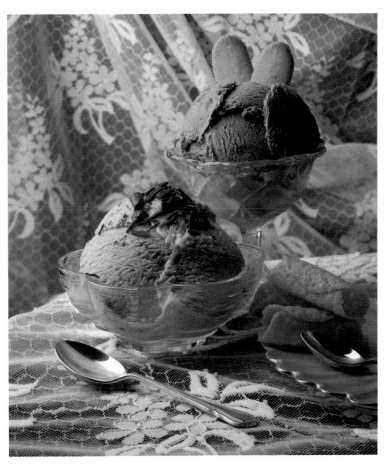

GINGER MERINGUE DAIRY ICE CREAM

125 g (4 oz) stem ginger
3 egg yolks
50 g (2 oz) sugar
300 ml ($\frac{1}{2}$ pint) milk
150 ml (5 fl oz) fresh double or whipping cream
75 g (3 oz) made meringues
stem ginger slices or chocolate leaves to decorate

1. Finely chop the drained ginger. Beat together the egg yolks and the sugar until pale. Stir in the warmed milk with the ginger; return to the pan.

2. Stir the custard over a gentle heat until it just coats the back of a spoon – do not boil. Pour out into a large bowl and cool. Freeze until mushy.

3. Beat the custard well to break down the ice crystals. Lightly whip the fresh cream, then fold into the custard. Freeze again until mushy and beat a second time.

4. Fold in the broken-up meringues and turn into a 900-ml (1½-pint) basin. Freeze until firm then closely cover basin. Return to the freezer for at least 6 hours.

5. When required unmould and decorate with ginger slices or chocolate leaves.

To freeze Pack at the end of stage 4.

Note: To make in a machine, agitate the mixture until the consistency of fresh whipped cream, fold in the meringues then continue as above.

Serves 6–8

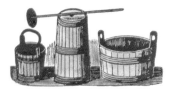

BUTTERSCOTCH DAIRY ICE CREAM

90 g (3½ oz) dark soft brown sugar
50 g (2 oz) English butter
300 ml ($\frac{1}{2}$ pint) warm milk
2 eggs
65 g (2½ oz) sugar
5 ml (1 tsp) vanilla flavouring
300 ml (10 fl oz) fresh whipping cream
shredded almonds, toasted, to decorate

1. Warm the brown sugar and butter until both have melted; bubble for 1 minute. Add the warm milk, heat gently until evenly blended, stirring.

2. Beat the eggs and sugar until well mixed, stir in the warm milk and vanilla flavouring. Strain back into the pan.

3. Stir over a low heat until the custard thickens slightly. Do not boil. Cool.

4. Lightly whip the fresh cream and mix into the custard. Pour into a freezer container to a depth of at least 5 cm (2 inches) and freeze until mushy. Beat, then return to the freezer until firm.

5. Transfer to the refrigerator to soften 45 minutes–1 hour before serving.

6. Spoon into sundae glasses. Decorate with browned shredded almonds.

To freeze Overwrap according to type of container.

Serves 8

Above, left to right:
PRALINE DAIRY ICE CREAM AND CHOCOLATE RAISIN DAIRY ICE CREAM
Praline is the French name for a delicious confection of nuts and carmelised sugar which is used to add a unique texture and flavour to many puddings and sweets. In this recipe for Praline Dairy Ice Cream, caramelised almonds add a rich flavour. Just before serving this delicious dairy ice is decorated with grated chocolate.

On the right is Chocolate Raisin Dairy Ice Cream, a luscious treat made with an Irish Cream Liqueur, plain dark chocolate, juicy raisins and, of course, fresh double cream.

ORANGE SHERBET

178-ml (6¼-oz) carton frozen orange juice

175 g (6 oz) caster sugar

45 ml (3 level tbsp) golden syrup

15 ml (1 tbsp) lemon juice

568 ml (1 pint) milk

300 ml (10 fl oz) fresh single cream

1. Turn out frozen, undiluted orange juice into a deep bowl. When beginning to soften add the sugar, golden syrup and lemon juice. Whisk until smooth.
2. Combine with the milk and cream and pour into a deep freezer container, cover and freeze. There is no need to whisk the mixture during freezing.
3. Transfer to the refrigerator to soften 45 minutes–1 hour before serving.
To freeze Overwrap according to type of container.
Serves 8

CHERRY YOGURT FROST

350 (12 oz) cherries, stoned

125 g (4 oz) caster sugar

300 ml (10 fl oz) natural yogurt

150 ml (5 fl oz) fresh double cream

2 egg whites

30 ml (2 level tbsp) icing sugar

10 ml (2 level tsp) arrowroot

1. Simmer the cherries with the caster sugar in 150 ml (¼ pint) water for 4–5 minutes. Strain off the juices and reserve. Reserve about six cherries for the sauce. Purée the remaining cherries, sieve and leave to cool slightly. Lightly whip the fresh cream. Stir the fresh cream and yogurt into the cherry purée.
2. Whisk the egg whites until stiff but not dry. Add the icing sugar and continue whisking until stiff peaks form. Gently fold into the fruit mixture. Pour the mixture into a freezer container and freeze until firm.
3. For the sauce, mix the arrowroot to a smooth paste with a little water. Stir into the reserved juices with the sliced cherries. Bring to the boil, reduce the heat and simmer until clear and thickened. Chill.
4. Transfer the cherry frost to the refrigerator to soften about 2 hours before serving. Spoon into glasses, top with cherry sauce.
To freeze Freeze sauce and cherry frost separately.
Serves 6

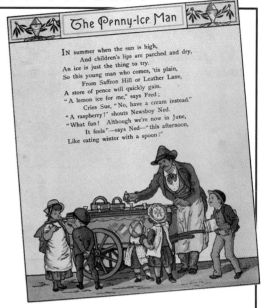

CRANBERRY YOGURT CRUSH

382-g (13½-oz) jar cranberry sauce

50 g (2 oz) caster sugar

450 ml (15 fl oz) natural yogurt

1. Stir all the ingredients together in a large bowl. Mix well.
2. Spoon the mixture into ice-cube trays fitted with square dividers and open freeze. This quantity will fill about three trays.
3. Place the trays in the freezer and leave until frozen.
4. Turn out cranberry cubes and pack in bags, return to the freezer. To serve, thaw slightly, then cut each cube into smaller squares. Pile into small glasses. A thin crisp biscuit makes the perfect accompaniment.
To freeze Overwrap according to type of container.
Serves 8

CHOCOLATE AND MINT FROST

300 ml (10 fl oz) fresh double cream

30 ml (2 tbsp) milk

50 g (2 oz) plain chocolate

15 ml (1 tbsp) finely chopped fresh mint

12 sponge fingers

chocolate leaves to decorate

1. Line a 600-ml (1-pint) basin with cling film.
2. Whip the fresh cream with the milk until stiff.
3. Break the chocolate into small pieces and place in a bowl over a pan of simmering water. Stir occasionally until melted.
4. Swirl the melted chocolate and chopped mint through the cream. Pour into the prepared basin then place in the freezer until frozen.

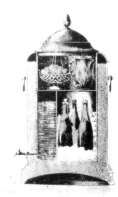

5. Arrange the sponge fingers on a serving plate, in the shape of a star. Turn out the frozen chocolate and mint frost from the mould and place on the sponge fingers. Decorate with chocolate leaves.
To freeze Cover the mould with freezer cling film.
Serves 8–10

BROWN BREAD DAIRY ICE CREAM

125 g (4 oz) fine brown breadcrumbs
50 g (2 oz) soft brown sugar
300 ml (10 fl oz) fresh double cream
150 ml (5 fl oz) fresh single cream
15 ml (1 tbsp) dark rum
50 g (2 oz) icing sugar, sifted

1. Spread the breadcrumbs on a baking sheet and sprinkle over the brown sugar. Bake in the oven at 200°C (400°F) mark 6 for about 10 minutes, stirring occasionally until the sugar caramelises and the crumbs are golden. Cool and break down with a fork.
2. Whisk together the fresh double and single creams until stiff. Gently fold in the rum and icing sugar.
3. Pour into a chilled shallow container and freeze for 1½–2 hours or until mushy in consistency.
4. Turn into a bowl and mash with a fork or whisk until smooth. Stir in the breadcrumbs. Spoon back into the container and freeze until firm.
To freeze Overwrap according to type of container.
Serves 4

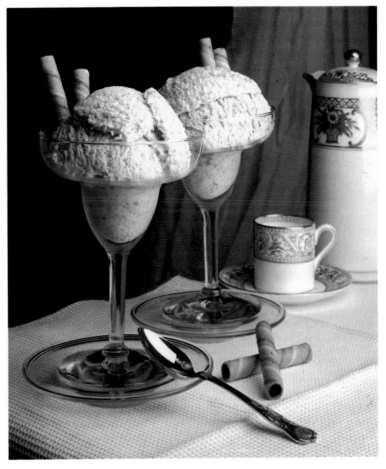

Above:
BROWN BREAD ICE CREAM
Spoil your family with this delicious frozen treat. This unusual ice cream is really a variation of the delicious Praline Ice Cream given on page 24. To give a rich texture and crunch, fine brown breadcrumbs are sprinkled with brown sugar and spread on a baking sheet to caramelise in the oven. This lovely caramel crunch is then stirred into a rich cream mixture flavoured with rum.

BEAUTIFUL BUTTER

Fresh golden butter is a must in all types of cooking for the unique flavour and texture it gives food. Butter is produced by churning cream and traditionally this was done by hand, although some farms used water wheels and some even had a dog churn. This was a large wooden wheel on which a dog ran to keep it turning. On market day the butter was taken to town in a basket kept cool with rhubarb leaves and decorated with primroses and other wild flowers.

Today butter is churned automatically in continuous butter-making machines. The pasteurised cream is churned at a controlled temperature in a stainless-steel vat until it forms into large masses of butterfat.

The butter is washed to remove the buttermilk, which is fed to livestock or used in the manufacture of cultured buttermilk or milk powder. Then the butter is salted and 'worked' or kneaded until it has the correct consistency and wrapped and packed ready for distribution. Butter to which a culture has been added is known as lactic butter, otherwise it is called sweetcream butter. Most English butters are slightly salted, although unsalted English butters, particularly good for butter icing and butter creams (see page 265), pastry making and confectionery, are also available.

The flavour and colour of butter vary according to the manufacture, the amount of salt added, the type of cattle and the time of year.

STORING AND FREEZING BUTTER
Store butter in a cool dark place – the refrigerator is best. Like fresh cream and milk it will pick up other flavours, so keep it covered and store it away from strong foods. If it is closely wrapped, butter can be frozen for 2–3 months, either in blocks or shaped into pats or moulds.

MAKING SAVOURY BUTTERS

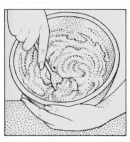

1 Creaming the butter with your chosen flavourings

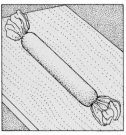

2 Forming the butter into a roll in greaseproof paper before putting it in the refrigerator to chill

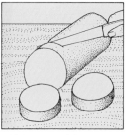

3 Slicing pats of savoury butter off the roll, as required

Below:
An end-over-end barrel churn, a design which became popular towards the end of the nineteenth century.

Bottom:
A rectangular box churn, also dating from the late nineteenth century.

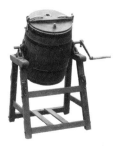

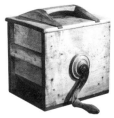

SAVOURY BUTTERS

Butter blends marvellously with other flavours, and savoury butters add exciting flavour and piquancy to a wide range of foods. They have been popular in English cookery since the seventeenth century and at that time were often made with oils extracted from herbs and spices.

Savoury butters are easy to prepare. The butter should be softened so that it is workable but not melting, and any herbs should be chopped very finely. When made, the butters should be formed into a roll and then chilled. To serve cut them into rounds about 1·25 cm (½-inch) thick and place on the hot food just before serving. Savoury butters are delicious on grilled and fried fish, meats, gammon steaks and beefburgers. Or they can be stirred through pasta and cooked vegetables, spread on hot breads or popped into jacket potatoes. Here is a mouthwatering selection to try.

MAÎTRE D'HÔTEL BUTTER

125 g (4 oz) English butter
30 ml (2 tbsp) finely chopped fresh parsley
5 ml (1 tsp) lemon juice
salt and freshly ground pepper

1. Whisk the butter until soft but not oily.
2. Add the seasonings and beat in well. Chill in the refrigerator in a small bowl, covered, or form into a long roll in greaseproof paper. To serve cut the roll into 1-cm (½-inch) slices and place on the meat or fish or use small knobs from the bowl.

Variations Use the same method as for Maître d'hôtel butter.

GARLIC BUTTER

125 g (4 oz) English butter
2 garlic cloves, skinned and crushed

SHRIMP BUTTER

125 g (4 oz) English butter
50 g (2 oz) peeled shrimps, finely chopped
5 ml (1 tsp) lemon juice

FRESH HERB BUTTER

125 g (4 oz) English butter
5 ml (1 tsp) chopped fresh tarragon
5 ml (1 tsp) chopped fresh parsley
5 ml (1 level tsp) finely grated onion

Note These herbs may be varied according to season.

ORANGE AND PARSLEY BUTTER

125 g (4 oz) English butter
grated rind of ½ orange
10 ml (2 tsp) orange juice
10 ml (2 tsp) chopped fresh parsley
freshly ground pepper

ANCHOVY BUTTER

125 g (4 oz) English butter
6 anchovies, drained and mashed

GREEN BUTTER

125 g (4 oz) English butter
50 g (2 oz) watercress, chopped

ONION BUTTER

125 g (4 oz) English butter
30 ml (2 level tbsp) finely chopped or grated onion

CURRY BUTTER

125 g (4 oz) English butter
10 ml (2 level tsp) curry powder

TOMATO BUTTER

125 g (4 oz) English butter
10 ml (2 tsp) tomato purée
pinch of caster sugar

PAPRIKA BUTTER

125 g (4 oz) English butter
5 ml (1 level tsp) yeast extract
2.5 ml (½ level tsp) paprika

HORSERADISH BUTTER

125 g (4 oz) English butter
30 ml (2 level tbsp) creamed horseradish

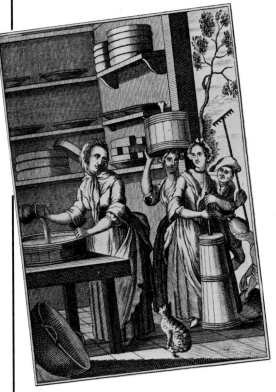

ALL ABOUT YOGURT

The nomadic tribes of Eastern Europe used to make a drink from fermented milk, which was the forerunner of the yogurt which we all eat in such great quantities today. The nomads' version was very acid because without refrigeration the milk just carried on fermenting. Most of us prefer a less acid flavour and firmer texture.

Yogurt is made from a skimmed milk base with added skimmed milk powder. The milk is pasteurised, then cooled and the special bacteria are added to cause fermentation. The milk is incubated in large tanks at a constant temperature until it thickens and then it is cooled. For flavoured yogurts, whole fruit in a syrup is stirred into the yogurt before it is filled into cartons.

Most yogurt produced in the UK is a low-fat product. As well as being a good source of protein, many natural varieties have Vitamins A and D added. If natural yogurt is too acid for your taste, you can add fruit, fruit juice, nuts, muesli, honey or any other flavouring you like.

Unless yogurt is pasteurised after preparation (it will say on the label) it will contain 'live' bacteria which remain dormant while kept cool. For this reason you should always buy yogurt from a refrigerated cabinet and keep it in the refrigerator. If it is kept somewhere warmer, the bacteria will become active again and produce more acid until the yogurt eventually separates. You can buy commercially frozen yogurt which should be thawed for 24 hours in the refrigerator. You can also freeze homemade yogurt for up to one month as long as it contains sugar. Manufactured flavoured yogurts can be treated in the same way.

MAKING YOGURT AT HOME

It is easy and cheap to make your own yogurt using pasteurised milk which has been boiled and quickly cooled, or with sterilised or UHT milk. First sterilise all your equipment with boiling water or a recommended sterilising solution.

1. Heat 568 ml (1 pint), less 30 ml (2 tbsp), milk to blood temperature.
2. Blend the reserved milk with 15 ml (1 tbsp) of natural yogurt until smooth and stir into the warm milk. Ensure that pasteurised yogurt is not used.
3. Pour into a wide-necked vacuum flask and leave for 6–8 hours.
4. Turn the warm yogurt into a basin, stand basin in cold water and whisk yogurt until cool.
5. Cover basin and refrigerate for 4–6 hours, during which time it will thicken up considerbly. Serve plain or flavoured. Keeps for up to a week in the refrigerator.

FOLKLORE IN THE DAIRY

The cow is so important to our food supply in Britain, that in the

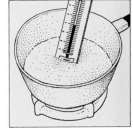

1 Heating the milk to blood temperature

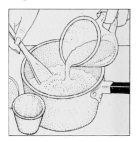

2 Blending in the natural yogurt

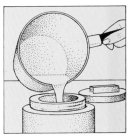

3 Pouring the mixture into a wide-necked vacuum flask

Above left:
Churning butter in an eighteenth-century dairy. Throughout the history of dairy farming, churns have been made in many different designs. In this engraving, the dairy maid is using an early type known as a 'plunger churn'. This cylindrical wooden churn, also shown below, bound with iron hoops stands about 3 feet high. The handle she plunges up and down is called 'the agitator'. Two other types of churn are shown opposite.

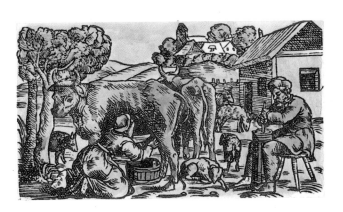

MAKING BUTTER SHAPES

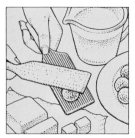

1 Shaping butter balls

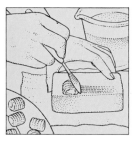

2 Preparing butter rolls

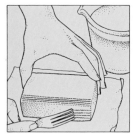

3 Making a decorative ridging on a butter block using a fork

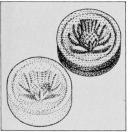

4 A butter mould should be wetted with cold water before the butter is pressed into it and chilled

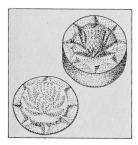

5 A sharp tap should release the chilled butter from the mould

countryside, the keeping of cows was often surrounded by folklore. Cattle were thought to be vulnerable to witchcraft, so rowan sprigs were often plaited round their horns or nailed in cowstalls to frighten witches away.

One good way to protect cows from enchantment was by dropping wax from Easter candles on their horns, or leaving the wax in the shape of a cross under the cowshed step.

The wise farmer chose his droving stick with an eye to the supernatural. Willow was unpopular, as it was thought to injure the cows, but hazel and rowan would fatten the animals and ash never cause an injury. A bough of holly thrown after a runaway cow would bring the errant beast back and a sprig in the cowshed was thought to bring good luck.

Many odd things were added to cattle's food to protect them from harm. In Worcestershire, Christmas mistletoe was given to the first cow to calve in the New Year and a little stolen hay was added to the Christmas Day feed, to bring good luck to the dairy. Shropshire cows were fed biblical texts with their hay.

A four-leaf clover hidden in the byre was reckoned to guard against evil, and cattle could be guaranteed to thrive in a field where the magical hawthorn grew. In Sussex, sick cattle were driven under an arched bramble spray, symbol of healthy rebirth, and hedgehogs and adders were killed on sight, because they supposedly sucked milk from the cows at pasture.

OLD BELIEFS ABOUT BUTTER

Many superstitions surrounded butter-making. The presence of silver in the dairy was always thought to bring good luck and in Yorkshire, dairymaids kept a crooked silver sixpence for a 'churn-spell' should the butter not come. A crown piece might be dropped into the

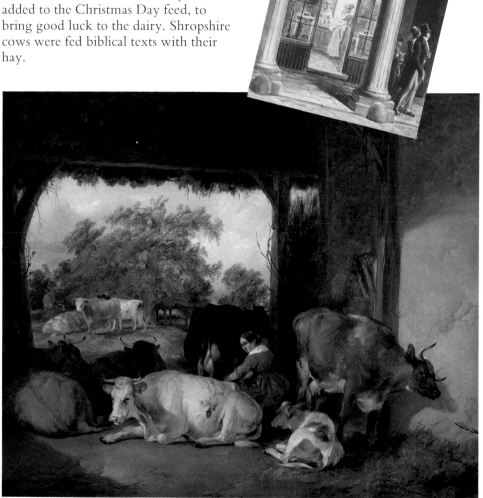

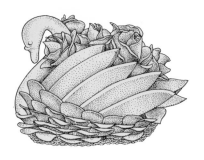

cream for the same reason, or a red-hot poker thrust into it. Many 'churn-spells' have been recorded which were chanted three times on days when it took a long time to produce butter solids from the cream. One runs like this:

'Come, butter, come,
Come, butter, come,
Peter stands at the gate,
Waiting for a buttered cake,
Come, butter, come.'

PRETTY PRINTS

One of the dairy maid's tasks was to shape the butter for sale. It was often sold in round pats, formed in wooden moulds that also measured the weight. Each pat was stamped with the pattern that identified the farm where the butter was made. Some of these stamps were very finely carved and often the design symbolised the type of farm. A swan meant a farm with water meadows; sprays of bog myrtle indicated a hill farm; corn sheafs, a corn-growing farm; and sometimes the farm's prize bull would have his portrait in the stamp.

Butter prints were made in hundreds of other delightful designs depicting squirrels, thistles and sometimes, even the cow herself, and today it is still quite possible to come across them in antique shops.

Competitions were held occasionally to test the skill of dairy maids from different farms. The women moulded large pieces of butter into intricate shapes – towers or baskets of fruit – and it was all done by eye, with no weighing or measuring allowed. These works of art would later be sold in shops or on stalls.

Butter prints started to go out of fashion at the end of the nineteenth century and Scotch hands took their place. These were wooden paddles with a ridged surface and were easy to use. The worker could still make patterns by criss-crossing the lines on the surface of the butter.

To use a butter print, make sure the top of the butter is level and press the dampened print firmly on to it. Leave in position and chill for several hours, or overnight. The print will lift off easily at serving time.

Left:
Butter sculpture, in which intricate shapes were skilfully moulded out of large blocks of butter, were an attractive feature of dairy shows in the nineteenth century. This beautiful swan was designed and carved out of butter by Mr John Blaney, a living butter sculptor who works at a dairy in Berkshire.

Opposite, top:
In early town dairies, such as this example in early nineteenth-century Regent Street, London, the milk was not ready-packed in bottles or cartons, but was collected by customers who brought their own jugs.

Opposite, below:
'Milking Time', a painting by Thomas Sydney Cooper (1803–1902) done in 1848. The British love of the countryside has not only expressed itself in landscape painting but in the strong tradition of cattle portraiture. From the eighteenth century onwards, cattle breeders often commissioned paintings of their prize animals. By the Victorian period, the general public were also keen on general scenes showing cattle. This particular artist was so popular as a cattle painter that he was nicknamed 'Cow Cooper'.

Some excellent examples of cattle portraiture are on view at the Museum of English Rural Life, Reading.

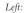

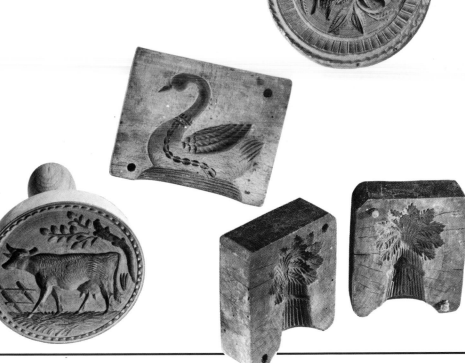

Left:
A selection of hand-carved wooden butter prints, traditionally used to stamp an attractive design on to butter and to indicate which farm the butter came from.

Like most of the woodware in the British dairy, butter prints were usually made of sycamore, a white wood which could stand up to frequent scrubbing without becoming rough or splintering.

In the West of England and Wales, the designs of butter prints were usually geometrical. In the rest of England, the prints gave clues about what sort of farm the butter came from. A swan, for example, indicates that the farm is near a river; a sheep indicates a sheep farm; a cow means that the farm is principally a dairy farm; a corn stook that it is mainly arable.

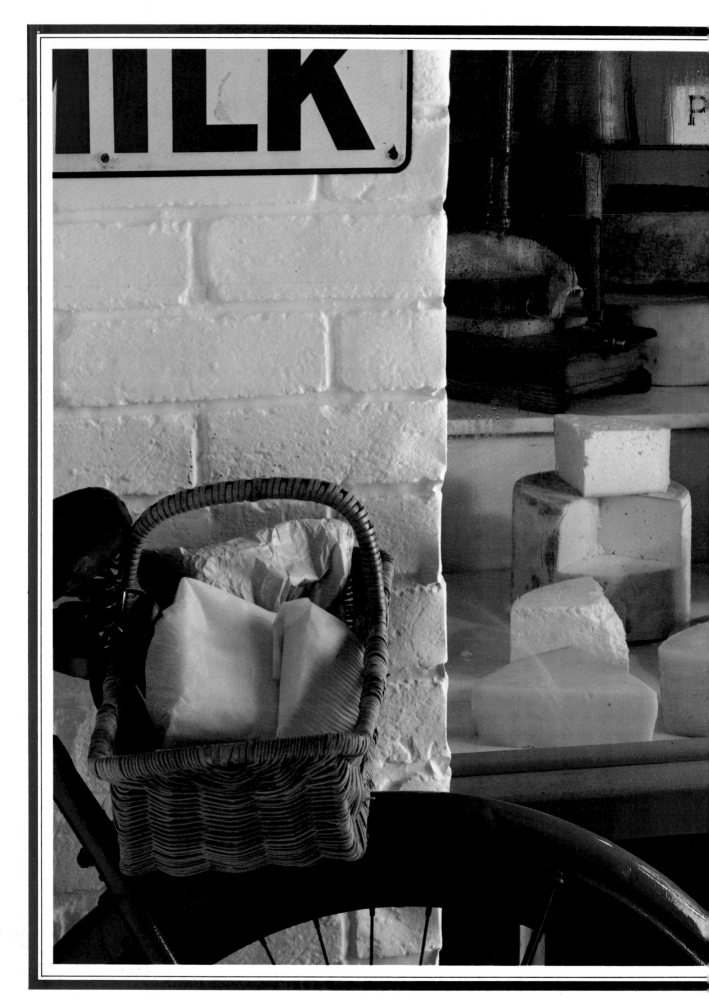

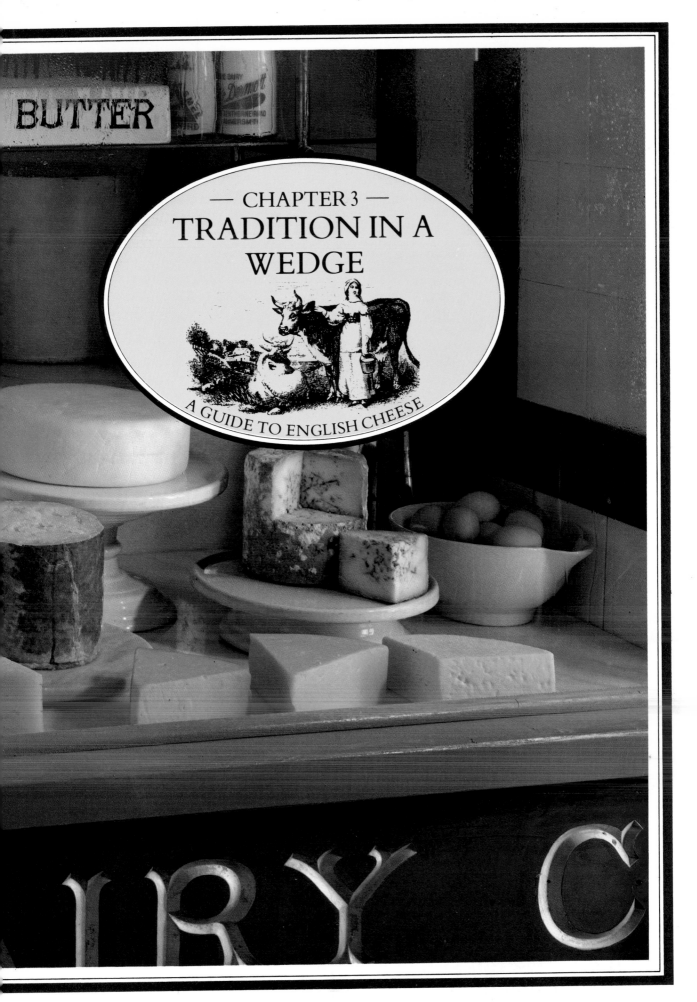

— CHAPTER 3 —
TRADITION IN A WEDGE

A GUIDE TO ENGLISH CHEESE

BUTTER

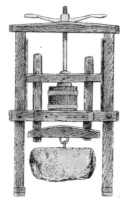

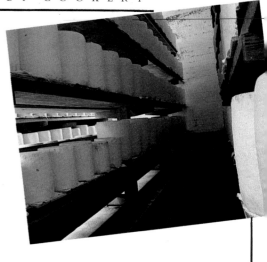

Above:
A wooden cheese press, an important piece of equipment in the making of traditional British cheese. When chopped curds had been placed in a mould lined with muslin, a press like this was used to force out the whey and to compress the texture of the curds. A step-by-step guide to cheesemaking is given opposite and on page 37.

Above right:
The cool interior of a farmhouse cheese store, the long narrow room lined with shelves where cheeses were left to mature. Cheese rooms like this were often built partly sunken into the ground to maintain an even temperature. For centuries, Cheddar cheeses were traditionally left to mature in the caves at Cheddar in Somerset.

One job of the dairy maid or farmer's wife was to turn the cheeses in the store room – a task which required physical stamina. To evenly distribute the water content, each cheese was turned every day for two weeks in winter and twice every day in summer. After the first two weeks, each cheese would then be turned every other day.

Right:
Key to the fine British cheeses shown on the preceding pages.

1 *Red Leicester*
2 *Wensleydale*
3 *Lancashire*
4 *Derby*
5 *English Cheddar*
6 *Caerphilly*
7 *Blue Stilton*
8 *Red Leicester*
9 *Double Gloucester*
10 *Cheshire*

Cheese is one of the best examples of fine British food. What began as a thrifty way of using up surplus milk on the farm has become one of our most valuable and versatile foods. Our cheeses with their splendid English – and Welsh – names, Cheddar, Cheshire, Caerphilly, Lancashire, Leicester, Double Gloucester, Derby, Wensleydale, Stilton, that come ringing down the centuries, are both excellent and unique. Nobody else in the world can touch us for the variety and quality of our hard cheeses, marvellous for eating, unbeatable for cooking. And just as each type has its own traditional shape, size and crust, each has its own personality and flavour.

We are very fortunate that our relatively small family of regional cheeses produces such a great range of flavours, aromas and textures with something to suit every palate. English and Welsh cheeses embrace the whole scale from mild to mature, sharp to mellow, and firm to crumbly.

Just as wine owes its character to the grape, the soil and the weather, so cheese is affected by the breed of cow, the quality of milk, the type of pasture, the geology of the region – especially the minerals in the ground – the seasons, the weather and the magic ingredients of the skill and pride of the cheesemaker who takes it through the various necessary and complicated stages. What our English and Welsh cheeses have in common is that they are firm cheeses, all made from full-cream cows' milk. They have varying maturing times, keep well, are perfect to serve from a cheeseboard, but have the sort of crumbling, grating and melting qualities needed for cooking.

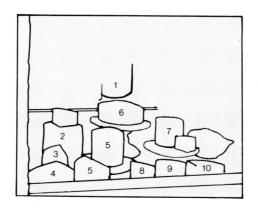

OUR COUNTRY HERITAGE

Who said cheese wasn't romantic? English and Welsh cheese are highly romantic. Poetic even. A good sturdy reliable food it might be, but its history is the history of England and Wales. It has all sorts of fascinating and deeply-rooted associations – with the rural past, the sweet country life of meadows and dairy maids, garlands, maypoles, haymaking, harvest, country markets and fairs, May Days and holidays; with architecture in the design of farmhouses with cheese rooms and dairies; with the Industrial Revolution and two World Wars; with the whole history of travelling – coaches, the railway, motor cars, pubs and inns; with women's work; with literature and folklore, and not least, with the enjoyment of food generally.

The story of cheese is embedded in the fabric of this country in the most fascinating way. Did you know, for instance, that the great cheesemaking traditions of the Yorkshire Dales were handed on from monks in the great abbeys of Jervaulx and Rievaulx; that dairy work on the farm was done by women: the farmer's wife, helped by a dairy maid hired from the village – 'the bigger the dairy maid, the better the cheese' says the old Derbyshire proverb; that one of the largest dairy companies in England had an express train as its trademark; that a Cheshire cat was in fact an old cheese measure; that the oldest cheese recipe – 1390 – was for adding grated cheese to soup, or that the reputations of Stilton and Cheshire cheese were made by travellers who tasted them at inns along the coaching routes?

The history of English and Welsh cheese goes back nearly 2,000 years and probably began with the making of ewes' milk cheese which certainly continued until medieval times. Even in the 1920s, ewes' milk was added to the cows' milk in the areas of Caerphilly where cheese was made. Cheesemaking is a work of art, a rural skill and a science in which tradition, technology, knowledge and intuition all play their part. Cheese has always been made to time-honoured methods and well-respected recipes, some of them secret and jealousy guarded. Such recipes were handed down from mother to daughter and often stated the best season for making a particular cheese. 'This cheese must be made between Michaelmas and All Hallows,' wrote one, or, 'This cheese must be made in May.' Almost every county had its own distinctive cheese with local variations, so that from the seventeenth to the nineteenth centuries this country was rich in local cheese all made in the farmhouse from the milk of cows grazing on local pastures. Some would be kept for family use, others sold at fairs or to middlemen who collected them from local farms and resold them in the towns. Stilton was expensive, Cheshire plentiful and cheap. Before the coming of the railways and the car, there was no other way of putting extra liquid milk to good use and profit, apart from making butter.

Since the mid-fifties we have seen not only the welcome return of classic English and Welsh cheeses, but many local and regional specialities like Sage Derby and Sage Lancashire, and the invention of a new soft blue cheese, Lymeswold. Farmhouse cheese is now made by only fifty farmers, mainly in Cheshire, Somerset and Lancashire. Modern creameries make all varieties of English and Welsh cheese (except Stilton), all the year round. The first cheese factory was started near Derby in 1870 and today, though engineering and science have taken the hard grind out of it, the essentials of cheesemaking remain the same.

Whether made on the farm or in the creamery there is still a need for a skilled cheesemaker to ensure the process results in a good cheese of a quality and standard to meet the preferences of the mild-cheese eater as well as those preferring a mature flavour.

It has always been a British tradition to end a meal on a savoury note with the cheese as a finale, often accompanied by fruit, but many now like to follow the French way and have cheese before the sweet so as to be able to go on drinking robust wine with it. Appreciating English cheeses is like appreciating wine: they all have their characteristic colour, fragrance, texture and flavour. Each has its own reputation and devoted admirers.

CHEDDAR: THE BIG CHEESE

This is our biggest cheese – it used to be made to a size up to 54 kg (120 lb) in weight – and many say it is our best. In Elizabethan times, Cheddar was made in the lush, rich pastures of the West Country around the Cheddar Gorge by local farmers. As the cheeses were very large they were left for a long time, from 2 to 5 years, before they were eaten.

Farmhouse Cheddar is made from the milk of one area and is ready to eat as early as 3 months, but at 9 months it is nicely mellow with a fully developed flavour. Creamery Cheddar is made from the milk of several areas, using as much as 682,000 litres (150,000 gallons) of milk a day, and producing 68,058 kg (50,000 lb) of cheese to sizes and weights to meet the needs of the wholesaler, caterer and consumer.

FIT FOR A QUEEN

The largest Cheddar on record, a giant 559 kg (11 cwt) and probably pressed under a mill-stone, was made from the milk of all the cows, 737 of them, in one

THE OLD WAY OF MAKING CHEESE
A coagulum forms after 'starter' and rennet are added to warm milk.

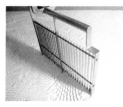

1 Cutting the coagulum

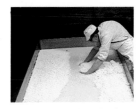

2 Separating curds and whey

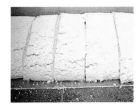

3 'Cheddaring' the curd

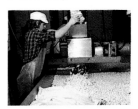

4 Milling and salting prior to filling moulds

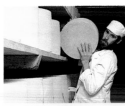

5 After pressing and dressing, the cheese is matured under controlled humidity and temperature over many weeks

Left:
A creamery is a building specially designed for the large-scale production of dairy foods. This is Longford Creamery, near Coventry, the first creamery to be built in England, which was opened on 4th May 1870.

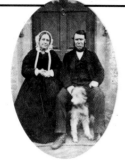

Above:
Joseph Harding and his wife, two of the great British cheesemakers. Joseph Harding was born at Marksbury, Somerset in 1805 and he was the first person to study and reform Cheddar cheesemaking. Until he codified the rules for cheesemaking into a scientific system, cheeses were made by ancient hit-and-miss methods of skill and good luck. Mrs Harding was also a first-rate cheesemaker and she passed on the craft to all of her seven sons and six daughters.

parish of Glastonbury as a wedding present for Queen Victoria who didn't want it back after she'd allowed it to go on exhibition. The farmers quarrelled over it and it ended up in Chancery and was never heard of again. In 1977 a Silver Jubilee Cheddar, more modestly tipping the scales at 36 kg (80 lb), was made in the same area for Queen Elizabeth II.

CHESHIRE: THE OLDEST CHEESE

The River Dee drains the north-west region of England and north-east Wales and Cheshire cheese has been made here since before Roman times. Cheshire is the oldest named cheese and was mentioned in the Domesday Book. Traditionally it gets its uniquely characteristic salty flavour from the salt beds underlying the soil of the region which makes it virtually impossible to imitate. It is known as the patriotic cheese as it can be red, white or blue. There is no difference in flavour between white and red Cheshire but many prefer the red, coloured with a vegetable dye, annatto. Blue Cheshire originally happened naturally, but today's blue-veined Cheshire with its characteristic flavour, is manufactured by only one farmhouse cheesemaker.

One of London's oldest eating houses, The Cheshire Cheese in Fleet Street, is an indication of how popular the cheese must have been in the eighteenth

Right:
The Cheshire Cheese pub, one of Britain's ancient inns still standing on Fleet Street, London.

century, the heyday of the great fairs in Chester, Shrewsbury and all the neighbouring market towns where the local cheeses were bought to be sold again in London.

Cheshire is a crumbly cheese. Prime condition for Cheshire is 4–8 weeks and Blue Cheshire 2–3 months.

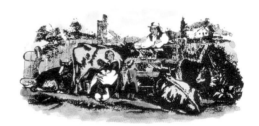

LANCASHIRE: THE TOASTIES' CHEESE

Lancashire is a soft-bodied cheese. Its crumbly texture makes it ideal for cooking. A young Lancashire cheese has a clean acid taste, whereas a mature cheese has quite a tang to it. Farmhouse Lancashire is unusual as one batch of curd is made during the evening and kept overnight, then added to freshly-made curds the next morning. Nowadays most Lancashire cheese made in creameries has similar characteristics to the traditional version, but is made from a single batch of curd giving a mild-flavoured crumbly cheese with a drier texture.

LEICESTER: RICH AND MELLOW

Traditionally, this is a firm, flat, wheel-shaped cheese whose dark russet colour from the addition of annatto dye makes it easy to identify. It originates from the region around Melton Mowbray which is also famous for delicious pork pies. Open textured and slightly flaky, Leicester has a rich mellow taste. It can be eaten at 2–3 months, but if kept longer it will develop a more nutty flavour.

DERBY: THE CHEESE WITH SAGE

Derby is a hard, mild, traditionally wheel-shaped cheese. It is good at 6–8 weeks for eating, and if left longer it develops a mature rich tangy flavour. Sage Derby is smaller and flavoured with rubbed sage leaves which give an attractive green marbling to the curd. It was sometimes made with a single layer of sage through the centre.

It was traditional to make special cheeses such as Sage Derby for harvest and Christmas eating on the farms and these were not usually for sale. Adding flavour like this was an old custom in many areas when wine, herbs, spices, chives, onions, cider, raisins, nuts, beer and garlic were used in or on the cheeses to give more variety to the diet. This custom is being revived today and most shops and supermarkets carry a range of flavoured cheeses.

DOUBLE GLOUCESTER: GREATLY ESTEEMED

A mild mellow cheese with a firm close texture, this cheese has a fine reputation going back to the sixteenth century. At one point it was said to be the most esteemed cheese in England. Gloucester was produced originally in its home county, a region rich in cheesemaking customs and using the milk only from Gloucester cows. Annatto is responsible for its orange colour. Double Gloucester gets its name from its size, which is twice that of Single Gloucester. Once known as the haymaking cheese, Single Gloucester is rarely seen now. It was made in May to be eaten in the hayfield with new baked bread and cider.

WENSLEYDALE: PRIDE OF THE YORKSHIRE DALES

Cheesemaking in the Yorkshire Dales goes back to Saxon times, and Wensleydale was originally made from ewes' milk by the monks of the great medieval abbeys such as Jervaulx in North Yorkshire. After the monasteries were dissolved by Henry VIII, the traditional recipe was used by generations of farmers' wives who adapted it for use with cows' milk.

Until the Second World War white and blue Wensleydale cheeses were made, but due to wartime restrictions blue cheesemaking was stopped. Today, a small amount of blue Wensleydale is still available. Wensleydale has a fairly close texture and is very crumbly, with

a mild slightly sweet flavour, and a delicious honeyed after-taste, after being matured for 3–5 weeks. It used to be sold at Michaelmas fairs for the Tyneside Christmas trade and has always been a popular cheese with Northern miners. The northern tradition of serving Wensleydale with apple pie or Christmas cake is reflected in the saying, 'Apple pie without cheese is like a lass without a squeeze!'

CAERPHILLY: THE MINERS' FAVOURITE

This fast-maturing cheese was named after the Glamorgan village of Caerphilly and is still traditionally made in South Wales, Somerset, Devon and Dorset. It is close textured, moist but flaky and has a mild, pleasant, slightly acid flavour. Caerphilly was preferred by miners because it remained moist down the mine and because a wedge was just the right size to carry underground.

STILTON: KING OF THE DINNER TABLE

This is a monarch among blue-veined cheeses, a connoisseur's cheese in a class of its own with a fine international reputation. Stilton belongs to the heart of England and has been made in the Vale of Belvoir and the beautiful Dove Valley region for generations. Stories about its origin vary slightly. The most popular version says it was a Mrs Paulet who first made the cheese 300 years ago. She supplied it to the Bell Inn, a coaching stop on the Great North Road at Stilton, and its reputation took off from there. Others say it was Mrs Paulet's mother, housekeeper at Quenby Hall, who first made the cheese. Well-satisfied customers of the Bell spread its fame and the secret recipe was handed down virtually unchanged. The recipe for this cheese is still closely guarded by a few makers who today form the Stilton Cheesemakers Association. Stilton is now a registered cheese which ensures that it can only be made in the three counties of Leicestershire, Nottinghamshire and Derbyshire. It is the only English cheese to have such a trademark.

Stilton is cylindrical in shape but its

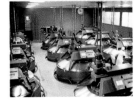

1 15,000-litre vats in which the coagulum forms

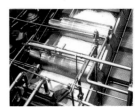

2 Curds travelling to the 'cheddaring' tower

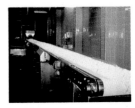

3 Milled curd on the way to press room

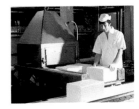

4 Cheese emerging from press and being cut into blocks

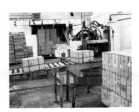

5 Boxed, vacuum-packed blocks ready for store

CUTTING A CHEESE

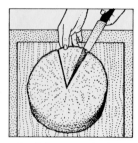

1 Carefully cutting the first wedge

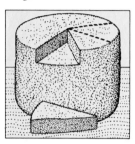

2 'Cut high, cut low' is still the way to slice a Stilton. This cheese should never be scooped out with a spoon as it is wasteful and looks unsightly

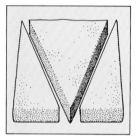

3 If your piece of cheese is pre-packed, it will look attractive on a cheeseboard if you cut it into a wedge

Below:
The Bell Inn, Stilton, Leicestershire.

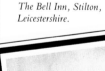

naturally rough crumbly brown crust and its white-to-creamy yellow body with the greeny-blue mould will vary according to its place and manufacturer. This cheese is at its best when fully ripe at 3–5 months when its beautifully creamy texture can vary from light moist and crumbly to smooth and firm.

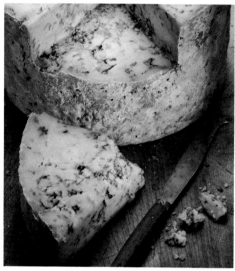

A whole Stilton should not be scooped or quarried out with a spoon; this practice is wasteful, dries it out and ruins the look of a fine whole cheese. When cutting a Stilton or any whole cheese, take a horizontal slice, and then cut that into a wedge-shaped slice – 'cut high cut low' is the best advice.

VARIATION ON A THEME

LOW FAT HARD CHEESE
Cheddar and Cheshire varieties are available with half the fat of the traditional cheeses.

VEGETARIAN CHEESE
Traditional hard cheeses made from rennet of microbial rather than animal origin.

NEW NAMES AND OLD FLAVOURS

Some of our traditional hard cheeses are now being made with additional and time-honoured flavourings. Red Windsor, for example, is Cheddar marbled with elderberry wine; Rutland is Cheddar with beer, garlic and parsley; Walton is a blend of Cheddar and Stilton with walnuts; Nutwood is Cheddar with cider, hazelnuts and raisins; Cheviot is Cheddar with chives; Charwood or Applewood is mature Cheddar smoked with an outer coating of paprika; Cotswold is Double Gloucester with chives and onions; Sherwood is Double Gloucester with sweet pickle; Huntsman is Double Gloucester layered with Blue Stilton, while Ilchester is Double Gloucester and mustard pickle!

SOFT CHEESES

These cheeses are soft to the touch and have a high moisture content.

UNRIPENED SOFT CHEESE
These may be purchased as full-fat, medium-fat, low-fat and skimmed-milk soft cheese, according to the fat content. In addition, cream cheese and double cream cheeses are available, having a minimum fat content of 45% and 65% respectively.

RIPENED SOFT CHEESE
Lymeswold is the first soft blue cheese to be produced commercially in this country. In fact it's the first new English cheese for many years.

COTTAGE CHEESE
This is an American-style soft cheese. Cottage cheese is slightly salted, made from skimmed milk with cream added, but it still has a fat content of between 2% and 10%. Acid and rennet produce a firm curd which is cut and drained. The characteristic granular texture is due to the slow gentle heating of the curd prior to washing and draining. The bland flavour and soft texture of this cheese makes it an ideal base to which pineapple, ham or chives are frequently added.

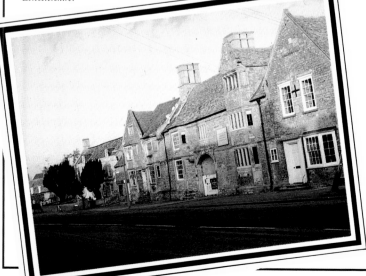

HOW TO BUY CHEESE

Freshly cut cheese should look fresh, with no dried areas or beads of fat on the surface. Cut, pre-wrapped cheese should have no evidence of mould, moisture or greasiness inside the packing. If there is, it has been stored at too high a temperature. To ensure pre-packed soft cheeses are eaten at their best, take notice of the 'sell by' or 'best before' date which is now legally required on the packaging.

It is advisable to buy only enough cheese for about a week at a time. However, for a large family or a party it may be more economical and convenient to buy a quarter, half or whole cheese, particularly if you have suitable storage space in the refrigerator or a cool larder.

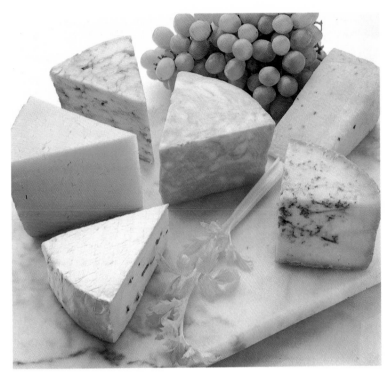

COOKING WITH CHEESE

One of the best things about cheese is its versatility, as it can be happily included in any meal and is useful as a snack at any time of the day. For breakfast cheese can be served with toast or sprinkled over eggs; for lunch it goes well in flans or with salad; and for dinners it can be used as a garnish for vegetables, in mousses or soufflés, or simply as a cheeseboard with fruit.

Cheese is easy to prepare, just slice or grate it, but when cooking with it, a little more care is needed. Cheese separates at relatively low temperatures, usually 65.5°C (150°F), and too much cooking causes the cheese to become leathery and unpalatable. Hard cheese cooks best if it is first shredded or grated. As cheese contains salt, dishes containing cheese need less salt added to them, so great care should be taken when seasoning cheese dishes.

HOW TO STORE IT

Cheese should be kept cool. A larder is ideal, but a refrigerator is used by the majority of people. Wrap cheese tightly in polythene, cling film or foil and bring it out of the refrigerator 1 hour before you want to eat it, so that it can come back to room temperature and develop its full flavour. Hard cheese will freeze well without any deterioration of flavour; cut it into 100–150-g (4–6-oz) pieces for easier thawing and wrap it in

film rather than foil. Use thawed cheese quickly as cheese which has been frozen tends to deteriorate more readily.

THE CHEESEBOARD

A good cheeseboard attractively presented should be every bit as tempting and appetising as the sweet trolley. When serving cheese at the end of a meal allow a good 50 g (2 oz) per head, as appetites tend to revive at the sight and smell of a fragrant cheese! For an informal meal where cheese is one of the main items, allow a good 125 g (4 oz) per head. A small selection of perhaps two or three quality cheeses is best. Use large freshly-cut wedges that vary in maturity, colour and texture and include a good blue-veined cheese. A whole small cheese in perfect condition always looks very impressive.

Your cheeseboard should allow plenty of room for cutting, but it should not be so big that it cannot be easily passed round the table. Serve cheese with crusty bread or biscuits, celery or grapes. Some people like to garnish a cheeseboard with watercress or parsley but an uncluttered cheeseboard is the most inviting – the cheese speaks for itself.

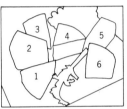

Above: When cheese is served in prime condition, accompanied by some crisp, fresh celery or fruit, a cheeseboard is a tempting sight which often sharpens appetites again, even after a hearty meal! In France cheese is usually served before the pudding, a custom which is rapidly catching on in Britain.

Key:
1 Lymeswold
2 Mature Cheddar
3 Sage Derby
4 Windsor Red
5 Cotswold
6 Blue Stilton

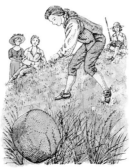

Above:
Cheese rolling, an ancient sport still held at Cooper Hill, between Gloucester and Cheltenham, on every Whit Monday.

GIVING A WINE AND CHEESE PARTY

A wine and cheese party is a happy and economical compromise between a cocktail party and a formal dinner. It suits most age groups, it is easily organised, and can be planned to suit any budget. All wines, but especially red wines, go well with cheese.

The main requirement for the party is as interesting an assortment of cheeses as you can buy, and suitable wines to accompany them.

The quantity of cheese required will depend somewhat on the extent of variety offered, but overall allow about 175 g (6 oz) per person. If the party takes place between meal times the requirement will be less; if it replaces an evening meal, perhaps more. For a small party a few well-selected cheeses in large pieces are preferable to a bewildering array of scrappy bits.

Arrange the cheeses separately on boards or plates to keep the flavours apart. If you are presenting large numbers of cheeses, label them; or group them geographically by regions of origin, or by types. You may have Lancashire and Wensleydale at the

northern end of the table, for example, followed by Cheshire, Derby, Leicester, Stilton, Caerphilly, Cheddar and Lymeswold. Or arrange them in alternating types and colours. In either case you might wish to show a tasting order: if you encourage your guests to proceed from the mildest to the strongest, cheese dips, soft or cottage cheese would come first.

It is a good idea to suggest which wine might best accompany each cheese, but this is of course only a guide as it is very much dependent on personal preference. A hock will be very suitable with the mild flavour of Wensleydale and Caerphilly while a light claret is perfect for white or red Cheshire and Double Gloucester. Tawny port or Oloroso sherry is very appropriate for a Blue Cheshire, a full claret or a red Burgundy for English Cheddar. A ruby port could be tried with Derby or White Stilton, but for a Blue Stilton, try tawny or vintage port or a red Burgundy. Claret or Madeira is good to accompany Leicester, while Lancashire calls for a light dry red wine, a medium dry sherry or ruby port.

Beer and cider are also natural accompaniments to English and Welsh

WINE TO SERVE WITH TRADITIONAL ENGLISH CHEESES

RED LEICESTER
Côtes de Bourg/*Bordeaux red*
Valpolicella/*Italian light dry red*
Mâcon Rouge/*Burgundy dry red*
Fruit wine/*mead*

DOUBLE GLOUCESTER
Médoc/*Bordeaux light red*
Dão/*Portuguese substantial dry white*
Barbaresco/*Italian dry red*
Fruit wine/*cherry*

ENGLISH CHESHIRE
Beaujolais/*light fruity red*
Bulls Blood/*Hungarian full-bodied red*
Corbieres/*French medium red*
Fruit wine/*redcurrant or dry apple*

LANCASHIRE
Manzanilla or Fino/*dry sherry*
Alsace White/*French fruity, dry white*
Fruit wine/*sweet apple*

ENGLISH CHEDDAR
Rioja Reserva Red/*Spanish dry red*
Chianti Classico/*Italian dry red*
Châteauneuf-du-Pape/*French full-bodied red*
Fruit wine/*elderberry*

BLUE STILTON
Port or Madeira
Barsac/*Bordeaux sweet white*
Barolo/*Italian dry red*
Oloroso/*dark, slightly sweet sherry*
Fruit wine/*elderberry*

DERBY
Bergerac/*Bordeaux light white*
California Red
Côtes du Rousillion/*French dry white, red or rosé*
Fruit wine/*elderberry*

WENSLEYDALE
Orvieto/*Italian dry white*
Anjou Rosé/*French rosé*
Laski Reisling/*German fruity white*
Fruit wine/*redcurrant*

CAERPHILLY
Moselle/*German white*
Provence Rosé/*dry rosé*
Soave/*Italian dry white*
Vinho Verde/*Portuguese slightly sparkling white*
Fruit wine/*gooseberry*

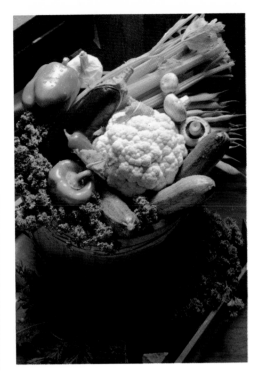

of raw foods – celery, green pepper, carrot, cucumber, small spring onions, florets of cauliflower, chicory leaves, wedges of fennel and some radishes. If wedges of apple or pear are to be served, first blanch them in boiling water for a few seconds to ensure that they keep their colour. Avoid sprinkling them with lemon juice as the acidity will mar the flavour of the cheese and wine.

Finally, make sure there is plenty of room round the tables so that guests can circulate easily and 'taste around' – this is more fun than queueing once to take a large lump of only one kind of cheese! With thoughtful planning and pleasing presentation your party fare should be even more attractive than the simple ploughman's lunch.

CHEESE CUSTOMS

As one of the world's leading cheese producers, Britain has many old customs connected with cheese. The sport of cheese rolling is an old annual custom that still survives in parts of the Cotswolds. The ceremony at Cooper Hill, between Gloucester and Cheltenham, traditionally held on Whit Monday, has very ancient origins connected with the villagers' rights to graze sheep on the hill and has taken place without a break since its beginnings. Nowadays it is held on Spring Bank Holiday Monday. The cheese, a Gloucester cheese of course, wheel-shaped and tough crusted but in any case protected by a strong wooden casing, is sent rolling and bouncing down a very steep slope at the top of which stands a flower-bedecked maypole. The youths of the neighbourhood line up on the hill top and dash after the cheese, 'measuring their length more than once and rolling a good part of the way like their quarry', according to one eyewitness. The winner keeps the cheese and there are money prizes for coming second and third. In Victorian times they raced after a cartwheel and won the cheeses as prizes.

Another Gloucestershire Whitsun custom is the Bread and Cheese Dole, first recorded in 1799 but probably going back much earlier and again connected with ancient rights. It takes

Left:
Vegetables and cheese are two foods which complement each other well, whether they are used raw or cooked.

A good selection of crunchy raw vegetables is the perfect accompaniment to fine English cheese at a wine and cheese party. For hot dishes try the delicious Cheesy Stuffed Aubergines on page 88 or the Courgettes Au Gratin on page 183.

cheese, and they are also more appropriate than wine for ready-flavoured cheeses such as cheese with added chives, onions, beer, herbs, wine or pickle. It is also wise to have fruit juices or soft drinks on hand in case guests prefer not to drink alcohol.

Chill the white wine for at least an hour before serving. Red wine is best served at room temperature and should be opened some 2–3 hours in advance of the party. It is usually sufficient to allow $\frac{1}{2}$ bottle of wine per person, but keep a few unopened bottles to one side as an emergency supply. Glasses can be usually hired from your local off-licence and some off-licences may be happy to offer the wine to you on a sale or return basis.

To accompany the cheeses remember to offer your guests a variety of fresh, crusty bread, including granary or another good wholemeal, some poppy-seeded plaits and best of all, some fresh homemade bread. For 15 people select four different large loaves. Serve portions of butter in pats, balls or curls in several dishes. For 15 people, allow 450 g (1 lb) but have more in reserve. Try to ensure that each cheese has its own knife – serrated for the hard cheeses, unserrated but sharp for the crumbly or sticky varieties.

To complement the texture of the cheeses, have a good selection of fingers place outside the parish church of St Mary's in St Briavels. After Evensong small pieces of bread and cheese are thrown into the air from large baskets for the waiting crowd. The parishioners paid a penny for this and it secured their right to cut and take wood from local woods.

At Randwick, near Stroud in Gloucestershire, the cheese rolling was more elaborate. Originally it belonged to May Day rites but became part of Rogation Day celebrations when blessings were asked on crops. Three cheeses, decked with flowers, were carried on litters into church, 'accompanied by shout, song and music'. Then they were taken into the churchyard, the decorations removed and they were rolled three times round the church anti-clockwise. Decked up again, they were put back in the litters and carried in procession to the village green where one was cut and distributed to the parishioners. The other two were kept for rolling down the hill at Wap Fair the following Saturday.

Cutting the cheese is a Christmas custom dating back to the early years of the Royal Hospital for Chelsea pensioners. English cheeses are presented and the oldest pensioner cuts one of them with the Regimental Sergeant Major's sword.

At one time it was always customary to have a special cheese for Christmas; as essential as cake or mince pies. Alison Uttley in *The Country Child* describes seeing them in the cheese room on the farm, 'Some of them were Christmas cheeses with layers of sage running through the middle like green ribbon.' In the North the cheese was always eaten with spice loaf.

In something very close to the New Year first-footing rites, the cheese at Eston in Cleveland plays a part in a Christmas Eve custom to bring good luck on the house. It is taken outside by the youngest member of the family and rolled over the step into the house right up to the table where it is placed on a dish and cut. In Northumberland cheese was sometimes part of a curious christening custom when a symbolic little parcel of life's necessities – bread, cheese, matches (to light your way) and salt – was carried by one of the

christening party and given to the first person of the opposite sex to the baby whom he or she met on the way to church.

WELSH RAREBIT

His intimate friends called him Candle-ends His enemies Toasted Cheese

You can't write about cheese without saying a special word about this most famous of toasted cheese dishes. It crops up again and again in old recipe books, records and stories, some well before Shakespeare's time, so it has obviously had a long history and is still going strong today. One modern cookery book lists ten variations, including Peruvian Rabbit, Way Down South Rabbit and Punjab Curry Rabbit. It has been referred to as the national dish of Wales, 'Davies' darling', 'the Welshman's delight'. Men always seem to have loved it – 'a favourite dish for a gentleman's supper'.

Is it rabbit or rarebit? Because it was made from the cheapest ingredients, bread and cheese, it was put about that the Welsh could afford nothing better and since they hadn't any rabbits of their own, nor any money to buy them from England, they invented this substitute called Welsh Rabbit. Another tale has it that when Welsh wives saw their menfolk returning from the hunt empty-handed they put cheese before the fire to melt as a substitute for the meat. Later rabbit was refined to rarebit, though some say even this is a corruption of rearbit, the savoury that came at the end of the meal. The Welsh must have been fonder of it than anyone else because it seems when too many of them got to heaven and caused overcrowding, St Peter went outside and shouted, 'Toasted Cheese'; whereupon all the Welshmen rushed out and St Peter locked the gate.

One thing you can't argue about is its wonderful taste. Mrs Beeton recommended Cheshire or Cheddar cheese for a good Welsh Rabbit, some prefer Lancashire or Double Gloucester and others say as long as it's a rich new cheese that will melt nicely without becoming stringy it will produce that unforgettable taste and smell.

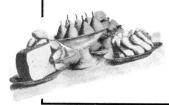

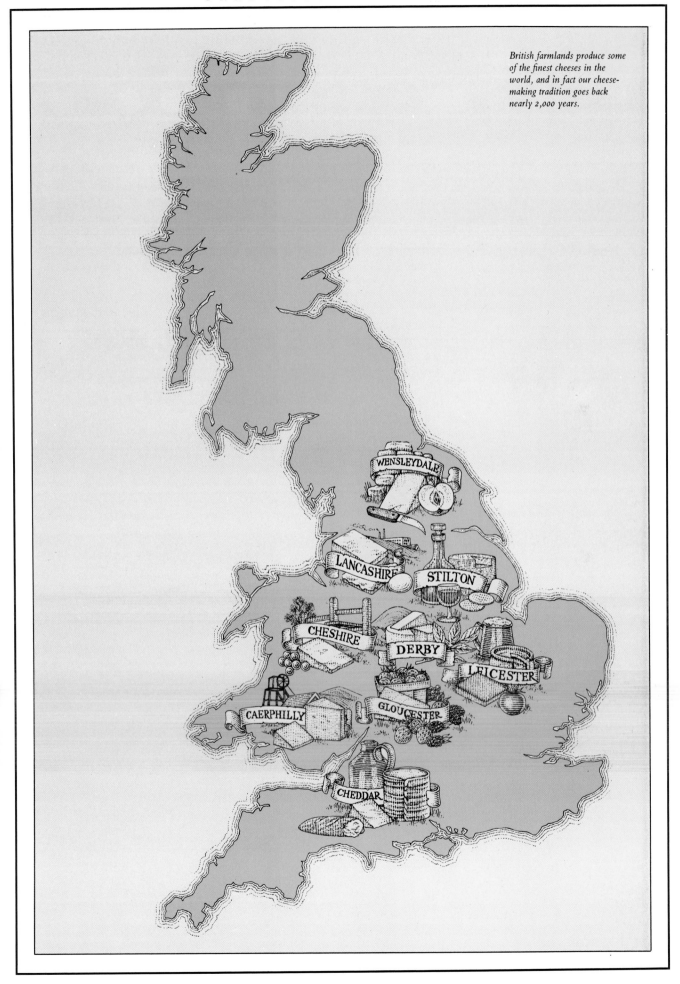

British farmlands produce some of the finest cheeses in the world, and in fact our cheese-making tradition goes back nearly 2,000 years.

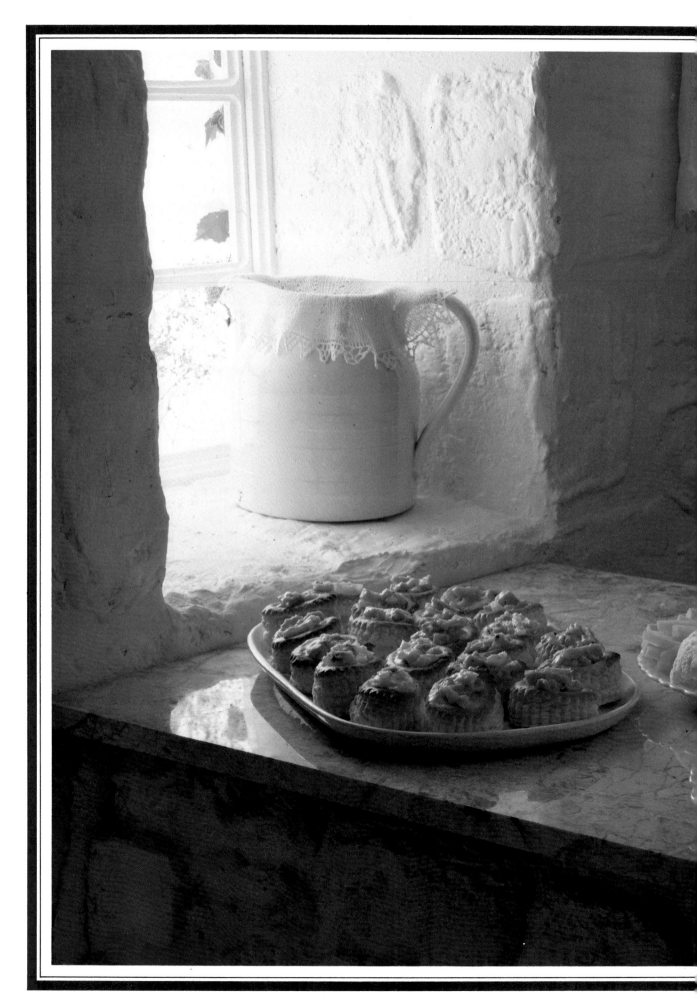

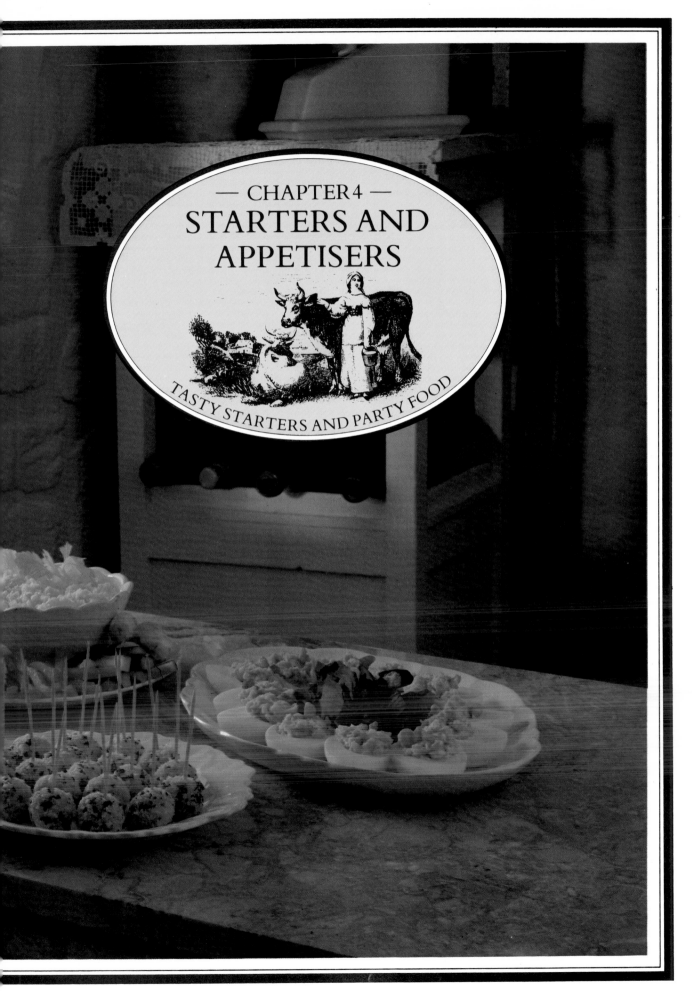

— CHAPTER 4 —
STARTERS AND APPETISERS

TASTY STARTERS AND PARTY FOOD

A fresh enticing starter not only sets the tone of the whole meal but paves the way for good things to come. Ideally it should be something a little bit special and unusual enough to generate some excitement. A good starter complements rather than competes with the main course. Make it simple, if the main course is rich and elaborate; or choose something cool and plain to begin with if your main course is spicy. A good starter shouldn't look or taste similar to what is to follow.

Starters can be part of a meal where your imagination and artistic flair come into play. Remember it's best to serve small portions, and to present them attractively with crisp eye-catching garnishes such as freshly chopped herbs or piquant lemon wedges, for example.

Even if the budget is tight the starter can be the place where a little luxury can be made to go a long way. A small amount of salmon, for instance, or prawns or Stilton can be stretched to provide an exotic first course. Cream, above all else, spells richness and luxury: use it in fillings and stuffings and in wonderful sauces which will transform otherwise humble foods like eggs, mushrooms and tomatoes. A good fruit and savoury combination, sharp and refreshing, like the Cheese and Apple Pears on page 54 are excellent when there's a rich sauce with the main course or a sweet made from fresh cream on the horizon.

Salads and cold starters that can be ready waiting while you deal with other parts of the meal are a good idea, but even last-minute frying of hot starters, such as Stilton Bites or Cheese and Ham Aigrettes, needn't be a worry if you are well organised – it's well worth a bit of a flurry to serve something hot or crisply brown from the grill.

Party dips should be really smooth as well as piquant and interesting. There's no point in serving something so bland and indifferent that nobody takes any notice of it. Dips should excite and intrigue and this chapter presents a mouthwatering selection for you to choose from. Serve the dips with raw fresh vegetables – preferably crunchy ones such as carrots, celery and cauliflower florets – and get your party off to a delicious start.

HOT STARTERS

STILTON BITES

50 g (2 oz) English butter

50 g (2 oz) flour

300 ml ($\frac{1}{2}$ pint) milk

175 g (6 oz) Blue Stilton cheese, grated

salt and freshly ground pepper

paprika

4 gherkins, roughly chopped

1 egg, beaten

50 g (2 oz) dry white breadcrumbs

1. Melt the butter in a pan, stir in the flour and cook gently for 1 minute, stirring. Remove pan from the heat and gradually stir in the milk. Bring to the boil slowly and continue to cook, stirring, until the sauce thickens, then add the cheese and seasonings and stir well.
2. Turn into a non-stick 17.5-cm (7-inch) square tin. Chill for several hours.
3. Remove from tin and cut into dice. Using floured hands, press a piece of gherkin into each dice. Carefully coat in egg and breadcrumbs.
4. Cook in hot deep fat or oil for several minutes until golden. Drain on absorbent kitchen paper and keep warm in a low oven.
Makes 60

SEAFOOD SCALLOPS

175 g (6 oz) haddock

150 ml ($\frac{1}{4}$ pint) dry white wine

small piece of onion

parsley sprig

bay leaf

350 g (12 oz) potato, peeled

50 g (2 oz) button mushrooms, wiped and sliced

25 g (1 oz) English butter

45 ml (3 level tbsp) flour

200 ml (7 fl oz) milk

50 g (2 oz) English Cheddar cheese, grated

50 g (2 oz) potted shrimps

salt and freshly ground pepper

1. Simmer the haddock in a saucepan with the wine, a small piece of onion, parsley and bay leaf for about 15 minutes.
2. Drain, reserving liquid. Add enough water to make up to 150 ml ($\frac{1}{4}$ pint). Skin and flake the fish. Boil the potatoes in a saucepan of boiling salted water until tender, drain and mash. Set aside.
3. Sauté the mushrooms in a knob of butter; set aside. In another pan, melt 25 g (1 oz) butter, stir in the flour and cook gently for 1 minute, stirring. Remove pan from the heat

and gradually stir in strained fish liquor and the milk. Bring to the boil slowly and continue to cook, stirring, until the sauce thickens, then add the flaked fish, mushrooms, cheese and potted shrimps. Adjust seasoning.

4. Pipe mashed potato around the edge of four scallop shells. Spoon the fish mixture into the centre and brown under a hot grill.

Serves 4

HADDOCK AND SHRIMP GRATIN

450 g (1 lb) haddock fillet, skinned

25 g (1 oz) English butter

1 medium onion, skinned and finely
    chopped

45 ml (3 level tbsp) flour

300 ml ($\frac{1}{2}$ pint) milk

45 ml (3 tbsp) dry white wine

184-g (6$\frac{1}{2}$-oz) can shrimps

75 g (3 oz) mature English Cheddar cheese

salt and freshly ground pepper

1. Cut the haddock fillet into twelve small strips. Fold strips in half and place two each in six individual ramekin or gratin dishes.
2. Melt the butter in a saucepan. Sauté the finely chopped onion until softened. Stir in the flour and cook gently for 1 minute, stirring. Remove pan from heat and gradually stir in the milk, wine and strained juices from the shrimps. Bring to the boil slowly and continue to cook, stirring, until the sauce thickens.
3. Remove pan from the heat and add the shrimps and 50 g (2 oz) grated cheese to the sauce. Season. Spoon a little into each ramekin. Scatter remaining cheese on top.
4. Cook in the oven at 190°C (375°F) mark 5 for 30 minutes. Serve immediately.

Serves 6

STILTON AND WALNUT CROÛTES

175 g (6 oz) Blue Stilton cheese, crumbled

50 g (2 oz) English butter, softened

50 g (2 oz) walnuts, chopped

salt and freshly ground pepper

15 ml (1 tbsp) brandy

1 small French loaf, cut into 20 slices

stuffed olives, sliced, to garnish

1. In a bowl, combine the crumbled Stilton with the softened butter. Add the walnuts, seasoning and brandy. Toast one side of the bread slices and spread the cheese mixture over the untoasted side.
2. Place under the grill until golden and the cheese is bubbling. Garnish with the sliced olives and serve immediately.

Makes 20

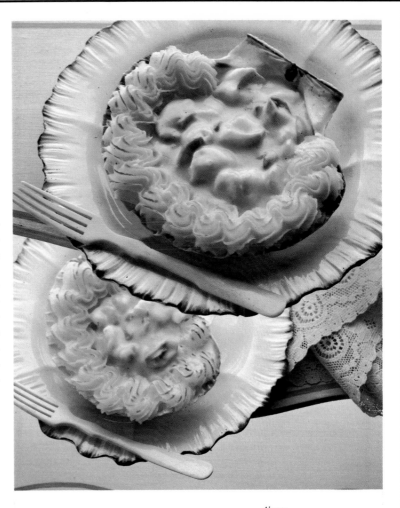

Above:
SEAFOOD SCALLOPS
This tempting hot starter combines haddock, mushrooms and potted shrimps in a delicious cheese sauce. It makes a spectacular opening to a dinner party when served on natural scallop shells edged with a swirl of piped potato and browned under the grill.

SOUFFLÉD CHEESE TARTLETS

65 g (2$\frac{1}{2}$ oz) English butter

115 g (4$\frac{1}{2}$ oz) flour

150 ml ($\frac{1}{4}$ pint) milk

75 g (3 oz) English Cheddar cheese, grated

1 egg, separated

salt and freshly ground pepper

1. In a bowl, rub 50 g (2 oz) butter into 100 g (4 oz) flour until the mixture resembles fine breadcrumbs.
2. Bind to a dough with a little cold water. Roll out on a floured surface and use to line twelve 5-cm (2-inch) patty tins.
3. Melt the remaining 15 g ($\frac{1}{2}$ oz) butter in a pan, stir in the remaining flour and cook gently for 1 minute, stirring. Remove the pan from the heat and gradually stir in the milk. Bring to the boil and continue to cook, stirring, until the sauce thickens, then add the cheese, egg yolk and seasonings.
4. Whisk the egg white until stiff and fold into the mixture. Spoon into the patty cases and bake in the oven at 200°C (400°F) mark 6 for 20–25 minutes until risen and golden. Serve immediately.

Makes 12

MAKING CHEESE
PALMIERS

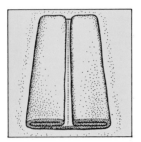

1 Folding the dough

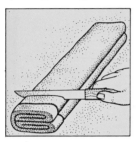

2 Cutting the folded dough
into slices

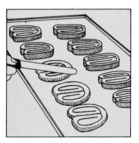

3 Flattening the Palmiers on
a greased baking sheet

Below:
CHEESE PALMIERS
Clever folding and slicing give
these delicious hot savouries
their impressive shape and
texture.

CHEESE D'ARTOIS

1 egg, beaten, plus beaten egg to glaze

25 g (1 oz) English butter, melted

50 g (2 oz) English Cheddar cheese, grated

salt and freshly ground pepper

227-g (8-oz) packet puff pastry, thawed

1. Mix the beaten egg, butter and cheese
until smooth and season well. Roll out the
pastry thinly into a 33-cm (13-inch) square,
cut it in half and place one half on a baking
sheet.
2. Spread the cheese mixture over the pastry
to within 0.5 cm ($\frac{1}{4}$ inch) of each edge.
Dampen the edges with the water and cover
with the remaining pastry. Glaze with beaten
egg and mark the pastry into fingers.
3. Bake in the oven at 200°C (400°F) mark 6
for about 10–15 minutes, until well risen and
golden brown. Cut into fingers before
serving.
Makes 20–24

CHEESE PALMIERS

227-g (8-oz) packet puff pastry, thawed

1 egg, beaten

75 g (3 oz) English Cheddar cheese, grated

salt and freshly ground pepper

paprika

1. Roll out the pastry to an oblong
30.5 × 25.5 cm (12 × 10 inches). Brush with
beaten egg.
2. Scatter over the grated cheese and
sprinkle with salt, pepper and paprika.
3. Roll up tightly lengthwise, rolling from
each side until the rolls meet in the centre.
Cut across into ten pieces.
4. Place cut side down on greased baking
sheet and flatten with a round-bladed knife.

5. Bake in the oven at 200°C (400°F) mark 6
for 15–18 minutes or until brown and crisp.
Ease off baking sheet and cool on a wire
rack.
Makes 10 palmiers

EGGS WITH
TARRAGON CREAM

4 eggs

120 ml (8 tbsp) fresh double cream

10 ml (2 tsp) chopped fresh tarragon

salt and freshly ground pepper

1. Butter four ramekin dishes. Break an egg
into each dish. Mix the fresh cream and the
tarragon in a basin; season.
2. Spoon 30 ml (2 tbsp) of the fresh cream
mixture over each egg and cover with foil.
Place the dishes in a thick-based shallow
pan (a frying pan is ideal) and add boiling
water to come three-quarters up the sides of
the dishes. Simmer gently for 8–10 minutes
until the egg whites are set but yolks are still
soft. Serve immediately.
Serves 4

CHOUX BUNS WITH
STILTON SAUCE

65 g (2$\frac{1}{2}$ oz) flour

pinch of salt

50 g (2 oz) English butter

2 eggs, beaten

75 g (3 oz) full fat soft cheese

50 g (2 oz) Blue Stilton cheese, crumbled

30 ml (2 tbsp) milk

25 g (1 oz) walnuts, finely chopped

1. Sift together the flour and salt. Put 150 ml
($\frac{1}{4}$ pint) water and butter into a saucepan.
Heat slowly until the butter melts, then bring
to a brisk boil.
2. Add the flour all at once, stirring quickly
until the mixture forms a soft ball and leaves
the sides of the pan clean. Cool slightly.
3. Gradually add the eggs, beating them in
until the mixture is smooth, shiny and firm
enough to stand in soft peaks. Place twenty
equal amounts on to a dampened and lightly
floured baking sheet.
4. Bake in the oven at 200°C (400°F) mark 6
for 20 minutes; cool.
5. Beat together the full fat soft cheese,
Stilton and milk; stir in the nuts.
6. Cut the puffs in half and fill the bottom
half with cheese mixture. Replace the tops
and serve immediately.
Makes 4–6

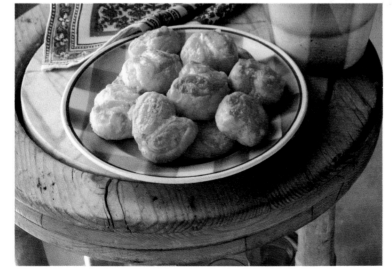

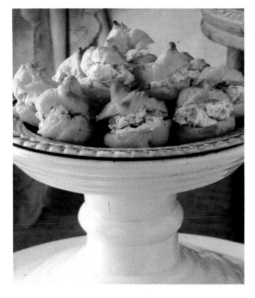

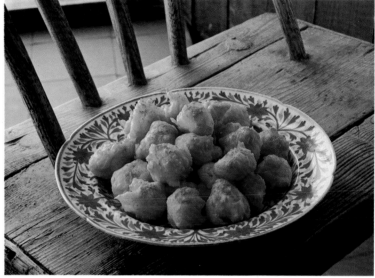

CHEESE AND HAM AIGRETTES

| 25 g (1 oz) English butter |
| 50 g (2 oz) flour |
| 2 eggs |
| 25 g (1 oz) English Cheddar cheese, grated |
| 25 g (1 oz) ham, chopped |
| 5 ml (1 level tsp) finely chopped onion |
| salt |
| cayenne pepper |
| vegetable oil for deep frying |

1. Bring the butter and 60 ml (4 tbsp) water to boiling point, and remove from heat.
2. Add the flour all at once stirring quickly until the mixture forms a soft ball and leaves the sides of the pan clean. Cool slightly.
3. Gradually add the eggs, beating them in until the mixture is smooth, shiny and firm enough to stand in soft peaks. Add the cheese, ham, onion and seasonings.
4. Mix well. Drop small teaspoonfuls of mixture into hot oil and fry each for about 4–5 minutes until golden brown.
5. Serve at once, sprinkled with the cayenne pepper.

Makes about 20

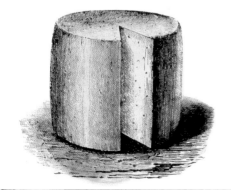

VEGETABLE PÂTÉ

| 125 g (4 oz) English butter |
| 1 medium onion, skinned and finely chopped |
| 1–2 garlic cloves, skinned and crushed (optional) |
| 2 sticks celery, cleaned and finely chopped |
| 30 ml (2 level tbsp) flour |
| 225 g (8 oz) button mushrooms, wiped and finely chopped |
| freshly ground pepper |
| 10 ml (2 level tsp) finely grated lemon rind |
| 15 ml (1 tbsp) lemon juice |
| 2.5 ml ($\frac{1}{2}$ level tsp) salt |
| 90 ml (6 tbsp) fresh double cream |
| 3 slices bread |
| 4–6 cocktail gherkins to garnish |

1. Place the butter in a frying pan and heat gently. Add the chopped onion and garlic and over a low heat cook without colouring, for about 5 minutes.
2. Toss the chopped celery and the flour together, and add to the pan together with the mushrooms. Continue cooking for a further 5–10 minutes, stirring frequently until all the ingredients are cooked.
3. Remove the pan from heat, add pepper to taste. Leave aside until the ingredients have cooled slightly. Add the lemon rind, juice and salt. Mash the ingredients in the pan until they are smooth, then stir in the fresh cream.
4. Spoon the pâté into 4–6 ramekin dishes and smooth the top. Cover each and chill overnight.
5. Just before serving, use a pastry cutter to stamp out 4–6 rounds of bread the same diameter as the ramekin dishes. Toast them lightly on both sides. Turn out the vegetable pâtés from the dishes on to the rounds of toast. Decorate each with a thinly sliced gherkin spread out as a fan.

Serves 4–6

Above left:
CHOUX BUNS WITH STILTON SAUCE
These light pastry buns, sliced and filled with a mixture of Stilton, cream cheese and walnuts, are certain to attract compliments when piled high to tempt your guests.

Above right:
CHEESE AND HAM AIGRETTES
These light, deep-fried morsels containing Cheddar cheese, chopped ham and onion, add a sophisticated note to party food for the more experienced cook.

CHEESE, SHRIMP AND MUSHROOM RAMEKINS

50 g (2 oz) mushrooms, wiped and sliced

47 g (1¾ oz) English butter

7 g (¼ oz) flour

150 ml (¼ pint) milk

3 eggs, hard-boiled

50 g (2 oz) English Cheddar cheese, grated

100 g (4 oz) shrimps, peeled

salt and freshly ground pepper

1. Fry the mushrooms in 15 g (½ oz) of the butter until soft.
2. Melt 7 g (¼ oz) butter for the sauce in a small pan, stir in the flour and cook gently for 1 minute, stirring. Remove pan from the heat and gradually stir in the milk. Bring to the boil slowly and continue to cook, stirring, until the sauce thickens.
3. Roughly chop the eggs and add to the sauce with 25 g (1 oz) cheese, the shrimps and fried mushrooms; season. Stir in the remaining butter and reheat without boiling.
4. Pour into buttered ramekin dishes. Sprinkle the remaining grated cheese on top and brown under a hot grill. Serve at once.
Serves 4

MUSHROOM AND CHEDDAR STARTER

65 g (2½ oz) English butter

1 onion, skinned and chopped

1 garlic clove, skinned and crushed

225 g (8 oz) mushrooms, wiped and thickly sliced

25 g (1 oz) flour

300 ml (½ pint) milk

salt and freshly ground pepper

50 g (2 oz) English Cheddar cheese, grated

15 ml (1 tbsp) fresh single cream

chopped fresh parsley to garnish

1. Melt 40 g (1½ oz) of the butter in a saucepan and fry the onion, garlic and mushrooms until tender.
2. Divide the mixture between four scallop shells or ramekin dishes.
3. Place the remaining 25 g (1 oz) butter, flour and milk in a saucepan. Heat, stirring continuously, until the sauce thickens and boils. Add seasoning, half the cheese and the fresh cream. Pour over the mushroom mixture. Sprinkle with the remaining cheese.
4. Bake in the oven at 190°C (375°F) mark 5 for 15 minutes, or brown under a hot grill.
5. Serve hot, garnished with parsley.

Variation
Replace mushrooms with skinned and sliced tomatoes, cooked broccoli or sliced hard-boiled eggs.
Serves 4

SEAFOOD PANCAKES

100 g (4 oz) wheatmeal flour

salt and freshly ground pepper

1 egg

568 ml (1 pint) milk

vegetable oil for frying

25 g (1 oz) English butter

25 g (1 oz) flour

175 g (6 oz) salmon, cooked

100 g (4 oz) peeled shrimps

50 g (2 oz) shelled cockles

1 drop of lemon juice

5 ml (1 tsp) tomato purée

50 g (2 oz) English Cheddar cheese, finely grated

parsley sprigs to garnish

1. Sift the wheatmeal flour and salt into a mixing bowl. Make a well in the centre and break in the egg. Gradually add 150 ml (¼ pint) milk, vigorously beating in the flour with a wooden spoon until a thick smooth batter is formed. Pour in 150 ml (¼ pint) milk, and beat again until quite smooth.
2. Heat a little oil in a frying pan and when it is very hot pour in a small amount of batter. Tip the pan quickly so that the batter runs over the bottom of the pan. Cook over a high heat until the underside is golden brown, then turn the pancake over either by tossing it, or by using a fish slice. Cook the other side until golden brown. Fry eight pancakes and keep warm.
3. Place the butter, flour and remaining 300 ml (½ pint) milk in a saucepan. Heat, stirring continuously, until the sauce thickens and boils. Add all the fish and cook for 3–4 minutes. Add lemon juice, tomato purée, salt, pepper and cheese.
4. Stuff the pancakes with the seafood

Below:
SEAFOOD PANCAKES
Combining shrimps, cooked salmon and cockles in a delicious cheese and tomato sauce, these tempting pancakes are an unusual hot starter which make a little seafood stretch a long way.

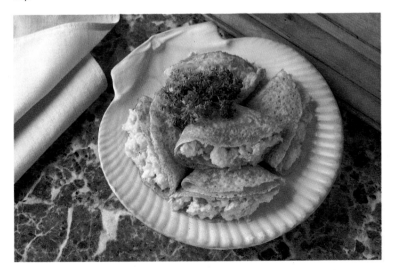

mixture and fold or roll up. Cover with foil and bake in the oven at 180°C (350°F) mark 4 for 20 minutes. Serve hot, garnished with parsley.
Makes 8

CELERY AND PRAWN SAVOURIES

1 onion, skinned and finely chopped
3 sticks celery, cleaned and chopped
25 g (1 oz) English butter
3 slices brown bread, crusts removed
100 g (4 oz) peeled prawns
75 g (3 oz) Lancashire cheese, grated
2 eggs, beaten
150 ml ($\frac{1}{4}$ pint) milk
salt
cayenne pepper
parsley sprigs to garnish

1. Sauté the onion and celery in butter without browning.
2. Cut the bread into 1-cm ($\frac{1}{2}$-inch) cubes, add to the vegetables in the saucepan and toss until coated with butter.
3. Lightly butter four large ramekin dishes. Divide a third of the bread mixture between each dish and use to cover the bases. Reserve four prawns for garnish and layer the rest with the cheese and the bread mixture, ending with a bread layer.
4. Beat together the eggs, milk, salt and pepper. Pour over the bread mixture.
5. Bake in the oven at 200°C (400°F) mark 6 for 35–40 minutes. Serve hot, garnished with parsley and remaining prawns.
Serves 4

STUFFED MUSHROOMS

12 large cup mushrooms, about 350 g (12 oz) total weight
4 sticks celery, cleaned
1 small onion, skinned
50 g (2 oz) walnuts
75 g (3 oz) English butter
75 g (3 oz) fresh breadcrumbs
60 ml (4 tbsp) chopped fresh parsley
30 ml (2 tbsp) lemon juice
salt and freshly ground pepper
1 egg, beaten
50 g (2 oz) English Cheddar cheese, grated
90 ml (6 tbsp) chicken stock

1. Wipe the mushrooms and pull out the stalks. Chop the stalks finely with the celery, onion and walnuts.
2. Heat the butter in a medium-sized frying pan and lightly brown the rounded sides of the mushrooms, a few at a time.
3. Remove from the pan, add the chopped

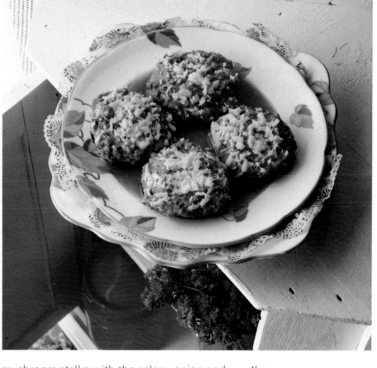

mushroom stalks with the celery, onion and walnuts. Fry quickly for 2–3 minutes, stirring occasionally.
4. Remove from the heat and stir in the breadcrumbs, parsley, lemon juice and seasoning, binding with the beaten egg.
5. Spoon into the mushroom caps and place side by side in a shallow ovenproof dish to just fit. Sprinkle a little cheese over each mushroom and pour the stock around the edges of the dish. Bake in the oven at 180°C (350°F) mark 4 for 20–25 minutes. Serve hot.
Makes 12

Above:
STUFFED MUSHROOMS
A light and tasty hot starter.
This recipe is ideal for busy
cooks as it can be prepared in
advance. Just add the stock and
pop the dish in the oven 20–25
minutes before serving.

SAVOURY VOL-AU-VENTS

four 397-g (14-oz) packets frozen puff pastry, thawed
beaten egg to glaze

1. Roll out each packet of pastry to an oblong 23 × 24.5 cm (9 × 9$\frac{1}{2}$ inches) and using a 7.5-cm (3-inch) round plain cutter, cut out five rounds from each packet.
2. Place on dampened baking sheets and brush with beaten egg. Using a 5-cm (2-inch) round plain cutter, cut part-way through the centre of each round.
3. Bake in the oven at 230°C (450°F) mark 8 for about 20 minutes until well risen and golden. Remove the soft centres from each vol-au-vent and cool the cases on a wire rack.
4. Before serving, fill with a cold filling (see page 52) and reheat in the oven at 180°C (350°F) mark 4 for about 15 minutes.
Makes 20

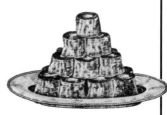

CUTTING
VOL-AU-VENT CASES

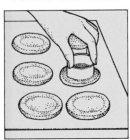

1 Cutting half-way through the pastry to mark the 'lid'

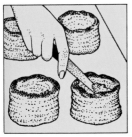

2 Removing the soft 'insides' when cooked

Below:
CHICKEN LIVER PÂTÉ
This smooth, creamy pâté, flavoured with a hint of garlic and brandy, is delicious when served with crusty French bread or with the crisp Melba toast given on page 84.

SPICED BACON AND CELERY FILLING

900 g (2 lb) smoked bacon joint

350 g (12 oz) celery, cleaned and trimmed

75 g (3 oz) English butter

2.5 ml (½ level tsp) ground ginger

2.5 ml (½ level tsp) ground cumin

2.5 ml (½ level tsp) ground coriander

75 g (3 oz) flour

900 ml (1½ pints) chicken stock

15 ml (1 tbsp) tomato purée

142 g (5 oz) natural yogurt

30 ml (2 tbsp) chopped fresh parsley

salt and freshly ground pepper

1. Cover the bacon joint with cold water and soak for 2–3 hours. Drain. Place in a saucepan, cover with cold water, bring slowly to the boil and simmer for about 1 hour, until tender.
2. Cut the bacon and celery into 2.5-cm (1-inch) matchstick strips.
3. Melt the butter in a large saucepan and sauté the celery with the ginger, cumin and coriander for 5 minutes.
4. Stir in the flour and cook gently for 1–2 minutes, stirring. Remove from the heat and gradually stir in the stock, tomato purée, yogurt and parsley. Bring to the boil and continue to cook, stirring, for 4–5 minutes. Stir in the bacon pieces and season. Leave until cold before filling the vol-au-vents.

Variation
Turkey or chicken leftovers can be substituted for some of the bacon.
Fills 20 7.5-cm (3-inch) vol-au-vents

CAULIFLOWER, CHEESE AND MUSHROOM FILLING

1.8 kg (4 lb) cauliflower, trimmed weight

100 ml (4 fl oz) dry white wine

75 g (3 oz) English butter

350 g (12 oz) onion, skinned and chopped

225 g (8 oz) mushrooms, wiped and thinly sliced

75 g (3 oz) flour

900 ml (1½ pints) milk

225 g (8 oz) English Cheddar cheese, grated

salt and freshly ground pepper

1. Cut the cauliflower into very small florets, boil for 2–3 minutes until barely tender. Drain well and cool.
2. In a small saucepan bring the white wine to the boil. Reduce over high heat until about 15 ml (1 tbsp) remains.
3. Melt the butter in a large saucepan. Sauté the onion and thinly sliced mushrooms until softened. Remove with a slotted spoon.
4. Stir the flour into the pan, adding extra butter if necessary. Cook for 2 minutes, stirring. Remove from the heat and gradually stir in the milk and reduced white wine. Bring to the boil, stirring, then simmer 4–5 minutes. Stir in cauliflower, mushrooms and onions. Simmer for a further 2 minutes. Reduce the heat, stir in the cheese. Season carefully. Leave until cold before filling the vol-au-vents.
Fills 20 7.5-cm (3-inch) vol-au-vents

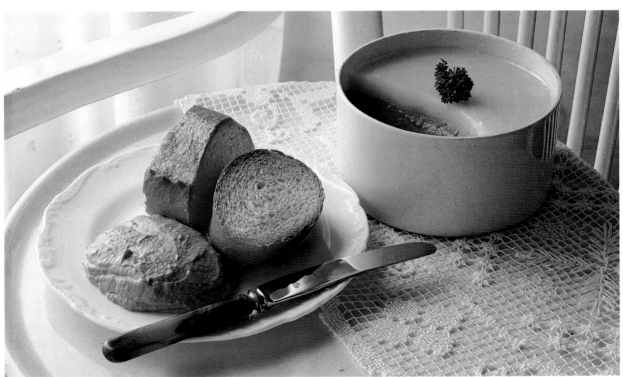

CHICKEN LIVER PÂTÉ

450 g (1 lb) chicken livers
50 g (2 oz) English butter
1 medium onion, skinned and chopped
1 garlic clove, skinned and crushed
75 ml (5 tbsp) fresh double cream
15 ml (1 tbsp) tomato purée
15 ml (1 tbsp) brandy
salt and freshly ground pepper
parsley sprigs to garnish

1. Clean the chicken livers and dry with absorbent kitchen paper.
2. Heat the butter in a saucepan, add the onion and garlic and cook for about 5 minutes until onion is soft. Add the chicken livers and cook for a further 5 minutes.
3. Cool and add the fresh cream, tomato purée and brandy; season well.
4. Purée the mixture in a blender and put into a serving dish. Chill in the refrigerator. Melted butter poured over the pâté will prevent it drying out. Garnish with parsley sprigs and serve with melba toast or crusty French bread.
Serves 8

SCHMALTZ HERRINGS

8 pickled rollmop herrings, drained
1 medium onion, skinned and thinly sliced
2 dessert apples, peeled, cored and sliced
lemon juice
142 ml (5 fl oz) soured cream
salt and freshly ground pepper
4 gherkins, finely chopped
cayenne pepper

1. Slice the herrings in rings and arrange them on a flat serving dish.
2. Place the onions over the fish. Toss the apples in a little lemon juice and place on top of the fish and onion.
3. Spoon over the soured cream mixed with the seasoning and gherkins. Sprinkle with a little cayenne pepper before serving.
Serves 4

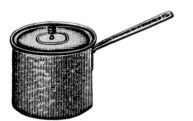

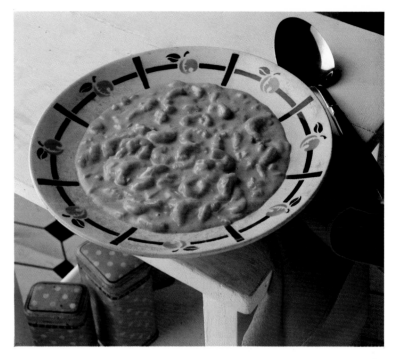

PRAWNS WITH CURRY MAYONNAISE

25 g (1 oz) English butter
1 small onion, skinned and finely chopped
5 ml (1 level tsp) flour
30 ml (2 level tbsp) curry powder
5 ml (1 tsp) tomato purée
2.5 ml ($\frac{1}{2}$ level tsp) salt
1.25 ml ($\frac{1}{4}$ level tsp) caster sugar
15 ml (1 level tbsp) apricot jam
150 ml ($\frac{1}{4}$ pint) mayonnaise
150 ml ($\frac{1}{4}$ pint) fresh single cream
juice of $\frac{1}{2}$ lemon
225–350 g (8–12 oz) peeled prawns

1. Melt the butter in a saucepan, add the onion and sauté very gently without browning for about 5 minutes until soft.
2. Stir in the flour and curry powder, and fry for 2–3 minutes. Stir in the tomato purée diluted with 60 ml (4 tbsp) water, together with salt, caster sugar and apricot jam.
3. Bring to the boil and simmer gently for about 5 minutes. Remove from the heat and strain the mixture into a basin.
4. Allow to cool. Stir in the mayonnaise, fresh cream and lemon juice.
5. Add the prawns to the sauce and serve with a rice salad.

Variation
This curry mayonnaise is also good with cooked chicken or hard-boiled eggs instead of prawns.
Serves 4

Above:
PRAWNS WITH CURRY MAYONNAISE
Prawns are always a popular starter and this piquant dish, which adds an exotic Eastern touch, is an unusual and delicious way of serving an old favourite.

STILTON CHEESE BALLS

225 g (8 oz) Blue Stilton cheese

75 g (3 oz) English butter, softened

15 ml (1 tbsp) chives, or spring onion tops, chopped

1 small stick celery, finely chopped

pinch of cayenne pepper

salt and freshly ground pepper

5 ml (1 tsp) cognac, or a few drops of Worcestershire sauce

40 g (1½ oz) fine dry breadcrumbs

30 ml (2 tbsp) finely chopped fresh parsley

1. Crumble the cheese into a bowl with the butter and beat to a smooth paste.
2. Beat in the chives or spring onion tops, celery, seasonings, and cognac or Worcestershire sauce. If mixture is very stiff, beat in a little more butter.
3. Check seasoning carefully. Roll into balls about 1 cm (½ inch) in diameter.
4. Mix the breadcrumbs and parsley on a plate. Roll the cheese balls in the mixture so that they are well coated. Chill.
5. Serve as they are, or pierced on a cocktail stick.
Makes about 24

CHESHIRE CHEESECAKE

25 g (1 oz) English butter

5 ml (1 level tsp) mustard powder

25 g (1 oz) flour

450 ml (¾ pint) milk

2 eggs, separated

15 g (½ oz) gelatine

175 g (6 oz) English Cheshire cheese, grated

salt and freshly ground pepper

8 cream cracker biscuits

8 anchovy fillets and 4 small pickled gherkins, sliced, to garnish

1. Butter a shallow 18-cm (7-inch) square cake tin. Melt the 25 g (1 oz) butter in a small saucepan with the mustard, stir in the flour and cook gently for 1 minute, stirring. Remove pan from the heat and gradually stir in the milk. Bring to the boil slowly and continue to cook, stirring until the sauce thickens.
2. Remove from heat and leave to cool. Stir the egg yolks into the sauce. Sprinkle gelatine over 30 ml (2 tbsp) water in a small bowl. Place the bowl over a pan of hot water and stir until dissolved, then stir into the sauce. Leave until almost set.
3. Whip the egg whites until stiff and fold into sauce with the grated cheese. Check

seasoning; pour into the tin and leave in a cool place for 15 minutes.
4. Cover the top with cream crackers, cut to fit, and leave to set firmly. Before serving, loosen edges with a knife and turn on to a serving plate with the crackers at the base. Garnish the top with anchovies, sliced gherkins and serve with additional crackers.
Serves 4–6

AVOCADO AND SEAFOOD CREAM

2 ripe avocados

15 ml (1 tbsp) lemon juice

53-g (2½-oz) can crab meat

1 small green pepper, seeded and chopped

1 small red pepper, seeded and chopped

15 ml (1 tbsp) mayonnaise

90 ml (3 fl oz) fresh double cream

2.5 ml (½ level tsp) mild chilli powder

salt and freshly ground pepper

1. Cut the avocados in half and remove the stones. Scoop out the flesh, keeping the skins, and mash with the lemon juice. Add the crab, peppers and mayonnaise.
2. Lightly whip the fresh cream and fold into the crab mixture. Add the chilli powder and seasonings.
3. Pile the mixture into the avocado skins and serve on a bed of lettuce with lemon wedges and hot buttered toast.

Variation
Any other variety of seafood, including fresh fish, could be used as an alternative to crab.
Serves 4

CHEESE AND APPLE PEARS

100 g (4 oz) English Cheddar cheese, grated

1 red dessert apple, chopped

25 g (1 oz) walnuts, chopped

25 g (1 oz) raisins

60 ml (4 tbsp) milk

Worcestershire sauce

salt and freshly ground pepper

2 dessert pears

lemon juice

1 tomato, sliced, to garnish

1. Place the cheese, apple, walnuts, raisins and milk in a bowl and mix well. Season

with a few drops of Worcestershire sauce, salt and pepper.

2. Cut the pears in half and scoop out the cores. Sprinkle with a little lemon juice and pile the cheese and apple mixture on the top of each pear half.

3. Serve each pear on individual plates on a bed of lettuce and garnish with tomato slices.

Serves 4

DELICIOUS DIPS

GARLIC DIP

1 medium onion, skinned and finely chopped

1 small garlic clove, skinned and crushed

142 ml (5 fl oz) soured cream

1. Combine the onion with the crushed garlic and soured cream.

2. Serve with crudités, cocktail biscuits, crisps, etc.

Serves 6

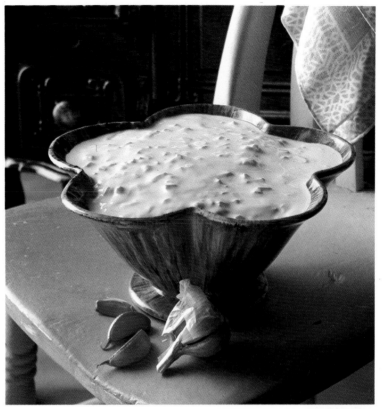

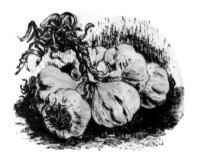

BLUE CHEESE DIP

142 ml (5 fl oz) soured cream

1 garlic clove, skinned and crushed

175 g (6 oz) Blue Stilton cheese, crumbled

juice of 1 lemon

salt and freshly ground pepper

snipped chives to garnish

1. Combine all the ingredients in a bowl and beat together well. Do not add too much salt as Stilton can be salty.

2. Put into a small dish and chill well. Garnish with snipped chives. Serve with savoury cocktail biscuits, pretzels, stuffed olives, etc.

Variation: Corn Dip
Omit the Stilton and garlic, adding instead 100 g (4 oz) cottage cheese and a 227-g (8-oz) drained can of corn niblets.

Serves 6–8

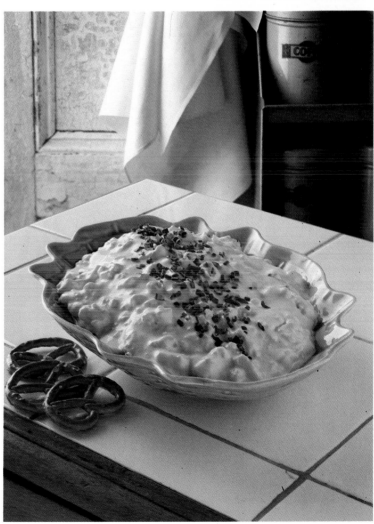

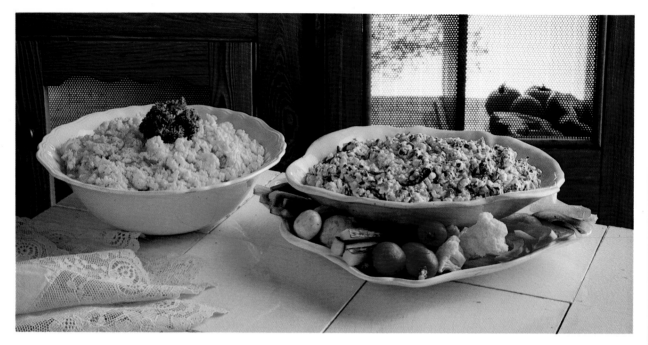

Above from left:
SPICY CHEESE AND
TOMATO DIP and
WATERCRESS DIP
Spiked with spicy
Worcestershire sauce and sharp
English mustard, the appetising
cheese and tomato dish is a great
party dip. So, too, is the
watercress-flavoured dip with its
sharp, tangy taste.

SPICY CHEESE AND TOMATO DIP

125 g (4 oz) Cheshire cheese, grated
50 g (2 oz) English butter, softened
1 small onion, skinned
5 ml (1 level tsp) mustard powder
15 ml (1 tbsp) tomato ketchup
30 ml (2 tbsp) fresh single cream
Worcestershire sauce
cayenne pepper
parsley sprig to garnish

1. In a bowl, beat together the cheese and softened butter with a wooden spoon.
2. Grate in the onion, add the mustard powder, tomato ketchup, fresh cream and a few drops of Worcestershire sauce. Season with a little cayenne pepper and mix well.
3. Put into a serving dish and chill. Garnish with a parsley sprig.
Serves 6

WATERCRESS DIP

225 g (8 oz) cottage cheese
60 ml (4 tbsp) milk
$\frac{1}{2}$ small onion, skinned and chopped
1 small garlic clove, skinned and crushed
$\frac{1}{2}$ bunch of watercress, washed and chopped
salt and freshly ground pepper

1. Beat the cheese with a wooden spoon and gradually add the milk until the mixture is smooth.
2. Stir the onion, garlic and watercress into the cheese.
3. Leave for at least 2 hours in a cool place to allow the flavours to infuse. Season and serve with crudités.
Serves 6

HERBY CHEESE DIP

15 ml (1 tbsp) chopped fresh mint
15 ml (1 tbsp) chopped fresh parsley
225 g (8 oz) English Cheddar cheese, grated
125 g (4 oz) cottage cheese
1 garlic clove, skinned and crushed
6 cocktail gherkins, chopped
salt and freshly ground pepper

1. Put the herbs and cheeses into a bowl and beat well until smooth. Add the garlic, gherkins and seasoning.
2. Chill well and serve with washed whole radishes, cucumber and celery sticks.
Serves 6

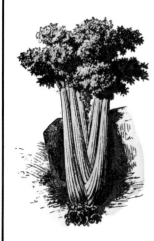

CHEDDAR CHEESE AND CELERY DIP

50 g (2 oz) English butter, softened
225 g (8 oz) English Cheddar cheese, grated
10 ml (2 level tsp) prepared mustard
100 g (4 oz) celery, cleaned and chopped
150 ml (5 fl oz) fresh double cream
salt and freshly ground pepper
nuts, chopped, to garnish

1. Beat the butter until smooth, then stir in the cheese, mustard and celery.
2. Gradually beat in the fresh cream; season.
3. Before serving, transfer to a bowl and sprinkle with chopped nuts.
Serves 6–8

ONION DIP

25-g (1-oz) packet thick onion soup mix
300 ml (½ pint) milk
150 ml (5 fl oz) fresh double cream
50 g (2 oz) ham, chopped
142 g (5 oz) natural yogurt
50 g (2 oz) Caerphilly cheese, grated
green olives, sliced, to garnish

1. Make up the soup following the packet instructions but using 300 ml (½ pint) milk. Allow to cool.
2. Whip the fresh cream until softly stiff and stir in the soup, ham, yogurt and cheese.
3. Chill well. Decorate with olives and serve with a selection of savoury biscuits, crisps and sticks of carrot and celery.

Variation

Use Cheddar, Red Leicester or Double Gloucester cheese in place of Caerphilly.

Serves 4 as a starter, 10 as a dip

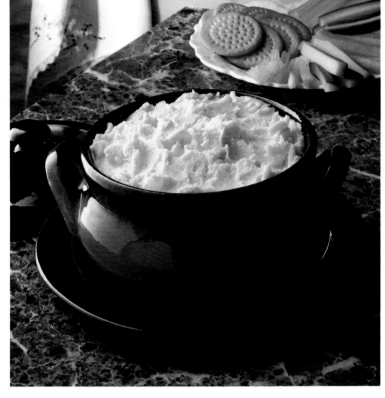

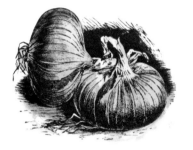

SAVOURY EGG STARTERS

ANCHOVY EGG APPETISER

Above:
POTTED CHEESE
This party dip combining grated Cheddar cheese, butter and a little sherry, is a traditional English starter. For centuries, English cooks have been using butter to 'pot' cheese, as well as fish, beef and game. Potted cheese can be served either as a party dip or with fingers of hot toast as the first course of a winter dinner.

POTTED CHEESE

100 g (4 oz) English butter
pinch of mace
salt and freshly ground pepper
225 g (8 oz) English Cheddar cheese, grated
15 ml (1 tbsp) milk
15 ml (1 tbsp) sherry

1. Beat together the butter and mace; season. Add the cheese a little at a time and beat well.
2. Stir in the milk and sherry to make a smooth mixture. Chill well.
3. Serve with a selection of savoury biscuits and crudités.

Variation

Use crumbled Blue Stilton cheese and port instead of Cheddar and sherry.

Serves 4

6 eggs, hard-boiled
56-g (2-oz) can anchovy fillets, drained
60 ml (4 tbsp) milk
100 g (4 oz) English butter
freshly ground pepper
30 ml (2 tbsp) lemon juice

1. Cut the eggs in half lengthways; remove the yolks and mash well with a fork.
2. Soak the anchovy fillets in milk for 20 minutes to remove excess salt.
3. Strain the anchovies, pound with the softened butter and plenty of black pepper until smooth.
4. Combine the yolks, butter mixture and lemon juice, correct the seasoning. Stuff into the egg whites, re-shaping into whole eggs.
5. Cover and chill well. Serve sliced on individual plates on a bed of lettuce. Accompany with wholemeal bread or rolls.

Serves 6

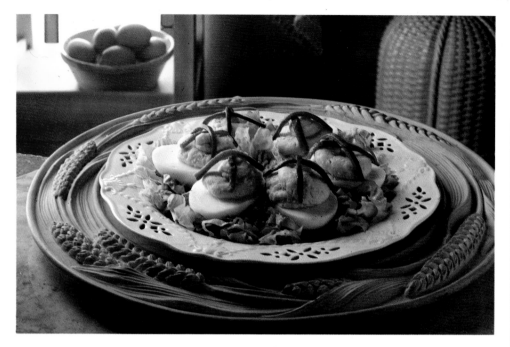

MUMBLED EGGS

8 eggs

10 ml (2 level tsp) mustard powder

salt and freshly ground pepper

50 g (2 oz) mushrooms, wiped and finely chopped

25 g (1 oz) English butter

50 g (2 oz) English Cheddar cheese, grated

15 ml (1 tbsp) fresh double cream

1. Beat the eggs with the mustard and seasoning; add the mushrooms.
2. Melt the butter in a saucepan over a low heat. Pour in the egg and mushroom mixture and stir until the eggs begin to set.
3. Sprinkle in the cheese and cook, stirring, for several minutes until well blended and the eggs are cooked.
4. Stir in the fresh cream and serve at once with buttered toast.
Serves 4

STILTON STUFFED EGGS

4 eggs, hard-boiled

30–45 ml (2–3 tbsp) fresh double cream

pinch of salt

50 g (2 oz) Blue Stilton cheese, crumbled

pinch of cayenne pepper

anchovy fillets to garnish

1. Cut the eggs in half lengthways; remove the yolks and mash well with a fork.
2. To the yolks, add the fresh cream, salt, cheese and a pinch of cayenne pepper. Mix well together. Spoon into a piping bag fitted with a 1-cm (½-inch) plain nozzle. Pipe the cheese mixture into the egg whites.

3. Garnish with thin strips of anchovy fillets, and serve on a bed of lettuce or watercress.

Variation
Walnut, Celery and Stilton Stuffed Eggs
Add 50 g (2 oz) finely chopped walnuts and 1 stick finely chopped celery to the cheese mixture.
Serves 4

CURRIED EGGS

4 eggs, hard-boiled

25 g (1 oz) English butter

1 onion, skinned and chopped

5 ml (1 level tsp) curry powder

25 g (1 oz) flour

300 ml (½ pint) milk

50 g (2 oz) sultanas

50 g (2 oz) cucumber, cubed

salt and freshly ground pepper

225 g (8 oz) long grain rice

green pepper to garnish

1. Cut the eggs in half lengthways and place in the centre of an ovenproof dish. Keep warm in a low oven.
2. Melt the butter in a saucepan and fry the onion until soft, stir in the curry powder and flour and cook gently for 1 minute, stirring. Remove the pan from the heat and gradually stir in the milk. Bring to the boil slowly and continue to cook, stirring, until the sauce thickens. Stir in the sultanas, cucumber and seasonings.
3. Cook the rice in boiling salted water for 9–10 minutes until tender and drain. Arrange in a ring around the eggs and pour the curry sauce over. Garnish with rings of green pepper.
Serves 4

SAVOURY MOUSSES AND SOUFFLÉS

HOT BLUE CHEESE AND CELERY MOUSSE

225 g (8 oz) celery, cleaned and thinly sliced

30 ml (2 tbsp) fresh single cream or top of milk

75 g (3 oz) Blue Stilton cheese

3 egg yolks

freshly ground pepper

4 egg whites

English butter

browned breadcrumbs to garnish

1. Cook the celery in the minimum of water in a covered pan for about 30 minutes, until really soft. Remove lid and boil to evaporate water completely.
2. In a blender, purée the celery with the cream and cheese until smooth. Pour into a bowl and cool slightly.
3. Beat in the egg yolks and black pepper. Whisk the egg whites until stiff and fold into the mixture.
4. Turn into a lightly buttered 1.4-litre (2½-pint) soufflé dish, cover with buttered foil.
5. Steam for about 30 minutes. Serve at once dusted with browned breadcrumbs.
Serves 4–6

CHILLED WALNUT AND STILTON SOUFFLÉS

25 g (1 oz) English butter

30 ml (2 level tbsp) flour

200 ml (7 fl oz) milk

200 ml (7 fl oz) chicken stock

100 g (4 oz) Blue Stilton cheese

salt and freshly ground pepper

paprika

150 ml (5 fl oz) fresh whipping cream

15 ml (3 level tsp) gelatine

75 g (3 oz) walnuts, chopped

3 egg whites

watercress sprigs to garnish

1. Tie a paper collar of greaseproof paper round the outside of six 150-ml (¼-pint) soufflé dishes to stand 5 cm (2 inches) above the rim.
2. Melt the butter in a saucepan, stir in the flour and cook gently for 1 minute, stirring. Remove from the heat and gradually stir in the milk and stock. Bring to the boil slowly and continue to cook, stirring until the sauce thickens.

3. Crumble in the cheese, season well and turn the mixture into a bowl to cool.
4. Whip the fresh cream until softly stiff and fold in.
5. Sprinkle gelatine over 45 ml (3 tbsp) water in a small bowl. Place the bowl over a pan of hot water and stir until dissolved, then stir into the cheese mixture. Chill until on the point of setting.
6. Fold in 50 g (2 oz) chopped walnuts with the stiffly whisked whites. Pour into the soufflé dishes. Chill until set. Garnish with the remaining walnuts and watercress.
Serves 6

SALMON AND TARRAGON MOUSSE

15 ml (3 level tsp) gelatine

1 chicken stock cube

25 g (1 oz) onion, skinned and finely chopped

1 garlic clove, skinned and crushed

1.25 ml (¼ tsp) chopped fresh tarragon

salt and freshly ground pepper

213-g (7½-oz) can salmon, drained and coarsely flaked

60 ml (4 tbsp) fresh double cream

cucumber and parsley or watercress sprigs to garnish

1. Sprinkle gelatine over 300 ml (½ pint) warm water mixed with stock cube in a small bowl. Place the bowl over a pan of hot water and stir until dissolved. Pour into blender and add all the remaining ingredients except the fresh cream and garnishes and liquidise for 1 minute.
2. Leave to cool in a bowl until just starting to set. Whip the fresh cream until stiff, then gently fold into the setting salmon mixture.
3. Turn the mousse into a 600-ml (1-pint) pudding basin or ring mould; cover with cling film and place in a refrigerator until firmly set.
4. Turn the mould out and garnish with a ring of cucumber slices round the base and a sprig of parsley or watercress in the centre. Serve with a salad or melba toast.
Serves 4–6

MAKING A SALMON MOUSSE

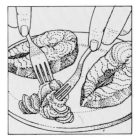

1 Flaking the cooked fish

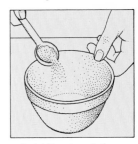

2 Sprinkling the gelatine over the warm liquid.

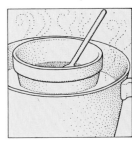

3 Dissolving the gelatine by placing the bowl over a pan of hot water

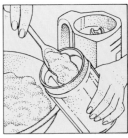

4 Liquidising all the ingredients except the fresh cream

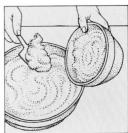

5 Folding the whipped cream into the salmon mixture

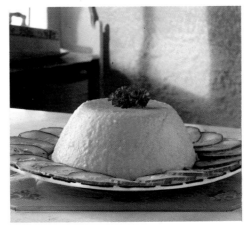

COOK'S TIP AVOCADOS are a delicious fruit. Unless you want a ripe avocado to eat that day, buy firm fruit and let them ripen at home at room temperature for 1 to 3 days. The avocado is ripe when it yields to gentle pressure. Ripe avocados can be stored successfully for 3 to 4 days on the lower shelf of the refrigerator. Remove from the refrigerator several hours before eating.

Just before serving, slice the avocado in half lengthways, making a cut that completely encircles the fruit and penetrates to the stone. Gently rotate the halves in opposite directions until they separate and ease out the stone.

Brush cut avocados with lemon juice to prevent discolouration.

AVOCADO MOUSSE

15 g ($\frac{1}{2}$ oz) gelatine
150 ml ($\frac{1}{4}$ pint) chicken stock
3 small or 2 large avocados
$\frac{1}{2}$ large onion
salt and freshly ground pepper
10 ml (2 tsp) Worcestershire sauce
150 ml ($\frac{1}{4}$ pint) mayonnaise
150 ml ($\frac{1}{4}$ pint) fresh double cream
cucumber slices to garnish

1 Sprinkle gelatine over 150 ml ($\frac{1}{4}$ pint) water in a small bowl. Place the bowl over a saucepan of hot water, and stir until dissolved.
2. Stir in the stock and set aside to cool for a few minutes.
3. Halve the avocados and remove the stones, scoop out the flesh with a fork and mash until smooth.
4. Grate the onion finely on to a plate, reserve 5 ml (1 tsp) of onion juice and discard onion flesh. Add this to the avocado flesh, season with salt, pepper and Worcestershire sauce.
5. Slowly pour the gelatine mixture into the avocado mixture and stir until just beginning to thicken. Then gently fold in the mayonnaise and the fresh cream, whipped until softly stiff.
6. Pour into a dampened 1-litre (1$\frac{1}{2}$-pint) mould and chill until firm. Just before serving, remove from the mould and place on a serving platter. Garnish with thinly sliced cucumber.

Serves 6

CUCUMBER CHEESE MOUSSE

1 cucumber
225 g (8 oz) full fat soft cheese
150 ml ($\frac{1}{4}$ pint) mayonnaise
15 g ($\frac{1}{2}$ oz) gelatine
2.5 ml ($\frac{1}{2}$ level tsp) salt
10 ml (2 level tsp) caster sugar
150 ml ($\frac{1}{4}$ pint) fresh double cream
watercress or parsley to garnish

1. Peel the cucumber, cut lengthwise and remove the seeds. Finely chop the flesh and leave to one side.
2. Blend the cheese until soft; stir in the mayonnaise. Sprinkle gelatine over 150 ml ($\frac{1}{4}$ pint) water in a small bowl. Place the bowl over a pan of hot water and stir until dissolved. Add the salt and caster sugar. Cool.
3. Whip the fresh cream until softly stiff. Stir the cooled gelatine mixture into the mayonnaise and cheese, add the cucumber and fold in the fresh cream. Mix thoroughly.
4. Pour the mixture into a dampened 1-litre (1$\frac{1}{2}$-pint) ring mould. Chill until firm. Turn out and garnish with watercress or parsley.

Serves 6

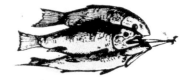

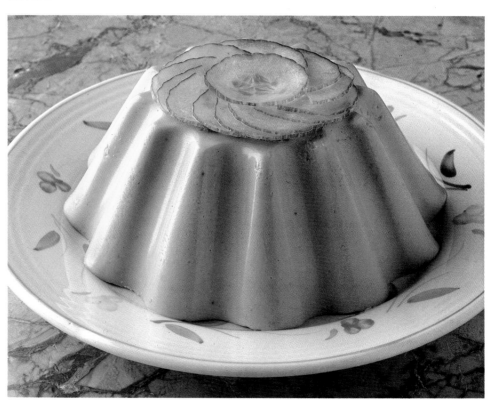

Right:
AVOCADO MOUSSE
Topped with a swirl of wafer-thin cucumber slices, this fresh green mousse is a spectacular way to serve avocados as a starter.

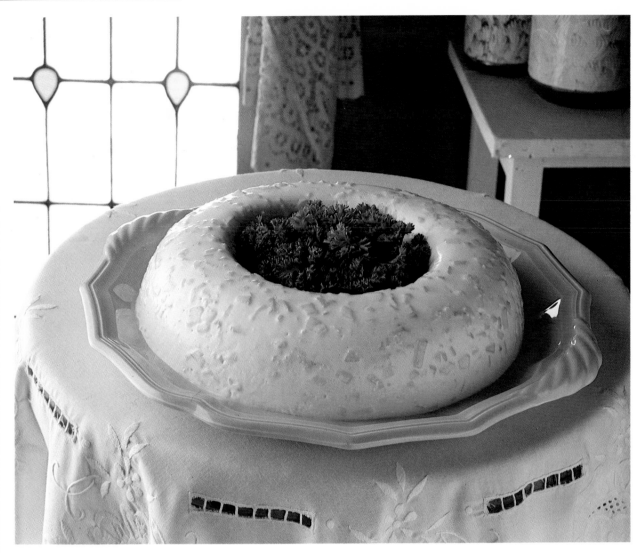

FISH PÂTÉ

75 ml (2½ fl oz) fresh double cream

45 ml (3 tbsp) mayonnaise

5 ml (1 tsp) horseradish sauce

225 g (8 oz) smoked mackerel fillets

5 ml (1 tsp) lemon juice

salt and freshly ground pepper

watercress

1. Whip the fresh cream and mix together with the mayonnaise and horseradish sauce. Flake mackerel and add this to the cream mixture. Stir in the lemon juice; season.
2. Place the watercress on a plate or in a small dish and spoon the pâté on top. Serve with brown bread and butter, or melba toast and lemon wedges.

Variation
In place of smoked mackerel, use kipper fillets or canned tuna fish.

SMOKED MACKEREL POTS

2 smoked mackerel fillets

15 g (½ oz) English butter

15 g (½ oz) flour

300 ml (½ pint) milk

40 g (1½ oz) English Cheddar cheese, grated finely

salt and freshly ground pepper

pinch of mustard powder

1. Remove the skin from the mackerel fillets and flake the fish into small pieces.
2. Melt the butter in a saucepan, stir in the flour and cook gently for 1 minute. Remove from the heat and gradually stir in the milk. Bring to the boil slowly and continue to cook, stirring, until the sauce is smooth.
3. Off the heat stir in 25 g (1 oz) cheese; season. Add the flaked fish and divide the mixture between four individual pots or dishes.
4. Sprinkle with the remaining cheese and place under a hot grill until golden and bubbling. Serve immediately.

Serves 4

Above:
CUCUMBER CHEESE MOUSSE
Trim the longer stalks from a generous bunch of fresh, clean parsley to garnish the centre of this delicious ring-shaped savoury mousse.

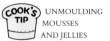

COOK'S TIP UNMOULDING MOUSSES AND JELLIES

Slide the tip of a round-bladed knife around the edge of a mould to loosen the sides of a set mixture.
Dip the mould into a basin of hot water for just a few seconds in order to release the bottom of the mixture.
Dry the mould and put a dampened serving plate upside down on top. Invert the plate and mould. Holding the mould on either side, shake gently to free the mixture. Place on the work surface and listen for the mould's release.
Using both hands, lift the mould carefully off the mixture so as not to spoil its shape.

STILTON SALAD RING

100 g (4 oz) Blue Stilton cheese, crumbled
150 ml (¼ pint) mayonnaise
10 ml (2 tsp) lemon juice
15 g (½ oz) gelatine
215-g (7½-oz) can red salmon, drained and flaked
50 g (2 oz) cucumber, chopped
50 g (2 oz) celery, cleaned and finely chopped
1 small onion, skinned and finely chopped
salt and freshly ground pepper

1. Mix the cheese with 15 ml (1 tbsp) of the mayonnaise, the lemon juice and 15 ml (1 tbsp) cold water. Beat thoroughly until smooth.
2. Dissolve the gelatine in 60 ml (4 tbsp) warm water, in a bowl over a pan of hot water. Stir half of the dissolved gelatine into the mixture.
3. Pour the cheese mixture into a 600-ml (1-pint) dampened ring mould and place in a refrigerator for about 15 minutes to set.
4. Meanwhile, mix the remaining ingredients together with the rest of the mayonnaise and the gelatine.
5. When the cheese mixture has set, spoon the salmon mixture over it and place in a refrigerator to set.
6. Remove the mould and turn on to a serving plate. Fill the centre of the Stilton ring with a tossed, mixed salad or with a bunch of trimmed watercress. Serve with brown bread and butter.
Serves 4–6

PRAWN AND CIDER MOUSSE

15 g (½ oz) English butter
15 g (½ oz) flour
300 ml (½ pint) cider
75 g (3 oz) English Cheddar cheese, grated
2 eggs, separated
30 ml (2 tbsp) tomato ketchup
30 ml (2 tbsp) chopped fresh parsley
salt and freshly ground pepper
225 g (8 oz) peeled prawns, roughly chopped
15 g (½ oz) gelatine
150 ml (5 fl oz) fresh double cream
cucumber and tomato slices to garnish

1. Melt the butter in a saucepan, stir in the flour and cook gently for 1 minute, stirring. Remove the pan from the heat and gradually stir in all but 45 ml (3 tbsp) of the cider. Bring to the boil slowly and continue to cook, stirring, until the sauce thickens.
2. Add the cheese, egg yolks, tomato ketchup, parsley and seasoning and stir the mixture until the cheese has melted. Stir in the prawns.

3. Sprinkle the gelatine over the reserved cider in a small bowl. Place the bowl over a pan of hot water and stir until dissolved.
4. Whip the fresh cream until softly stiff. Stir into the cheese mixture, and then add the gelatine, mixing well.
5. Whisk the egg whites until stiff and gently fold into the mixture. Pour into a large dish or individual dishes.
6. Put in refrigerator to set. Garnish with slices of cucumber and tomato.
Serves 4

SMOKED MACKEREL MOUSSE

300 ml (½ pint) milk
1 onion, skinned and sliced
1 carrot, peeled and sliced
bay leaf
10 ml (2 level tsp) gelatine
25 g (1 oz) English butter
30 ml (2 level tbsp) flour
275 g (10 oz) smoked mackerel fillets
1 small onion, skinned and roughly chopped
15 ml (1 tbsp) creamed horseradish
142 g (5 oz) natural yogurt
15 ml (1 tbsp) lemon juice
salt and freshly ground pepper
2 egg whites
watercress sprigs or lemon slices to garnish

1. Place the milk in a saucepan with the onion, carrot and bay leaf and bring slowly to the boil. Take off the heat, cover the pan and leave to infuse for 30 minutes.
2. Meanwhile, sprinkle gelatine over 30 ml (2 tbsp) water in a small bowl and leave to soak for at least 10 minutes.
3. Melt the butter in a small pan, stir in the flour and cook gently for 1 minute, stirring. Remove the pan from the heat and gradually strain on the infused milk, stirring until smooth. Bring to the boil slowly and continue to cook, stirring, until the sauce thickens.
4. Remove from the heat and stir in the soaked gelatine until dissolved. Pour out into a bowl and cool.
5. Flake the mackerel, discarding the skin. Place the cool sauce, fish, onion and horseradish in a blender and liquidise until smooth. Pour out into a bowl and stir in the yogurt, lemon juice and seasoning to taste.
6. Whisk the egg whites until softly stiff, then fold them gently through the fish mixture.
7. Spoon into six ramekin dishes and refrigerate to set. Garnish with watercress sprigs or a twist of lemon; serve chilled with warm brown French bread.

Variation: Fresh Haddock Mousse
Substitute fresh haddock, skinned and poached, for the smoked mackerel and use 150 ml (¼ pint) mayonnaise instead of natural yogurt.
Serves 6

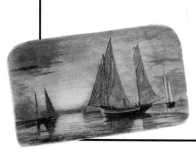

COCKTAILS FROM THE DAIRY

COOK'S TIP SHAKING COCKTAILS
If you don't have a proper shaker, use a glass jam jar or other screw-topped container.

BRANDY ALEXANDER

⅓ glass of brandy

⅓ glass of crème de cacao

⅓ glass of fresh single cream

1. Shake and strain into a cocktail glass.

GRASSHOPPER

⅓ glass of crème de menthe

⅓ glass of crème de cacao

⅓ glass of fresh single cream

1. Shake and strain into a glass.

EVERTON BLUE

¼ glass of gin

¼ glass of blue curaçao

¼ glass of crème de banane

¼ glass of fresh single cream

lemon juice

Grenadine

1. Shake all the ingredients except Grenadine and strain into a champagne glass. Add a dash of Grenadine so that the drink is blue at the top and red at the bottom.

HAMLET

⅓ glass of plum liqueur

⅓ glass of white crème de menthe

⅓ glass of fresh single cream

1. Shake well and strain into a wine glass.

IRISH COFFEE

30 ml (2 tbsp) Irish whiskey

hot strong black coffee

10 ml (2 level tsp) demerara sugar

15–30 ml (1–2 tbsp) fresh double cream

1. Stir whiskey and sugar in a wine glass of hot coffee.
2. Float the fresh cream on top by pouring over the back of a warm spoon. Do not stir.

WINTER MILK PUNCH

1 litre (2 pints) milk

25 g (1 oz) ground almonds

100 g (4 oz) sugar

5 ml (1 level tsp) finely grated orange rind

2 egg whites

60 ml (4 tbsp) rum

90 ml (6 tbsp) brandy

1. Pour the milk into a large pan with the almonds, sugar and the grated orange rind.

Bring just to the boil and remove from the heat.
2. Whisk the egg whites until stiff. Add to the hot milk mixture with the rum and brandy.
3. Whisk gently until the punch is frothy. Ladle into cups and serve.

Serves 8

HOT COFFEE FOAM

2 eggs, separated

15 ml (1 level tbsp) caster sugar

30 ml (2 tbsp) coffee liqueur

300 ml (½ pint) hot strong black coffee

300 ml (½ pint) hot milk

grated nutmeg

1. Beat the egg yolks and sugar together until very thick and pale in colour. Gently whisk in the liqueur, coffee and milk.
2. Beat the egg whites stiffly and divide equally between four cups. Pour the hot coffee mixture into the cups over the egg whites.
3. Sprinkle each lightly with nutmeg. Serve immediately.

Serves 4

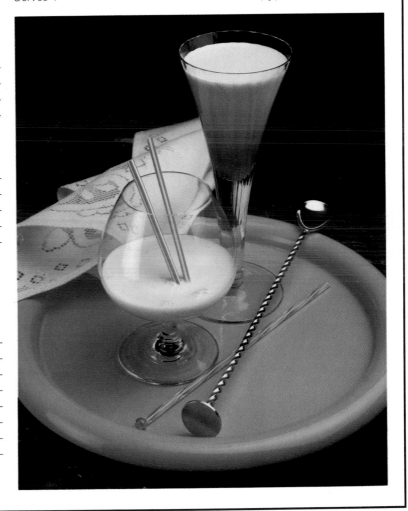

Below:
BRANDY ALEXANDER (left) and EVERTON BLUE.

COOK'S TIP TO CRUSH ICE, wrap some cubes in a clean cloth or a strong polythene bag and knock forcefully against a hard surface, or hit with a wooden rolling pin. Do not use a blender, as this will damage the blades.

MILK POSSET

568 ml (1 pint) milk

45 ml (3 tbsp) white wine or sherry

a squeeze of lemon juice

sugar

pinch of ground ginger and grated nutmeg

1. Heat the milk until it froths.
2. Add the wine or sherry and stir in the strained lemon juice and sugar.
3. Serve sprinkled with ginger and nutmeg.
Serves 2

SPECIAL CREAM CHOCOLATE

100 g (4 oz) plain chocolate

2.5 ml ($\frac{1}{2}$ level tsp) ground cinnamon

568 ml (1 pint) milk

150 ml (5 fl oz) fresh whipping cream

1. Add the chocolate and cinnamon to the milk in a saucepan. Heat gently until dissolved, then bring to the boil.
2. Whip the fresh cream until softly stiff and whisk most of it into the milk. Pour into four cups or glasses and top with the rest of the cream and a pinch of cinnamon or grated chocolate.
Serves 4

Below: clockwise from the top SPECIAL CREAM CHOCOLATE, IRISH COFFEE (page 63) and EMERALD COOL.

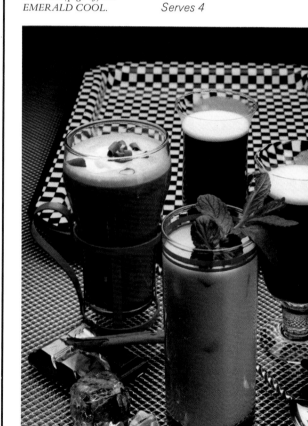

BRAZILIAN BANANA MILKSHAKE

568 ml (1 pint) cool fresh milk

30–45 ml (2–3 level tbsp) drinking chocolate

142 g (5 oz) natural yogurt

1 banana, mashed

30 ml (2 tbsp) rum (optional)

walnuts, chopped, to garnish

1. Liquidise all the ingredients in a blender or whisk until smooth.
2. Pour into four glasses; serve sprinkled with chopped nuts.
Serves 4

HOT MILK MOCHA

300 ml ($\frac{1}{2}$ pint) milk

10 ml (2 level tsp) drinking chocolate

5 ml (1 level tsp) instant coffee

15 ml (1 tbsp) fresh double cream

1. Boil the milk and pour into cups.
2. Add the drinking chocolate and coffee and stir well.
3. Swirl in the fresh cream and serve.
Serves 2

COCKTAIL SHAKES

These are easy – just mix a dash of spirit or liqueur with the other ingredients, shake and serve over ice.

LATIN LOVER

1 glass of cool fresh milk

Campari

dry vermouth

PINA COLADA

$\frac{1}{2}$ glass of cool fresh milk

$\frac{1}{4}$ glass of pineapple juice

coconut liqueur

white rum

maraschino cherries and pineapple slices to decorate

PUBLICAN'S POSSET

1 glass of cool fresh milk

brandy

sherry

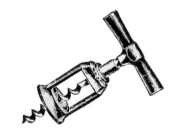

RED SUNSET

1 glass of cool fresh milk

mandarin brandy

RHUMBA

1 glass of cool fresh milk

dark rum

lemon or lime slices and cherries to decorate

BRANDY REVIVER

1 glass of cool fresh milk

brandy

crème de cacao

COFFEE COLA

½ glass of cool fresh milk

¼ glass of Coca Cola

coffee liqueur

CARIBBEAN KISS

1 glass of cool fresh milk

crème de cacao

coffee liqueur

CHERRY SPARKLE

½ glass of cool fresh milk

¼ glass of soda water

cherry brandy

HIGHLAND FLING

1 glass of cool fresh milk

whisky

ORANGE COCKTAIL

1 glass of cool fresh milk

orange-flavoured liqueur

dash of orange juice

orange slices to decorate

EMERALD COOL

1 glass of cool fresh milk

crème de menthe

mint sprigs to decorate

BANANA DAIQUIRI

1 glass of banana-flavoured milk

white rum

banana liqueur

TICKLED PINK

1 glass of strawberry-flavoured milk

kirsch

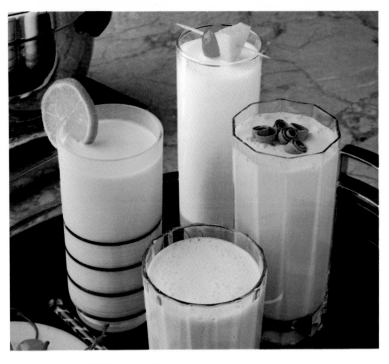

Above: clockwise from the top
PINA COLADA,
CHOCOLATE
CHARMER,
GRASSHOPPER (page 63)
and RHUMBA.

GOLDEN ISLE

1 glass of banana-flavoured milk

brandy

toasted coconut to decorate

CHOCOLATE CHARMER

1 glass of chocolate-flavoured milk

brandy

grated chocolate to decorate

CHOCOLATE MINT JULEP

1 glass of chocolate-flavoured milk

mint liqueur

chopped nuts and mint leaves to decorate

COFFEE MOCHA

1 glass of chocolate-flavoured milk

coffee liqueur

CALYPSO

1 glass of coffee-flavoured milk

dark rum

lemon or lime slices and cherries to decorate

HAWAIIAN PUNCH

1 glass of pineapple-flavoured milk

white rum

coconut liqueur

STRAWBERRY FARE

1 glass of strawberry-flavoured milk

Drambuie

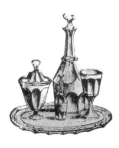

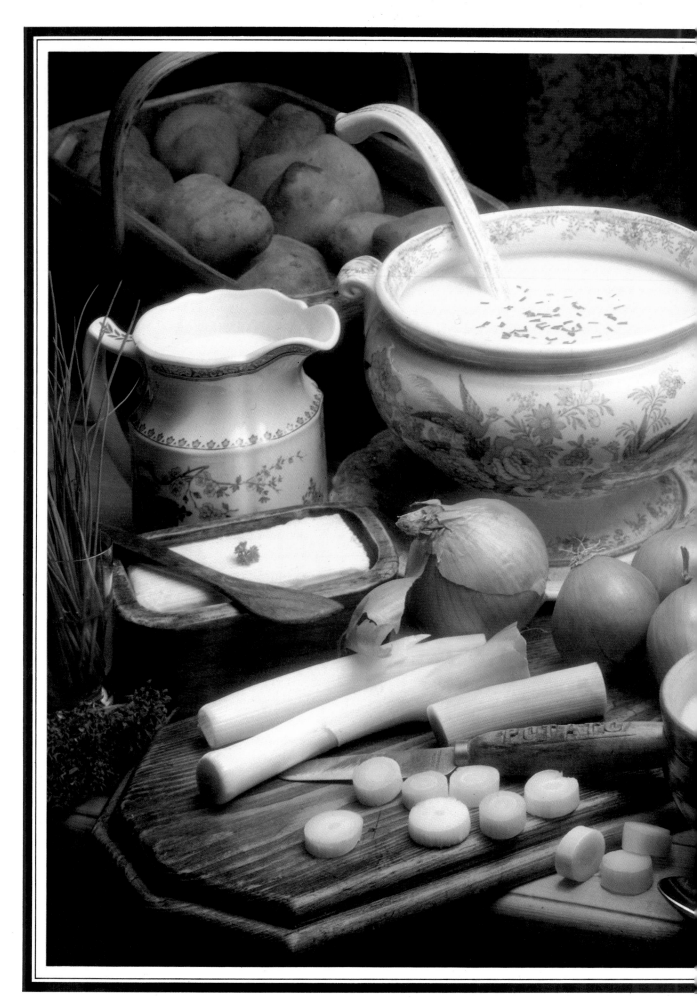

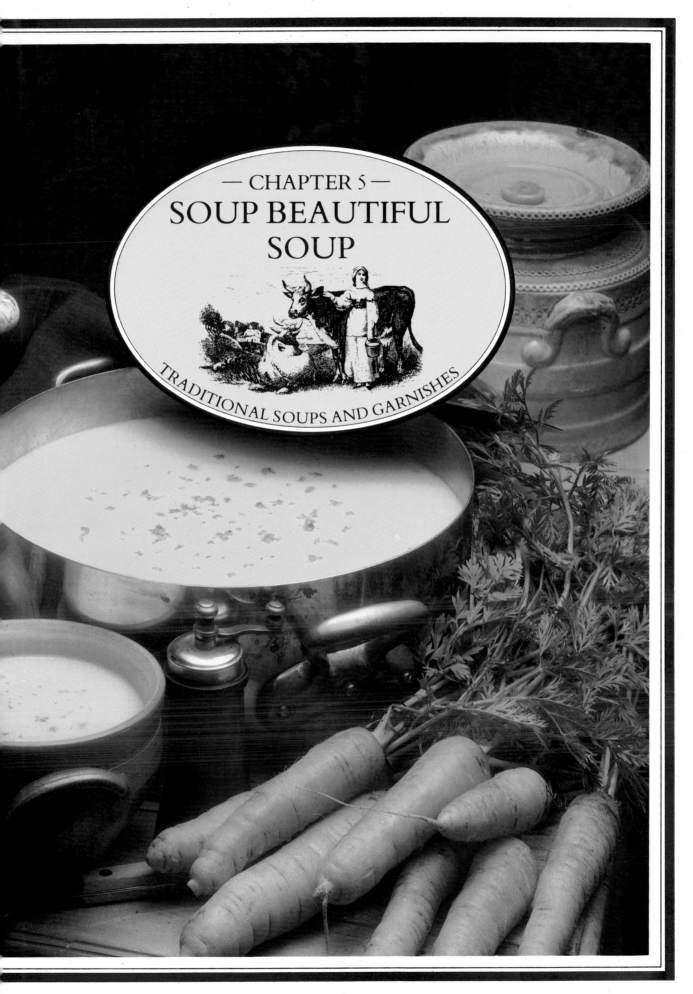

— CHAPTER 5 —
SOUP BEAUTIFUL SOUP

TRADITIONAL SOUPS AND GARNISHES

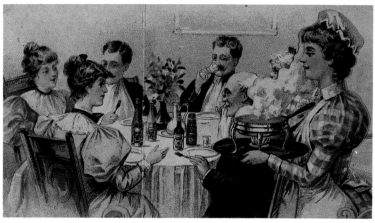

Above:
Over the centuries there have been many fashions and ups and downs in the popularity of soups, as our eating and cooking habits changed. Today, we have a wonderful range of traditional soups to try, all of them based on fine British produce. From the delicate Lettuce Soup (opposite) to the rich Smoked Fish Chowder on page 77, there is a delicious homemade soup to suit every taste and budget.

COOK'S TIP ALL SOUPS FREEZE WELL. If egg yolks or fresh cream are included in the recipe, however, they must be added after reheating. Pour the cold soup into rigid containers, seal well and freeze. Either thaw at room temperature or heat immediately to boiling point.

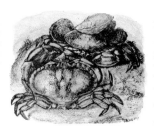

Delicious homemade soup is welcome any time, ladled from a tureen as a heart-warming first course on a cold winter's evening, or served chilled from a bowl nestling in chipped ice as a refreshing start to a sophisticated summer meal. Good homemade soup is always delicious and far, far better than any of the commercial versions. Like home-baked bread, once you have tasted it there is no going back! Real tomato, real mushroom, real asparagus – there's no mistaking the true flavours.

Soup has always been a basic part of traditional English food. We are great lovers of soup in this country and it has always been a warming part of our diet. Today, we are lucky to be able to draw on a wonderful repertoire of traditional soup recipes based on vegetables, fish, meat and game. One of our oldest is Watercress Soup on page 76 for which recipes date back to the seventeenth century. As with all other nourishing vegetable soups, the secret of making this is to let the vegetables gently soften in good English butter in a *covered* pan to bring out their unique flavour. Good soup must taste distinctly of the things it is made of: don't let the flavours become confused.

The thickness of soup is a matter of personal choice and as soup is such a versatile dish, it can be easily adjusted to your own preference. When thinned down with milk or cream, a thickish 'main meal' soup can be transformed into a perfect light appetiser. If you are serving soup as a starter, it is worth remembering that too generous a helping can be an embarrassment and can spoil the appetite for subsequent courses. Amounts should be based on 200 ml ($\frac{1}{3}$ pint) per serving.

OLD-FASHIONED ENGLISH SOUPS

SHROPSHIRE PEA SOUP

50 g (2 oz) English butter
1 small onion, skinned and finely chopped
900 g (2 lb) fresh peas, shelled
1.1 litres (2 pints) chicken stock
2.5 ml ($\frac{1}{2}$ tsp) caster sugar
2 large sprigs of fresh mint
salt and freshly ground pepper
2 egg yolks, size 2
150 ml (5 fl oz) fresh double cream
sprig of fresh mint to garnish

1. Melt the butter in a large saucepan, add the onion and cook for 5 minutes until soft. Add the peas, stock, sugar and sprigs of mint. Bring to the boil and cook for about 30 minutes.
2. Put the soup through a fine sieve or purée in a blender. Return to the pan and add the seasoning.
3. In a bowl beat together the yolks and fresh cream and add to the soup. Heat gently, stirring, but do not boil otherwise it will curdle.
4. Transfer to a soup tureen and garnish with a sprig of fresh mint.
Serves 6

DEVONSHIRE CRAB SOUP

25 g (1 oz) English butter
1 small onion, skinned and finely chopped
1 celery stick, cleaned and chopped
75 g (3 oz) long grain rice
568 ml (1 pint) milk
meat of 1 cooked crab, or 225 g (8 oz) frozen or canned crab meat, drained and flaked
300 ml ($\frac{1}{2}$ pint) chicken stock
salt and freshly ground pepper
5 ml (1 tsp) anchovy essence
30 ml (2 tbsp) brandy
150 ml (5 fl oz) fresh double cream
chopped fresh parsley to garnish

1. Melt the butter in a large saucepan, add the onion and celery and cook for 10 minutes until soft. Add the rice and milk, cover and cook for 15 minutes until the rice is cooked. Cool slightly.

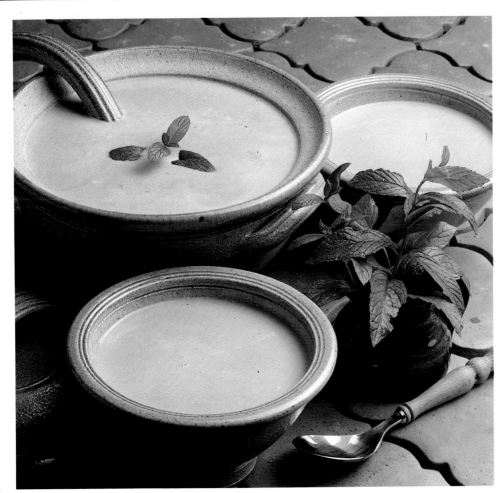

Left:
SHROPSHIRE PEA SOUP
This classic English soup tastes fresh from the country vegetable garden. Peas were brought to this country by the Romans and the green velvety-smooth texture of this versatile vegetable is enriched in this recipe with egg yolks and fresh cream.

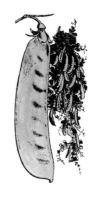

Below:
DEVONSHIRE CRAB SOUP
Whether made from freshly cooked or pre-packed crab meat, this richly flavoured soup brings the breezy tang of the English seaside to your table.

2. Pass the soup through a sieve or purée in a blender. Return to the pan together with the crab meat. Add the stock, seasoning, anchovy essence and reheat.
3. Add the brandy and fresh cream but do not boil. Transfer to a soup tureen, sprinkle with chopped parsley and serve very hot accompanied with melba toast and butter.
Serves 6

LETTUCE SOUP

50 g (2 oz) English butter
350 g (12 oz) lettuce leaves
125 g (4 oz) spring onions, trimmed
15 ml (1 level tbsp) flour
600 ml (1 pint) chicken stock
150 ml (¼ pint) milk
salt and freshly ground pepper

1. Melt the butter in a deep saucepan. Sauté the roughly chopped lettuce and spring onions until very soft. Stir in the plain flour then add the stock. Bring to the boil, cover and simmer for 45 minutes to 1 hour.
2. Cool the soup. Purée in a blender or rub through a sieve. Return to the saucepan and add the milk and seasonings. Reheat to serving temperature.
Serves 4

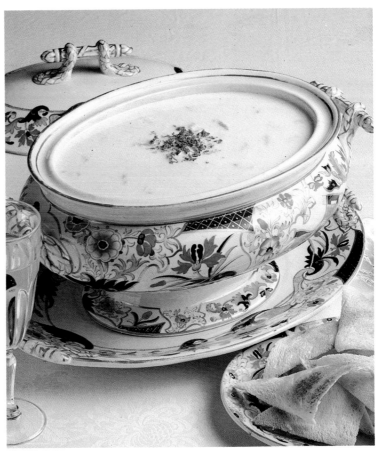

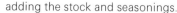

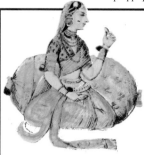

MULLIGATAWNY SOUP

1 medium onion, skinned and finely chopped
125 g (4 oz) carrot, peeled and finely chopped
125 g (4 oz) swede, peeled and finely chopped
1 small dessert apple, peeled and finely chopped
50 g (2 oz) streaky bacon, finely chopped
50 g (2 oz) English butter
25 g (1 oz) flour
15 ml (1 level tbsp) mild curry paste
15 ml (1 level tbsp) tomato purée
30 ml (2 level tbsp) mango chutney
1.4 litres (2½ pints) beef stock
5 ml (1 tsp) dried mixed herbs
pinch of ground mace
pinch of ground cloves
salt and freshly ground pepper
50 g (2 oz) long grain rice
150 ml (5 fl oz) fresh double cream

Below:
MULLIGATAWNY SOUP
The English have always been fond of highly spiced food, a taste which can be traced back in our cooking to medieval times and which can be seen today in our pungent commercially prepared sauces and mustards.

This tasty curried broth belongs to the early nineteenth century and is part of the heritage of the British Raj. English people who spent years in India grew to love the local spicy food and brought back their favourite recipes which were adapted in the Victorian kitchen.

Try this soup accompanied by the large spicy crisps called Poppadoms for another exciting taste of India.

1. Melt the butter in a large saucepan and fry the onion, carrot, swede, apple and bacon until lightly browned.
2. Stir in the flour, curry paste, tomato purée and chutney. Cook for 1–2 minutes before adding the stock and seasonings.
3. Bring to the boil, skim and simmer, covered, for 30–40 minutes. Sieve the soup or purée in a blender.
4. Return the soup to the pan, bring to the boil, add the rice and boil gently for about 12 minutes, until the rice is tender.
5. Adjust seasoning. Stir in the fresh cream, reserving a little. Do not boil. Pour into a tureen or bowls and swirl with cream.
Serves 6

STILTON SOUP

50 g (2 oz) English butter
1 onion, skinned and finely chopped
2 celery sticks, cleaned and sliced
40 g (1½ oz) flour
45 ml (3 tbsp) dry white wine
900 ml (1½ pints) chicken stock
300 ml (½ pint) milk
100 g (4 oz) Blue Stilton cheese, crumbled
50 g (2 oz), English Cheddar cheese, grated
salt and freshly ground pepper
60 ml (4 tbsp) fresh double cream
croûtons to garnish

1. Melt the butter in a saucepan, add the vegetables, and fry gently for 5 minutes. Stir in the flour and cook for 1 minute. Remove from the heat, stir in the wine and stock, return to the heat, bring to the boil, and simmer for 30 minutes.
2. Add the milk and cheeses, stirring constantly; season. Stir in the fresh cream.
3. Rub through a sieve or purée in a blender and reheat without boiling. Serve garnished with croûtons.
Serves 4–6

CREAMY AND MAIN MEAL SOUPS

CREAM OF ARTICHOKE SOUP

900 g (2 lb) Jerusalem artichokes
2 slices of lemon
25 g (1 oz) English butter
1 medium onion, skinned and chopped
30 ml (2 level tbsp) cornflour
450 ml (¾ pint) milk
15-30 ml (1–2 tbsp) lemon juice
15–30 ml (1–2 tbsp) chopped fresh parsley
5–10 ml (1–2 level tsp) salt
freshly ground pepper
60 ml (4 tbsp) fresh single cream

1. Wash and peel the artichokes. Place in a large saucepan with 900 ml (1½ pints) cold salted water and lemon slices. Bring to the

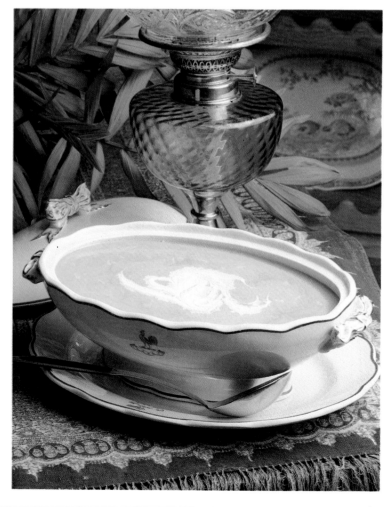

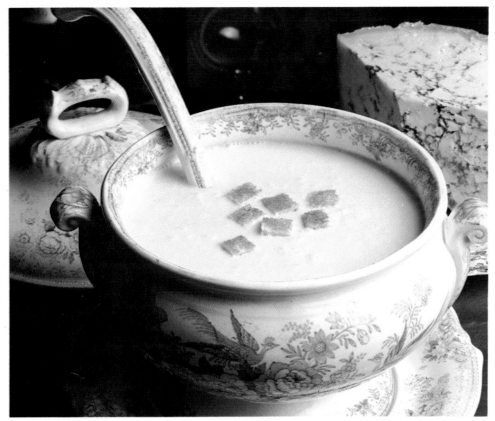

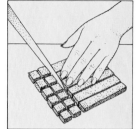

1 Cutting the croûtons from slices of bread from which the crusts have been trimmed

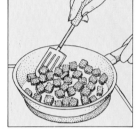

2 Frying the croûtons in butter to a crisp golden brown

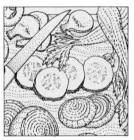

3 When fresh vegetables are used as a soup garnish, they must be sliced very thinly or cut into fine matchstick strips called julienne.

boil and simmer gently for 25 minutes until tender.

2. Drain, reserving the cooking liquid, and make up to 600 ml (1 pint) with water. Mash the artichokes. Discard the lemon slices.

3. Melt the butter in a clean pan, add the onion and cook for about 5 minutes until soft but not coloured. Remove the pan from the heat, stir in the cornflour and gradually add the reserved artichoke cooking liquid and milk.

4. Add the artichokes and bring to the boil, stirring. Cook for 2–3 minutes.

5. Cool the soup. Purée in a blender or rub through a sieve and return to the saucepan. Stir in the lemon juice, parsley, seasoning and fresh cream.

6. Reheat gently but do not boil. Garnish with croûtons.

Serves 6

CREAM OF ONION SOUP

25 g (1 oz) English butter

450 g (1 lb) onions, skinned and thinly sliced

568 ml (1 pint) milk

salt and freshly ground pepper

20 ml (4 level tsp) cornflour

45 ml (3 tbsp) fresh single cream

parsley sprigs to garnish

1. Heat the butter in a saucepan, add the onions, cover and cook gently until softened, shaking the pan occasionally to prevent browning. This is known as sweating.

2. Add the milk, 300 ml ($\frac{1}{2}$ pint) water and seasoning and bring to the boil, stirring. Reduce the heat and simmer covered for about 25 minutes, until the onion is tender.

3. Blend the cornflour with 45 ml (3 tbsp) water, stir into the soup and bring to the boil. Cook gently for a few minutes until slightly thickened, stirring. Add the fresh cream, check seasoning and reheat without boiling. Garnish with parsley sprigs.

Serves 4

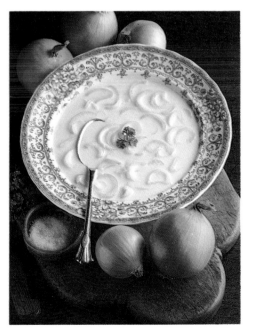

Above:
STILTON SOUP
Here two fine cheeses, Blue Stilton and English Cheddar, prove their versatility in this unusual and nourishing soup which gives a hearty welcome on a winter's evening.

Left:
CREAM OF ONION SOUP
A strong-flavoured warming soup which, when served with hot toast and butter, can be a quick winter meal in itself. Traditionally, a rich onion soup like this was often served to ward off a cold.

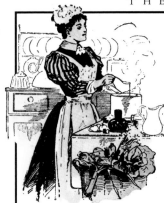

CREAM OF LEMON SOUP

25 g (1 oz) English butter

2 medium onions, skinned and thinly sliced

75 g (3 oz) carrot, peeled and thinly sliced

75 g (3 oz) celery, cleaned and thinly sliced

2 lemons

1.1 litres (2 pints) chicken stock

2 bay leaves

salt and freshly ground pepper

150 ml (5 fl oz) fresh single cream

snipped fresh chives and lemon slices to
garnish

1. Melt the butter in a large saucepan, add the vegetables; cover the pan and cook gently for 5–10 minutes, or until the vegetables are beginning to soften.

2. Meanwhile, thinly pare the lemons using a potato peeler. Blanch the rinds in boiling water for 1 minute; drain. Squeeze the juice from the lemons to give 75–90 ml (5–6 tbsp).

3. Add the lemon rind and juice to the pan with the stock, bay leaves and seasoning. Bring slowly to the boil, cover the pan and simmer gently for about 40 minutes, or until the vegetables are very soft.

4. Cool the soup a little, remove the bay leaves, then rub through a sieve or purée in a blender. Return the soup to a clean pan, reheat gently, stirring in the cream. Do not boil. Adjust seasoning and serve garnished with snipped chives and lemon slices.

Serves 6

Right:
*CREAM OF LEMON
SOUP*
The combination of chicken and lemon goes back to the seventeenth century when both oranges and lemons were expensive luxuries. Over the centuries, lemons became associated with chicken, and oranges with duck. A rich, jellied, homemade chicken stock is by far the best for this delicious soup.

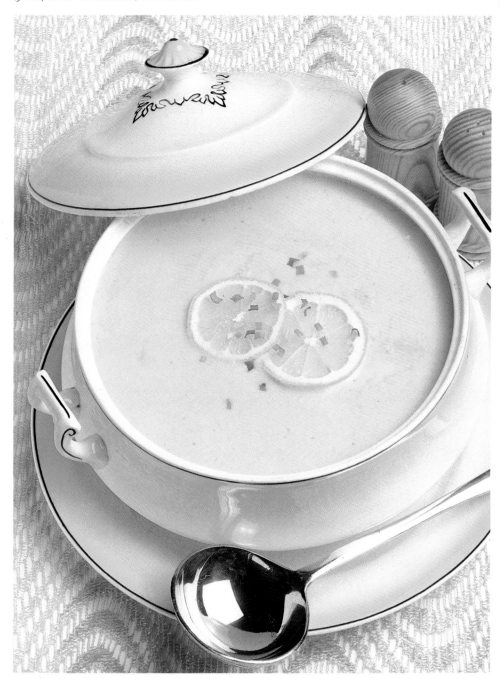

CREAM OF PARSLEY SOUP

25 g (1 oz) English butter
125 g (4 oz) fresh parsley, roughly chopped
1 medium onion, skinned and sliced
50 g (2 oz) celery, cleaned and sliced
20 ml (4 level tsp) flour
1 litre (1¾ pints) chicken stock
salt and freshly ground pepper
60 ml (4 tbsp) fresh single cream

1. Melt the butter in a large saucepan and add the parsley, onion and celery. Cover the pan and cook gently until the vegetables are quite soft. Shake the pan from time to time.
2. Stir in the flour until smooth, then mix in the stock. Season and bring to the boil.
3. Cover the pan and simmer for about 25 minutes. Cool a little then rub through a sieve or purée in a blender. Reheat, adjust seasoning and stir in the fresh cream just before serving.
Serves 4

WALNUT AND MUSHROOM SOUP

350 g (12 oz) button mushrooms
1 small onion, skinned and finely chopped
50 g (2 oz) English butter
15 ml (1 level tbsp) flour
450 ml (¾ pint) chicken stock
450 ml (¾ pint) milk
50 g (2 oz) walnuts, chopped
2.5 ml (½ level tsp) salt
freshly ground pepper
150 ml (5 fl oz) fresh single cream or top of milk

1. Wipe and chop the mushrooms, reserving a few finely sliced mushrooms for garnish. In a saucepan, soften the onion in the melted butter, add the chopped mushrooms and fry for 2 minutes.
2. Remove from the heat, stir in the flour, stock, milk, walnuts and seasoning. Bring to the boil. Simmer, covered, for about 30 minutes.
3. Purée the soup, add the finely sliced mushrooms and fresh cream, return to the pan and cook slowly for a further 5 minutes, adjusting seasoning. Do not boil. Serve hot.
Serves 6

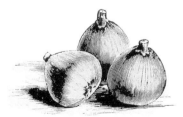

CREAM OF ALMOND SOUP

40 g (1½ oz) blanched almonds
750 ml (1¼ pints) milk
¼ medium onion, skinned and thinly sliced
2 sticks celery, cleaned and finely chopped
25 g (1 oz) English butter
15 g (½ oz) flour
salt and freshly ground pepper
grated nutmeg
60 ml (4 tbsp) fresh single cream
15 g (½ oz) blanched almonds, toasted, to garnish

1. Chop 40 g (1½ oz) of the almonds finely, and bring them to the boil in half the milk with the onion and the celery. Simmer for 30 minutes, then sieve or purée in a blender.
2. Melt 15 g (½ oz) butter in a pan; remove from the heat. Stir in the flour, and gradually blend in the remaining milk. Stir in the heated milk and almonds, return to the heat and simmer for 10 minutes.
3. Add the salt, pepper and a little grated nutmeg. Stir in the fresh cream and heat the soup but do not boil.
4. Cut the remaining almonds into thin slivers, and in the remaining butter quickly fry until lightly golden brown.
5. Pour the soup into a tureen or individual dishes and serve sprinkled with browned almonds.
Serves 4

CREAM OF SPINACH SOUP

50 g (2 oz) English butter
175-g (6-oz) packet frozen spinach (leaves or chopped spinach), thawed
1 medium onion, skinned and finely chopped
25 g (1 oz) flour
300 ml (½ pint) chicken stock
568 ml (1 pint) milk
salt and freshly ground pepper
pinch of grated nutmeg
30 ml (2 tbsp) fresh single cream

1. Melt the butter in a large saucepan and gently sauté the spinach and onions for 5–6 minutes. Add the flour and stir thoroughly; remove from the heat.
2. Add stock, return to the heat and boil, stirring continuously until the mixture thickens. Carefully blend in the milk and bring back to the boil, stirring. Cover and simmer for 15–20 minutes; season.
3. Sieve the soup or purée in a blender, and, if necessary, thin with milk. Reheat gently.
4. Pour into a warmed soup tureen or individual dishes and stir in the fresh cream just before serving.
Serves 6

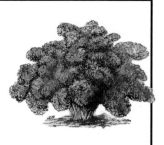

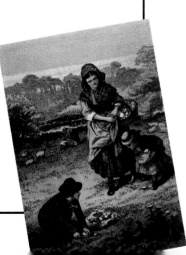

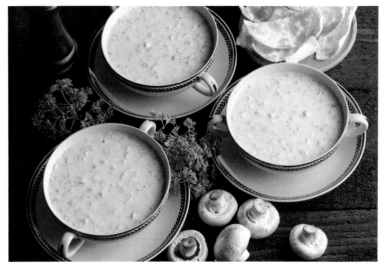

Above:
MUSHROOM SOUP
This delicious soup, finished with fresh cream, brings the open-air goodness of the woods and fields to your table.

CAULIFLOWER CHEESE SOUP

1 medium cauliflower
salt
50 g (2 oz) English butter
25 g (1 oz) flour
300 ml (½ pint) milk
100 g (4 oz) English Cheddar cheese, finely grated

1. Cut the cauliflower florets from the stalk and reserve. Cook the stalk gently in boiling salted water for 45 minutes. Drain and reserve the water; rub the stalk through a sieve or purée in a blender.
2. Melt the butter in a saucepan and sauté the florets. Remove the cauliflower and set aside. Stir the flour into the butter, and add 300 ml (½ pint) of reserved cauliflower water. Cook, stirring continuously until the mixture thickens. Pour in the milk and bring to the boil.
3. Add florets and puréed stalk to the soup. Gently stir in all but 30 ml (2 tbsp) cheese. Pour into soup tureen and serve, sprinkled with the remaining cheese.
Serves 4

MUSHROOM SOUP

25 g (1 oz) English butter
25 g (1 oz) flour
300 ml (½ pint) chicken stock
300 ml (½ pint) milk
15 ml (1 tbsp) chopped fresh parsley
100 g (4 oz) mushrooms, wiped and finely chopped
salt and freshly ground pepper
15 ml (1 tbsp) lemon juice
30 ml (2 tbsp) fresh cream

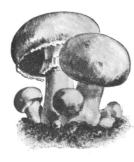

1. Place all the ingredients except lemon juice and fresh cream in a large saucepan. Bring to the boil, whisking continuously,

over a moderate heat. Cover and simmer for 10 minutes.
2. Remove from the heat and add the lemon juice and fresh cream, stirring well.
3. Pour into a tureen or individual dishes, and serve immediately with melba toast.
Serves 4

PRAWN BISQUE

25 g (1 oz) English butter
45 ml (3 level tbsp) flour
750 ml (1½ pints) fish or chicken stock
juice of ½ lemon
150 ml (¼ pint) dry white wine
225 g (8 oz) peeled prawns
150 ml (5 fl oz) fresh double cream
salt and freshly ground pepper
fresh prawns and chopped fresh parsley to garnish

1. Melt the butter in a saucepan, add flour and cook for 2–3 minutes. Remove from the heat and gradually stir in the stock. Bring to the boil and continue to stir until the soup thickens. Add the lemon juice, dry white wine and prawns and simmer for 2 minutes. Remove from the heat.
2. Add the fresh cream and seasoning and reheat, but do not boil.
3. Serve garnished with whole, fresh prawns and chopped fresh parsley.
Serves 4–6

CURRIED PARSNIP SOUP

40 g (1½ oz) English butter
1 medium onion, skinned and sliced
700 g (1½ lb) parsnips, peeled and finely diced
5 ml (1 level tsp) curry powder
2.5 ml (½ level tsp) ground cumin
1.4 litres (2½ pints) chicken stock
salt and freshly ground pepper
150 ml (5 fl oz) fresh single cream
paprika to garnish

1. Heat the butter in the base of a large pan and fry the onion and parsnip together for about 3 minutes.
2. Stir in the curry powder and cumin and fry for a further 2 minutes.
3. Add the stock, bring to the boil, reduce heat and simmer covered for about 45 minutes, until the vegetables are tender.
4. Cool slightly, then use a perforated draining spoon to place the vegetables in a blender, add a little stock; purée until smooth.
5. Return to the pan. Adjust seasoning, add the fresh cream and reheat to serving temperature but do not boil. Serve sprinkled with paprika.
Serves 6

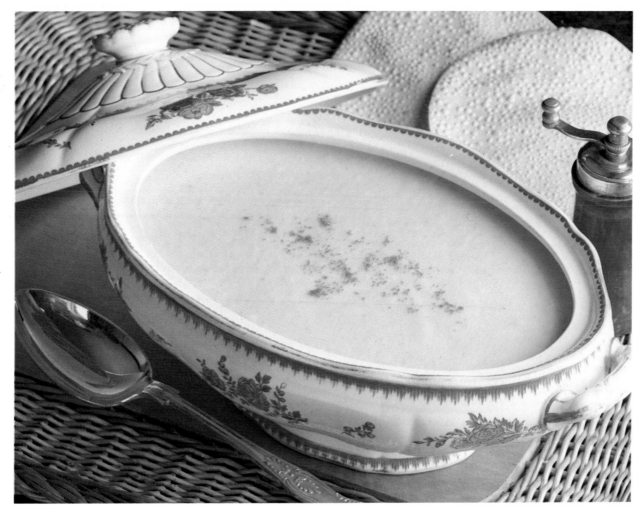

MUSHROOM AND WATERCRESS SOUP

50 g (2 oz) English butter

40 g (1½ oz) plain flour

600 ml (1 pint) chicken stock

450 ml (¾ pint) milk

225 g (8 oz) mushrooms, wiped and finely chopped

30 ml (2 tbsp) chopped watercress

salt and freshly ground pepper

croûtons to garnish

1. Melt the butter in a saucepan, add the flour and cook gently for 3–4 minutes.
2. Blend in the chicken stock and heat, stirring continuously until the soup thickens and boils.
3. Add the milk, mushrooms and watercress. Cook for 5 minutes; season. Serve hot garnished with croûtons.

Variation

In place of the mushrooms and watercress, substitute 1 chopped onion fried in melted butter, and 450 g (1 lb) chopped spinach, added with the milk.

Serves 4

SPINACH AND ORANGE SOUP

100 g (4 oz) English butter

1 kg (2.2 lb) fresh leaf spinach, cleaned, trimmed and roughly chopped

2 medium onions, skinned and finely chopped

2 oranges

60 ml (4 level tbsp) flour

900 ml (1½ pints) chicken stock

900 ml (1½ pints) milk

10 ml (2 level tsp) salt

freshly ground pepper

shreds of orange rind, blanched

1. Melt the butter in a large heavy-based pan, add the vegetables and grated rind of both oranges (retaining a few pared strips for the shreds). Cover with a piece of wet greaseproof paper and the lid; sweat for about 25 minutes, or until soft.
2. Stir in the flour, stock and milk off the heat. Return to the heat, bring to the boil, season and simmer for 15 minutes.
3. Purée the soup, then reheat for serving, adding the orange juice at the last minute. Garnish with the orange rind.

Serves 6–8

Above:
CURRIED PARSNIP SOUP
This unusual soup makes use of one of our most neglected vegetables. Although parsnips are traditionally roasted with beef, which they complement perfectly, British cooks have rarely made full use of them. Try this tasty and satisfying soup with its hint of exotic Indian spices.

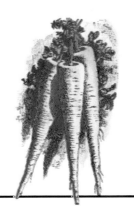

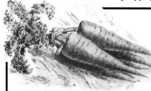

CARROT SOUP

50 g (2 oz) English butter

350 g (12 oz) carrots, peeled and diced or grated

2 leeks or onions, cleaned and sliced

450 ml (¾ pint) chicken stock

salt and freshly ground pepper

150 ml (¼ pint) milk

90 ml (6 tbsp) fresh single cream

chopped fresh parsley to garnish

1. Melt the butter in a large pan and fry the carrots and leeks or onions for 5–10 minutes.
2. Add the stock and seasoning and simmer for another 15–20 minutes. Sieve or purée the soup in a blender and return to the pan. Alternatively, cook vegetables for a further 10 minutes then beat with a wooden spoon. This gives a soup with more texture.
3. Stir in the milk and fresh cream; adjust seasoning and heat, but do not boil. Pour into a hot soup tureen and sprinkle with parsley.
Serves 4

WATERCRESS SOUP

2 bunches of watercress

25 g (1 oz) English butter

1 small onion, skinned and finely chopped

350 g (12 oz) potatoes, peeled and diced

450 ml (¾ pint) chicken stock

300 ml (½ pint) milk

salt and freshly ground pepper

142 g (5 oz) natural yogurt or 150 ml (5 fl oz) fresh single cream

1. Wash the watercress and reserve a few sprigs to garnish. Cut away any coarse stalks. Chop the leaves and remaining stalks.
2. Melt the butter in a large saucepan, and gently fry the onion and watercress for about 15 minutes until soft. Add the potatoes, stock, milk and seasoning. Bring to the boil and simmer gently for 30 minutes, stirring occasionally.
3. Rub the soup through a sieve or purée in a blender. Reheat gently with 60 ml (4 tbsp) of yogurt or fresh cream but do not boil.
4. Pour into a soup tureen or individual bowls, serve garnished with chopped watercress sprigs. Serve the remaining yogurt or fresh cream separately.
Serves 4

Below:
WATERCRESS SOUP
The earliest recipes for this traditional English soup are found in seventeenth-century cookery books. Gently cooking the watercress in good English butter is the secret of its rich and wholesome flavour.

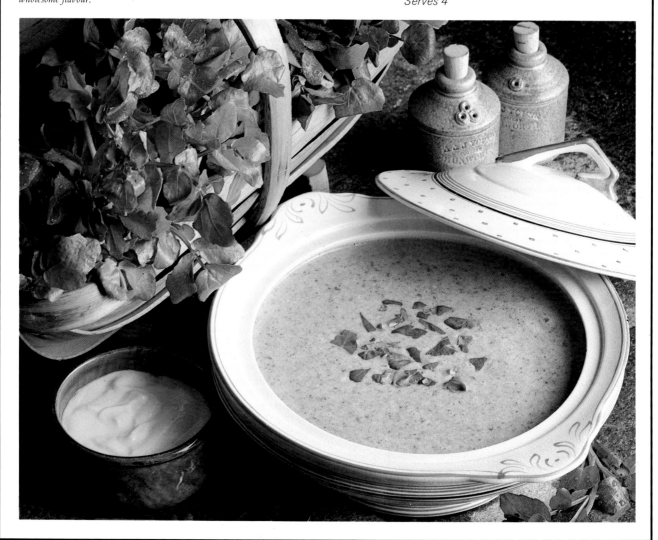

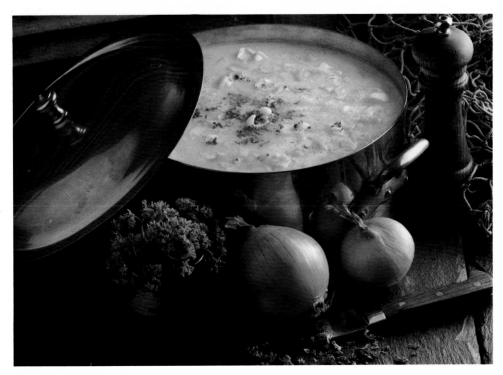

MAIN MEAL SOUPS

SMOKED FISH CHOWDER

450 g (1 lb) smoked haddock fillet

*225 g (8 oz) potatoes, peeled and cut into
1-cm (½-inch) dice*

2 medium onions, skinned and sliced

50 g (2 oz) English butter

30 ml (2 level tbsp) flour

*175 g (6 oz) carrot, peeled and coarsely
grated*

150 ml (¼ pint) fresh single cream

salt and freshly ground pepper

chopped fresh parsley to garnish

1. Simmer the fish in 1.1 litres (2 pints)
water for 10 minutes until tender. Drain,
reserving the liquid. Flake coarsely,
discarding skin and any bones.
2. Sauté the onion in the butter until soft,
then stir in the flour. Gradually add the
strained fish stock and bring to the boil,
stirring. Add the potatoes and the coarsely
grated carrot. Simmer for about 10 minutes
until the vegetables are tender.
3. Stir in the fresh cream and flaked fish.
Season well and heat to serving
temperature. Do not boil. Garnish with lots
of chopped parsley.

Variation
Corn Chowder
Substitute 100 g (4 oz) streaky bacon and a
350-g (11½-oz) can drained sweetcorn for
the fish.
Serves 4

WHITE BEAN SOUP

175 g (6 oz) haricot beans

*1 medium onion, skinned and finely
chopped*

1 small garlic clove, skinned and crushed

1.4 litres (2½ pints) chicken stock

2.5 ml (½ tsp) dried rosemary

125 g (4 oz) Red Leicester cheese, grated

salt and freshly ground pepper

croûtons to garnish

1. Place the beans in a bowl and cover with
boiling water. Leave for 2–3 hours. Drain
well.
2. Place the onion in a large saucepan with
the garlic, beans and stock. Add the dried
rosemary. Bring to the boil, cover and
simmer gently for 1–1½ hours or until the
beans are tender.
3. Purée half the stock in a blender with half
the beans or rub through a sieve.
4. Return the puréed soup to the pan, add
the cheese and adjust seasoning. Bring to
serving temperature. Serve accompanied
with crisp, fried croûtons.
Serves 4

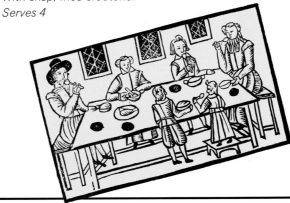

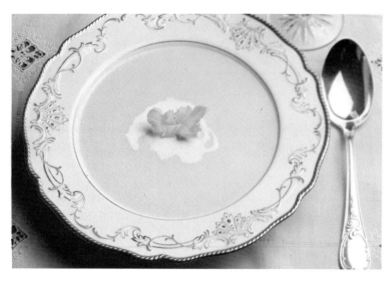

Above:
CREAM OF CELERY SOUP
Celery did not come into general use in England until the early nineteenth century. Since then, its crisp nutty flavour has been much appreciated in soups and sauces, and raw, as a traditional accompaniment to fine English cheese.

When buying celery, it is useful to remember that the whiter the celery stalks, the more flavour they will have.

ASPARAGUS AND CHEESE SOUP

275-g (10-oz) can asparagus
125 g (4 oz) potato, cooked
30 ml (2 tbsp) soured cream
150 ml ($\frac{1}{4}$ pint) milk
450 ml ($\frac{3}{4}$ pint) chicken stock
25 g (1 oz) mature English Cheddar cheese

1. Using a blender, purée together the asparagus, potato, soured cream and milk.
2. Pour into a saucepan with the chicken stock and heat gently. Grate the cheese straight into the pan, adjust seasoning and serve with warm, crusty bread.
Serves 2

CREAM OF CELERY SOUP

25 g (1 oz) English butter
1 head of celery, cleaned and finely chopped
2 onions, skinned and chopped
1 rasher of bacon, chopped
100 g (4 oz) cottage cheese, sieved
300 ml ($\frac{1}{2}$ pint) chicken stock
300 ml ($\frac{1}{2}$ pint) milk
salt and freshly ground pepper
75 ml (3 fl oz) fresh single cream
celery leaves to garnish

1. Melt the butter in a saucepan and soften the celery, onion and bacon gently for 5 minutes.
2. Stir in the cottage cheese, stock, milk and salt and pepper. Bring to the boil and simmer for 30 minutes; then sieve or purée in a blender. Reheat and add half the fresh cream.
3. Pour into a soup tureen or individual dishes and float the remaining cream on the top of each, with a few celery leaves. Serve immediately.
Serves 4

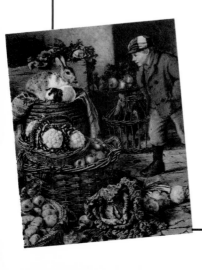

CREAM OF VEGETABLE SOUP

50 g (2 oz) English butter
225 g (8 oz) carrots, peeled and finely diced or grated
175 g (6 oz) swede, peeled and finely diced
2 small leeks, cleaned and finely chopped
25 g (1 oz) flour
450 ml ($\frac{3}{4}$ pint) chicken stock
salt and freshly ground pepper
150 ml ($\frac{1}{4}$ pint) milk
90 ml (6 tbsp) fresh single cream
chopped fresh parsley to garnish

1. Melt the butter in a large saucepan and fry the carrots, swede and leeks for 5–10 minutes.
2. Stir in the flour. Add stock, salt and pepper and simmer for another 15–20 minutes, before adding the milk and fresh cream. Adjust seasoning and heat gently. Do not boil.
3. Pour into warmed bowls and sprinkle with parsley. Serve with warmed crusty bread or rolls.
Serves 4

HARVEST VEGETABLE SOUP

25 g (1 oz) English butter
450 g (1 lb) carrots, peeled and diced
1 medium onion, skinned and sliced
2 medium potatoes, peeled and diced
1 small green pepper, seeded and chopped
50 g (2 oz) lentils
salt and freshly ground pepper
$\frac{1}{2}$ bay leaf
40 g (1$\frac{1}{2}$ oz) flour
450 ml ($\frac{3}{4}$ pint) milk
100 g (4 oz) English Cheddar cheese, grated
croûtons to garnish

1. Melt the butter and fry the carrots, onion, potatoes and green pepper until softened.
2. Add 450 ml ($\frac{3}{4}$ pint) water, lentils, salt, pepper and bay leaf and simmer for 30 minutes.
3. Mix the flour with a little of the milk and gradually blend in the rest. Stir well into the soup until it thickens. Simmer for 5 minutes then stir in 75 g (3 oz) cheese.
4. Pour into a serving dish, garnish with the remaining cheese and sprinkle with croûtons. Serve immediately.

Variation
Vegetable and Oatmeal Broth
Substitute 25 g (1 oz) medium oatmeal and 225 g (8 oz) swede for the lentils and potatoes.
Serves 4

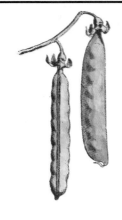

GREEN PEA AND BACON CHOWDER

1 medium onion, skinned and finely chopped

225 g (8 oz) streaky bacon, diced

25 g (1 oz) English butter

225 g (8 oz) potatoes, peeled and cut into 1-cm (½-inch) cubes

30 ml (2 level tbsp) flour

600 ml (1 pint) chicken stock

568 ml (1 pint) milk

salt and freshly ground pepper

450 g (1 lb) fresh peas, shelled (enough to yield 225 g (8 oz) peas)

50 g (2 oz) English Cheddar cheese, grated

snipped fresh chives and fresh single cream to garnish

1. In a large saucepan fry the onion and bacon together in the hot butter until golden. Stir in the potato and continue cooking for 2 minutes.
2. Add the flour to the pan, stirring, cook for 1 minute and gradually stir in the stock and milk. Season well. Bring to the boil, cover and simmer for 15–20 minutes until the potato is tender.
3. Add the peas, bring back to the boil and continue simmering, covered, for another 10–15 minutes until the peas are cooked.
4. Serve chowder sprinkled with grated cheese, snipped chives and a swirl of fresh cream. Accompany with buttered oat cakes or brown baps.

Serves 4

CHEESE AND ONION SOUP

25 g (1 oz) English butter

2 onions, skinned and cut into rings

2 sticks celery, cleaned and chopped

25 g (1 oz) flour

568 ml (1 pint) milk

300 ml (½ pint) chicken stock

salt and freshly ground pepper

pinch of grated nutmeg

2 slices bread

175 g (6 oz) English Cheddar cheese, grated

chopped fresh parsley to garnish

1. Melt the butter in a large saucepan. Lightly fry the onion rings and chopped celery without browning.
2. Add the flour and cook for 1–2 minutes. Gradually beat in the milk, stock and seasonings. Heat, whisking continuously, until the soup comes to the boil and thickens. Simmer for 5 minutes.
3. Meanwhile, toast the bread on one side. Sprinkle 50 g (2 oz) grated cheese on the untoasted side and grill until the cheese melts. Cut into small squares.
4. Remove the soup from the heat and stir in the remaining grated cheese. Pour into warmed soup bowls or a tureen and float toasted cheese on top.

Serves 4

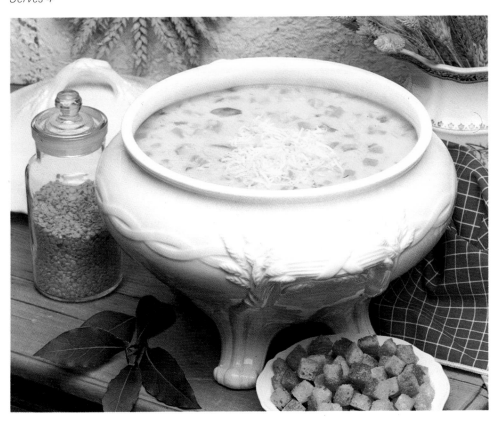

Left:
HARVEST VEGETABLE SOUP
Topped with fine English Cheddar and sprinkled with croûtons, this nourishing vegetable soup is warming and welcoming as the autumn evenings draw in. For step-by-step croûtons see page 71.

Opposite:
PRAWN AND AVOCADO SOUP
Fresh mouthwatering prawns and succulent avocados comple.nent each other perfectly as a popular starter. Here they are combined in an original way, as a delicious chilled summer soup.

LEEK AND POTATO SOUP

2 medium leeks, cleaned
1 small onion, skinned and finely chopped
25 g (1 oz) English butter
350 g (12 oz) potatoes, peeled and finely sliced
600 ml (1 pint) chicken stock
5 ml (1 level tsp) salt
freshly ground pepper
1 blade of mace
300 ml (10 fl oz) fresh double cream
30 ml (2 tbsp) snipped fresh chives or finely chopped watercress to garnish

1. Finely chop the white part of the leeks.
2. Melt the butter gently in a saucepan, add the leeks and onion and fry without browning for 7–10 minutes. Add the potatoes to the pan with the stock, salt and pepper and mace.
3. Bring to the boil, lower heat and cover pan. Simmer very gently for 20–30 minutes, or until the vegetables are tender.
4. Rub the soup through a fine sieve or purée in a blender. Chill thoroughly. Just before serving stir in the fresh cream. Transfer to individual soup bowls and serve sprinkled with chives or watercress.
Serves 4–6

PRAWN AND AVOCADO SOUP

2 large ripe avocados
30 ml (2 tbsp) lemon juice
600 ml (1 pint) chicken stock, cold
300 ml (½ pint) milk
salt and freshly ground pepper
Worcestershire sauce
75 ml (2½ fl oz) mayonnaise
75 ml (2½ fl oz) fresh single cream
15–30 ml (1–2 tbsp) tomato ketchup
50 g (2 oz) peeled prawns, chopped
5 ml (1 level tsp) chopped onion

1. Mash the flesh of the avocados with the lemon juice.
2. Whisk in the stock and milk and season with salt, pepper and Worcestershire sauce. If the soup is too thick, dilute with a little extra milk. Chill well.
3. Mix together the mayonnaise and fresh cream. Stir in the tomato ketchup, chopped prawns, onion and Worcestershire sauce; season.
4. Serve soup in bowls and swirl a spoonful of prawn sauce into each.
Serves 8

Below:
CHILLED SUMMER SOUP
On a very hot day serve this fresh green soup in cups nestling in larger bowls of chipped ice.

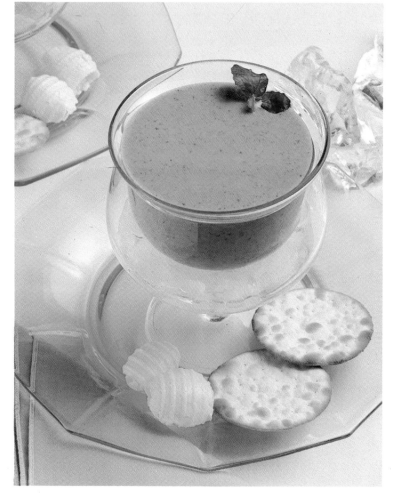

ICED SOUPS

CHILLED SUMMER SOUP

900 g (2 lb) peas, shelled
1 large bunch watercress
50 g (2 oz) English butter
1 medium onion, skinned and thinly sliced
1.1 litres (2 pints) milk
salt and freshly ground pepper
150 ml (5 fl oz) fresh single cream

1. Trim off 'hairy' watercress roots and wash the rest well. Drain and roughly chop the watercress reserving a few sprigs for garnish.
2. Melt the butter in a saucepan, add the watercress and onion, cover and cook gently for about 15 minutes, without browning.
3. Remove from the heat and stir in the milk, peas and seasoning. Bring to the boil, stirring.
4. Cover and simmer gently for about 30 minutes, until the peas are really soft. Cool slightly, rub through a sieve or purée in a blender.
5. Pour into a large bowl. Adjust seasoning, cool. Stir in the fresh cream and chill well before serving. Garnish with watercress sprigs.
Serves 6

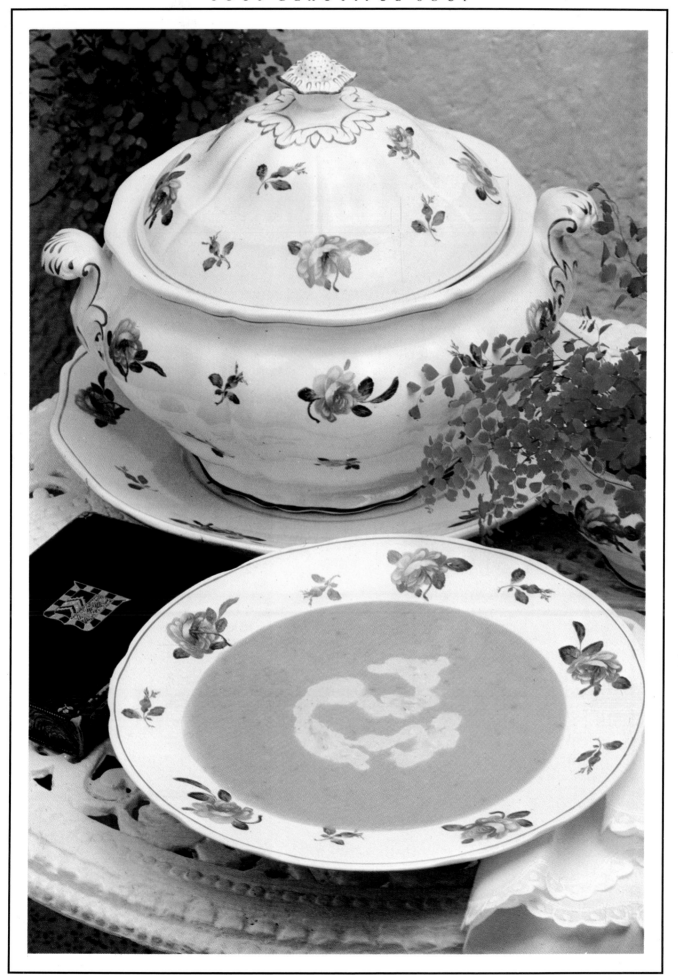

CHILLED MUSHROOM AND LEMON SOUP

450 g (1 lb) open mushrooms, wiped

grated rind and juice of 1 lemon

1 garlic clove, skinned and crushed

salt and freshly ground pepper

5 ml (1 level tsp) dried thyme or 15 ml (1 tbsp) chopped fresh thyme

900 ml (1½ pints) chicken stock

150 ml (5 fl oz) fresh single cream

parsley sprigs to garnish

1. Reserve one or two mushrooms for garnish and roughly slice the rest. Put in a flat dish and marinate with lemon rind and juice, garlic, seasoning and herbs for several hours, turning occasionally.
2. In blender, purée the mushrooms and the marinade with the stock. Stir in the fresh cream and adjust seasoning.
3. Chill well before serving. Garnish with the remaining mushrooms, very finely sliced, and parsley sprigs.

Serves 6–8

ICED CUCUMBER AND YOGURT SOUP

1 large cucumber

300 ml (10 fl oz) natural yogurt

½ small green pepper, seeded and finely chopped

1 garlic clove, skinned and crushed (optional)

30 ml (2 tbsp) wine vinegar

15 ml (1 tbsp) fresh chives, snipped

salt and freshly ground pepper

300 ml (½ pint) milk, chilled

30 ml (2 tbsp) finely chopped fresh parsley

1. Grate the unpeeled cucumber on a medium grater. Transfer to a bowl and stir in the yogurt.
2. Add the green pepper and garlic (if used) to the cucumber mixture with vinegar and chives.
3. Season with salt and pepper and chill very thoroughly. Just before serving stir in the milk.
4. Ladle into individual soup bowls, sprinkling each with chopped parsley, and serve chilled.

Serves 4–6

Below:
CHILLED MUSHROOM AND LEMON SOUP
Served really cold, and not just tepid, this smooth, sharp-tasting purée of mushrooms has the consistency of fresh single cream. If you prefer only a hint of garlic, rub a cut clove round the inside of the bowl in which the soup will be chilled, and omit the crushed garlic clove in the marinade.

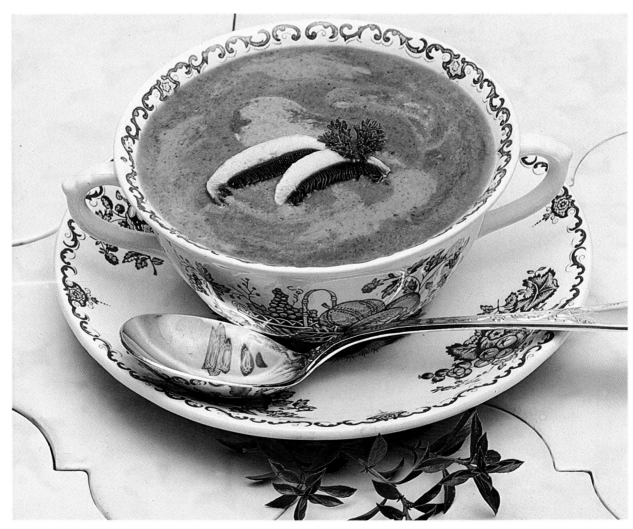

BORTSCH

6 small raw beetroot, about 1 kg (2¼ lb), peeled

2 medium onions, skinned and chopped

1.1 litres (2 pints) beef stock

salt and freshly ground pepper

30 ml (2 tbsp) lemon juice

90 ml (6 tbsp) dry sherry

142 ml (5 fl oz) soured cream

chopped fresh chives to garnish

1. Grate the beetroot coarsely and put in a pan with the onion, stock and seasoning. Bring to the boil and simmer, covered, for 45 minutes.
2. Strain, discard the vegetables and add the lemon juice and sherry to the liquid. Adjust seasoning. Serve well chilled with a whirl of soured cream and chopped chives.
Serves 4

ICED TOMATO SOUP

450 g (1 lb) ripe tomatoes

1 small onion, skinned and sliced

20 ml (4 level tsp) tomato purée

411-g (14½-oz) can chicken consommé

4 fresh basil leaves or 5 ml (1 tsp) dried basil

10 g (½ oz) fresh breadcrumbs

142 ml (5 fl oz) soured cream

1. Roughly chop the tomatoes; purée in a blender in two batches with the onion, tomato purée, consommé and basil.
2. Rub through a nylon sieve into a saucepan and heat gently to remove frothy texture; season well.
3. Add the breadcrumbs to the soup, and chill well before serving. Garnish with swirls of stirred soured cream.
Serves 4

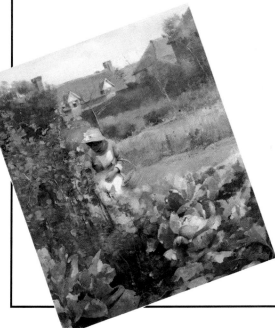

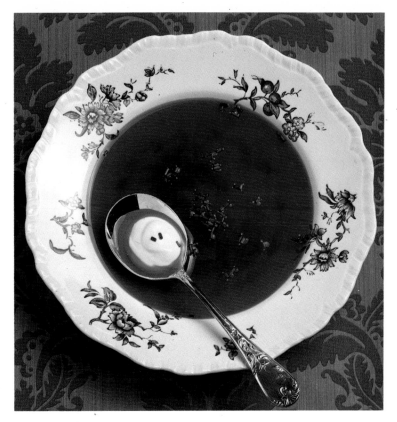

Above:
BORTSCH
Ruby-red and topped with a delicious swirl of soured cream, this traditional Russian soup, which takes its colour from beetroot, makes a spectacular start to an autumn meal.

CHILLED SKATE SOUP

450 g (1 lb) skate

1 medium onion, skinned and thinly sliced

125 g (4 oz) celery, cleaned and sliced

45 ml (3 tbsp) lemon juice

2 bay leaves

salt and freshly ground pepper

300 ml (½ pint) milk

142 ml (5 fl oz) soured cream

25 g (1 oz) lump fish roe (caviar-style)

snipped fresh chives to garnish

1. Rinse the skate and place in a medium-sized saucepan with the thinly sliced onion and sliced celery. Pour over 600 ml (1 pint) water with 30 ml (2 tbsp) lemon juice, bay leaves and seasoning.
2. Bring slowly to the boil, cover the pan and simmer gently until the fish begins to flake away from the bone.
3. Lift the fish from the soup and flake it, discarding the skin and bone.
4. In a blender, purée the pan ingredients (discarding bay leaves) with the fish and milk until smooth. Adjust seasoning, taste and add remaining lemon juice if necessary.
5. Chill well before serving with stirred soured cream and caviar swirled through each portion. Garnish with snipped chives.
Serves 6

Right: clockwise from top
ANCHOVY TWISTERS,
BABY LOAVES WITH
TARRAGON BUTTER,
MUSTARD BAKE-UPS,
PEANUT SABLÉS,
PIQUANT PALMIERS,
PAPRIKA NIBLETS,
PARSLEY AND ONION
DROPS, MELBA TOAST
Served warm from the oven,
one of these delicious savoury
accompaniments turns a hearty
homemade soup into a
memorable meal.

SOUP ACCOMPANI-MENTS

These tasty accompaniments can be placed alongside your soup to turn it into a hearty main meal. Try any of the following.

PEANUT SABLÉS

Rich, short and very savoury, a dish of sablés makes a popular partner to most soups. They keep well in the freezer, and since they can be stored in an airtight container for up to two weeks, it is worth making a bumper batch. Refresh them on the day. Tip-line the baking sheet with greaseproof paper to avoid the base and edges being over-baked.

125 g (4 oz) English butter
175 g (6 oz) flour
125 g (4 oz) Red Leicester cheese, grated
beaten egg to glaze
50 g (2 oz) salted peanuts, chopped

1. Rub the butter into the flour and add the cheese. Stir well, season and bind to a firm dough with 30 ml (2 tbsp) water. Knead lightly.
2. Roll out to a 20.5-cm (8-inch) square. Trim to neaten. Place on a baking sheet, cut into four strips, spaced apart. Glaze with beaten egg.
3. Press in the peanuts. Cut the strips into fingers and triangles, separate out.
4. Bake in the oven at 180°C (350°F) mark 4 for about 20 minutes. Set to cool on wire racks.

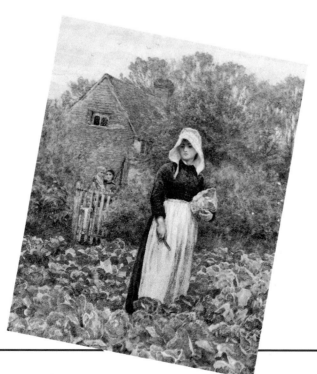

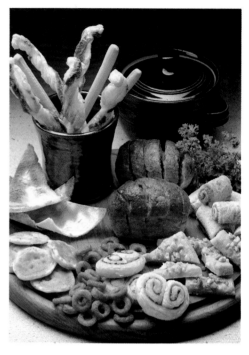

PIQUANT PALMIERS

Really quick to make, they look as though you've spent hours producing them.

277-g (8-oz) packet frozen puff pastry, thawed
60 ml (4 level tbsp) tomato purée
freshly ground pepper

1. Roll out the pastry to an oblong about 30.5 × 25.5 cm (12 × 10 inches). Lightly spread it with tomato purée, and season with the freshly ground pepper.
2. Roll up from the two narrow edges so that the rolls meet in the centre. Trim off the edges and slice into twelve pieces. Place cut-side down on greased baking sheets, leaving room to spread. Press down lightly with the heel of the hand to flatten a little.
3. Bake in the oven at 220°C (425°F) mark 7 for about 12 minutes.

MELBA TOAST

Homemade melba toast has the edge on the bought packaged variety. It's nicest served while still a little warm, in a basket or on a napkin-lined plate. If it is made a short time ahead, store it in an airtight container, then refresh it for a short time in the oven.

slices of thick cut ready-sliced bread, white or brown

1. Preheat the grill and toast the bread on both sides. Using a serrated knife, cut off the crusts and slide the knife between the toasted edges to split the bread.
2. Cut each piece into four triangles, place again under grill, untoasted side uppermost until golden and the edges curl.

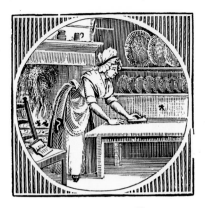

ANCHOVY TWISTERS

Made in no time with a packet of bought pastry, these salty feather-light sticks emerge golden from the oven. Eat them when fresh.

227-g (8-oz) packet frozen puff pastry, thawed

beaten egg to glaze

two 50-g (1¾-oz) can anchovies

1. Roll out the pastry to a 20.5-cm (8-inch) square. Glaze it with beaten egg and cut it into 2-cm (¾-inch) wide strips.
2. Lay the drained anchovies in the centre of each strip, pressing lightly to make them stick.
3. Lightly grease a 28-cm (11-inch) swiss-roll tin. Lift the strips and twist them along their length several times. Lay them across the short side of tin and attach the edges over the rim (this stops untwisting). Repeat with each strip.
4. At this stage you can leave the twisters loosely covered in a cool place. Bake them in the oven at 200°C (425°F) mark 7 for about 12 minutes. Cool. Halve to serve.

MUSTARD BAKE-UPS

If it is a little on the thick side, roll out the sliced bread once or twice; this makes the texture more pliable. Before baking, store wrapped in the fridge for a couple of days, or in the freezer for up to a month.

white bread, thinly sliced

English butter

whole-grain mustard

1. Generously butter the bread. Spread it with the mustard, and cut off the crusts. Roll up each slice inside damp greaseproof paper and refrigerate for at least 1 hour to firm up.
2. Remove paper, halve each roll lengthwise and place seam-side down on baking sheets. Bake in the oven at 220°C (425°F) mark 7 for about 12 minutes, until golden and crisp. Serve hot.

PAPRIKA NIBLETS

These make a pleasant change from croûtons and taste excellent with cream soups.

white bread, sliced

paprika

1. Using two small cutters, one a little larger than the other, stamp out rings from the slices of bread. Fry them quickly in hot oil until golden. Drain, sprinkle with the paprika and serve.

BABY LOAVES WITH TARRAGON BUTTER

As an accompaniment to main meal soups, use the small individual brown loaves which many bakers sell, to make an interesting alternative to hot garlic bread.

175 g (6 oz) English butter

10 ml (2 tsp) dried tarragon

squeeze of lemon juice

4 small individual brown loaves

1. Beat together the butter, tarragon and lemon juice. Slash the loaves diagonally four or five times and spread the cut surfaces generously with tarragon butter.
2. Place the loaves on a baking sheet and lightly cover with foil. Warm them through in the oven at 180°C (350°F) mark 4 for about 10 minutes. Serve immediately.
Makes 4

PARSLEY AND ONION DROPS

These are favourites when time permits them to be made really fresh and served straight from the pan.

1 small onion, skinned and chopped

25 g (1 oz) English butter

30 ml (2 tbsp) chopped fresh parsley

salt and freshly ground pepper

½ quantity drop scone batter, without sugar (see page 241)

1. Sauté the onion in butter.
2. Add the sautéed chopped onion with plenty of chopped parsley and seasoning to the drop scone batter.
3. Fry the mixture in tiny spoonfuls, flipping them over once bubbles appear.

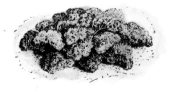

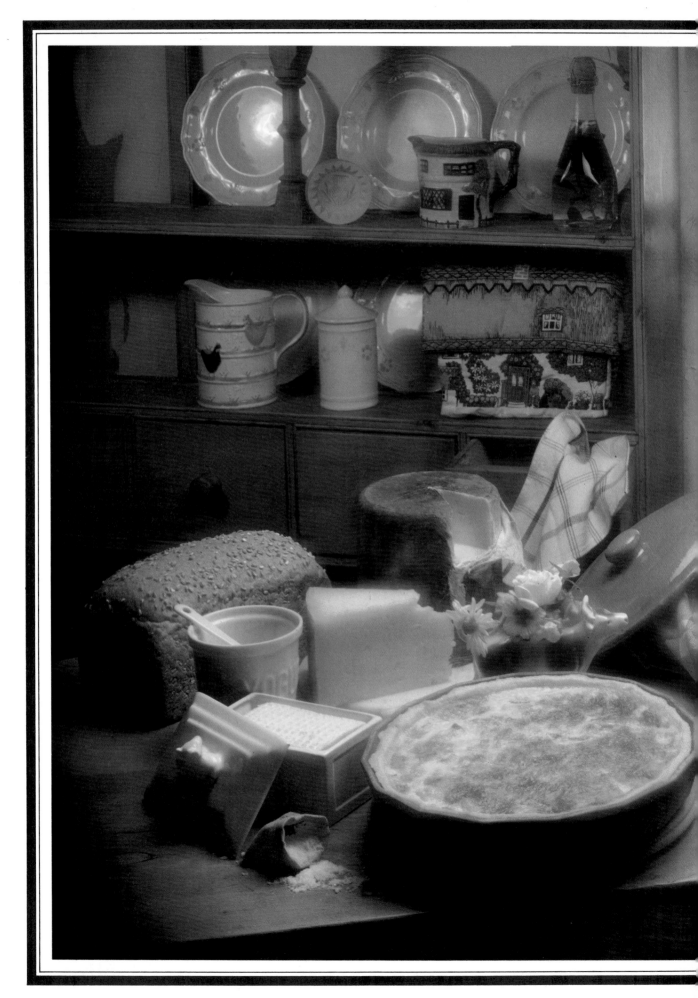

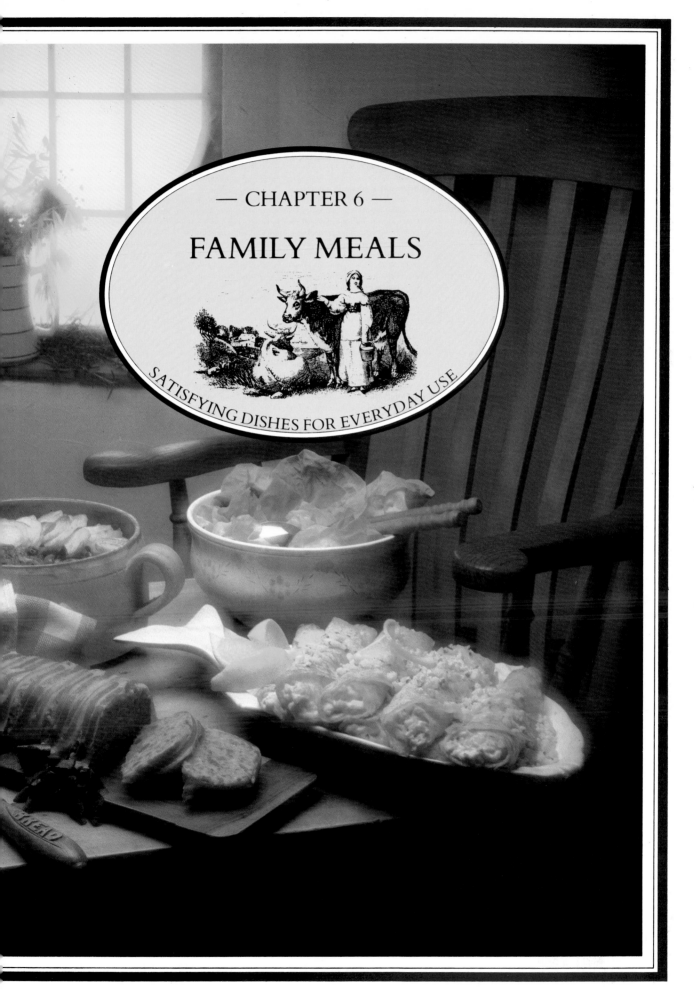

— CHAPTER 6 —

FAMILY MEALS

SATISFYING DISHES FOR EVERYDAY USE

Family meals are a challenge, but an exciting one and no problem if you make inventive use of good nourishing economical foods like cheese, milk, eggs, fresh vegetables in season, the cheaper kinds of meat and fish, and the pulses and pastas. Butter and fresh cream are delicious and nourishing and a little goes a long way.

Cheese is one of the great mainstays of family cooking and a main meal with cheese need never be dull. Witness the continuing popularity of favourites like cheese soufflé, the more substantial cheese pudding, the meal-in-itself called Lancashire 'foot'.

Casseroles make comfortable meals. There's no clockwatching involved and they can safely be left to simmer quietly for hours, the longer the better in most cases. They are marvellous for feeding a family with staggered mealtimes.

Pasta is a godsend for fast meals as it is quick to prepare and very versatile when combined with a wide range of mouthwatering sauces. Cheese does wonders for pasta and so does a beautifully creamy sauce.

Then there is the whole useful range of savoury flans and quiches, which you can have hot or cold with vegetables or baked potatoes and salad.

This chapter presents recipes for comfortable homely food with nothing grand or glamorous about it. This is food that doesn't need fussing over, either in the preparation or the eating and it is not extravagant with either ingredients or fuel. These are well-liked economical dishes capable of almost endless variations, all well balanced, highly nutritious and thoroughly enjoyable.

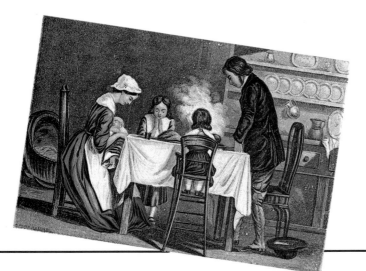

FAMILY SUPPER DISHES

CHEESY STUFFED AUBERGINES

2 medium aubergines, stalks removed
50 g (2 oz) ham, chopped
15 ml (1 tbsp) chopped fresh parsley
1 tomato, skinned and chopped
50 g (2 oz) fresh breadcrumbs
½ onion, skinned and grated
salt and freshly ground pepper
175 g (6 oz) English Cheddar cheese, grated
chopped fresh parsley to garnish

1. Cut the aubergines in half lengthways and scoop out the flesh to leave a 0.5-cm (¼-inch) shell. Roughly chop the flesh.
2. Make the stuffing by combining the ham, parsley, tomato, breadcrumbs, onion, seasoning and 50 g (2 oz) cheese with the aubergine flesh.
3. Place the aubergine shells in a baking dish and fill with the mixture. Sprinkle with the remaining cheese. Cover with foil.
4. Bake in the oven at 200°C (400°F) mark 6 for 20 minutes, then uncover and cook for a further 5–10 minutes until crisp and golden. Serve hot, garnished with chopped parsley.
Serves 4

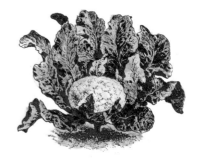

CHEESE KEBABS

225 g (8 oz) English Cheddar cheese
½ cucumber
4 tomatoes, quartered
8 pineapple chunks
coleslaw and mayonnaise to serve

1. Cube the cheese into 12 pieces. Dice the cucumber into 12 pieces.
2. Arrange 3 pieces of cheese, 4 pieces of tomato, 3 pieces of cucumber and 2 pieces of pineapple on each kebab skewer. Serve on a bed of coleslaw accompanied by mayonnaise.
Serves 4

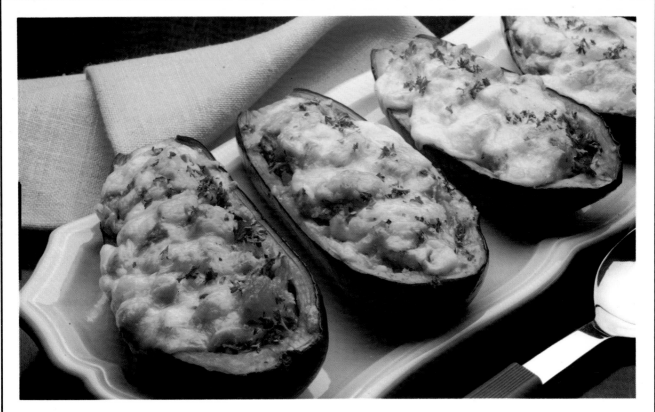

CAULIFLOWER CHEESE

1 cauliflower, trimmed

40 g (1½ oz) English butter

45 ml (3 level tbsp) flour

300 ml (½ pint) milk

100 g (4 oz) English Cheddar cheese, grated

salt and freshly ground pepper

1. Cook the cauliflower in fast boiling salted water until just tender, then drain and place in an ovenproof dish.
2. Melt the butter in a pan, stir in the flour and cook gently for 1 minute. Remove pan from the heat and gradually stir in the milk. Bring to the boil and continue to cook, stirring, until the sauce thickens, then add 75 g (3 oz) cheese and seasoning to taste.
3. Pour the sauce over the hot cauliflower, sprinkle with the remaining cheese and brown under a hot grill.

Serves 4

MACARONI CHEESE

175 g (6 oz) shortcut macaroni

40 g (1½ oz) English butter

60 ml (4 level tbsp) flour

568 ml (1 pint) milk

salt and freshly ground pepper

pinch of nutmeg, or 2.5 ml (½ level tsp) prepared mustard

175 g (6 oz) mature English Cheddar cheese, grated

30 ml (2 tbsp) fresh breadcrumbs

1. Cook the macaroni in a saucepan of fast boiling salted water for 10 minutes and drain well.
2. Meanwhile, melt the butter in a pan, stir in the flour and cook gently for 1 minute. Remove pan from the heat and gradually stir in the milk. Bring to the boil and continue to cook, stirring, until the sauce thickens, then remove from the heat and add seasonings, 100 g (4 oz) cheese and the macaroni.
3. Pour into an ovenproof dish and sprinkle with the remaining cheese and breadcrumbs.
4. Place on a baking sheet and bake in the oven at 200°C (400°F) mark 6 for about 20 minutes, until golden and bubbling, or brown under a very hot grill.

Serves 4

Above:
CHEESY STUFFED AUBERGINES
Originally from tropical Asia, aubergines are now grown anywhere in the world where it is warm and sunny. Stuffed aubergines are old favourites in Italy and the countries of the eastern Mediterranean. This dish is perfect for lunch with a green salad, crusty bread and a bottle of red wine.

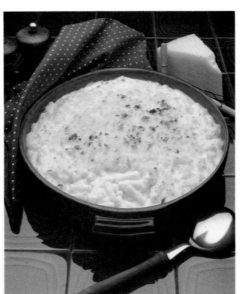

Left:
MACARONI CHEESE
Surprisingly, macaroni, or 'macrows' as it used to be called, has been eaten in Britain since the fourteenth century. This dish – a favourite of the Victorians – is simple to make and an excellent standby.

Right:
LEEKS IN CHEESE SAUCE
The leek, or 'porleac', was one of only two vegetables mentioned by Hywel Dda, a Welsh prince of the tenth century, in his laws. In this dish, the leeks are wrapped in ham, covered in sauce and then grilled until golden and bubbly.

Below:
CHEESE FONDUE
After an exhausting day on the slopes of the Swiss Alps, skiers weave their way homewards to enjoy the traditional warming ritual of a fondue. Here, too, participants must display some dexterity – if you lose your bread in the fondue you must pay a forfeit. Serve our cheese version next time you entertain and you'll find it's a wonderful ice-breaker!

CHEESE FONDUE

1 garlic clove, skinned and crushed

150 ml (¼ pint) dry cider or dry white wine

225 g (8 oz) mature English Cheddar cheese, grated

10 ml (2 level tsp) cornflour

freshly ground pepper

pinch of grated nutmeg

1 liqueur glass brandy or kirsch

1. Rub the inside of a fondue pot or flameproof dish with the garlic. Pour in the cider or wine, place the dish over a gentle heat and warm the liquid.
2. Add the cheese gradually and continue to heat gently, stirring, until all the cheese has melted.
3. Add the cornflour and seasonings, blended to a smooth paste with the brandy or kirsch, and continue cooking for a further 2–3 minutes. When the fondue reaches a very smooth consistency, it is ready to serve.
4. Fondue is traditionally served in the centre of the table, kept warm over a spirit lamp. Crusty cubes of bread are speared on long-handled forks and dipped into it.
Serves 4

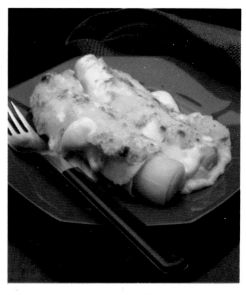

LEEKS IN CHEESE SAUCE

8 medium leeks, cleaned and trimmed

50 g (2 oz) English butter

75 ml (5 level tbsp) flour

568 ml (1 pint) milk

100 g (4 oz) English Cheddar cheese, grated

salt and freshly ground pepper

8 thin slices of ham or bacon

fresh breadcrumbs

1. Put the whole leeks into a saucepan of boiling salted water and boil gently for 20 minutes, until soft. Drain and keep warm.
2. Meanwhile, melt about three-quarters of the butter in a pan, stir in the flour and cook gently for 1 minute, stirring. Remove the pan from the heat and gradually stir in the milk. Bring to the boil and continue to cook, stirring, for about 5 minutes, then add 75 g (3 oz) cheese and seasoning to taste.
3. Wrap each leek in a slice of ham or bacon, place in an ovenproof dish and coat with sauce. Top with breadcrumbs and the remaining cheese. Dot with the remaining butter and brown under the grill.
Serves 4

GRANDMA'S CHEESE PUDDING

1.1 litres (2 pints) milk

125 g (4 oz) fresh breadcrumbs

450 g (1 lb) English Cheddar cheese, grated

8 eggs

5 ml (1 level tsp) French mustard

salt and freshly ground pepper

1. Bring the milk to the boil in a saucepan, place the breadcrumbs in a bowl and pour milk over. Stir in the cheese.
2. In a bowl lightly beat eggs with mustard and with milk and breadcrumbs. Season.
3. Butter a large, shallow 2.8-litre (5-pint)

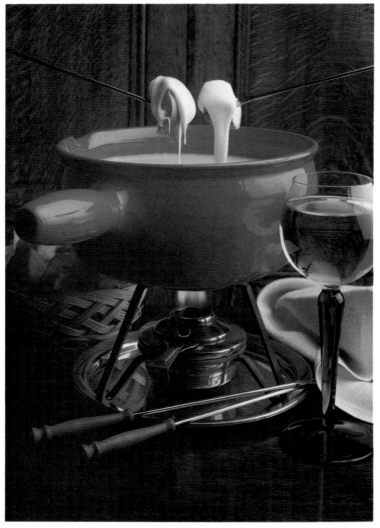

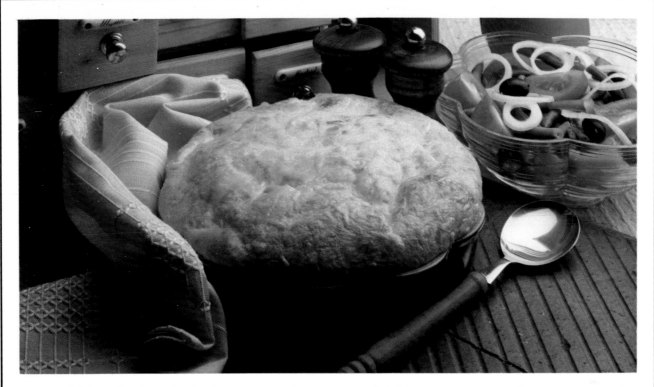

ovenproof dish well and pour in the cheese pudding mixture. Bake in the oven at 180°C (350°F) mark 4 for about 45 minutes, until lightly set and golden.

4. Serve at once with a crisp, garlic-dressed salad of green beans, green pepper, tomato, onion, anchovies and black olives.

Serves 8

LANCASHIRE 'FOOT'

1 medium onion, skinned and finely chopped
15 g (½ oz) English butter
225 g (8 oz) Lancashire cheese, crumbled
5 ml (1 level tsp) prepared mustard
397-g (14-oz) packet frozen puff pastry, thawed
1 egg, beaten

1. In a frying pan fry the onion in butter until transparent. Transfer to a bowl and combine with cheese and mustard.

2. Cut the pastry into eight pieces. Roll each one into an oval shape (the pastry should be fairly thin). Cut each oval in half lengthwise; at one end roll a little of the pastry to the side to give a 'foot' shape.

3. Spoon the cheese mixture over half the pieces, leaving a margin around the edges. Dampen these edges with egg, cover with the other pieces of pastry. Seal the edges and knock up. Brush the tops with more egg.

4. Place on baking sheets. Bake in the oven at 220°C (425°F) mark 7 for about 20 minutes. Serve warm with baked tomato halves or a tomato salad.

Makes 8

SMOKED MACKEREL GOUGÈRE

350 g (12 oz) smoked mackerel fillets
1 medium onion, skinned and sliced
150 g (5 oz) English butter
175 g (6 oz) flour
150 ml (¼ pint) milk
45 ml (3 tbsp) cider
30 ml (2 level tbsp) natural yogurt
salt and freshly ground pepper
4 eggs, beaten
75 g (3 oz) English Cheddar cheese, grated
15 ml (1 level tbsp) dry breadcrumbs

1. Flake the mackerel flesh, discarding skin and any bones.

2. To make the sauce, fry the onion in 25 g (1 oz) of butter until soft and golden. Add 25 g (1 oz) flour with the milk, stirring briskly, and simmer for 3 minutes. Remove from the heat, stir in the cider, yogurt, fish and seasoning (be cautious with salt). Cover and refrigerate.

3. For the choux paste, melt the remaining butter in 300 ml (½ pint) water. Bring to the boil, take off the heat and beat in remaining flour until just smooth. Beat in eggs, a little at a time, and then the cheese.

4. Spoon the choux paste around the sides of a 1.1-litre (2-pint) shallow ovenproof dish. Cover and refrigerate.

5. When required, spoon sauce into centre of choux paste, sprinkle with breadcrumbs and bake in the oven at 200°C (400°F) mark 6 for 40–45 minutes until risen and golden.

Serves 4

Above:
GRANDMA'S CHEESE PUDDING
A simple dish which looks elegant and tastes delicious, it is made from fresh eggs, milk and Cheddar. Cheese puddings have long been popular with farmers in the Midlands and East Anglia.

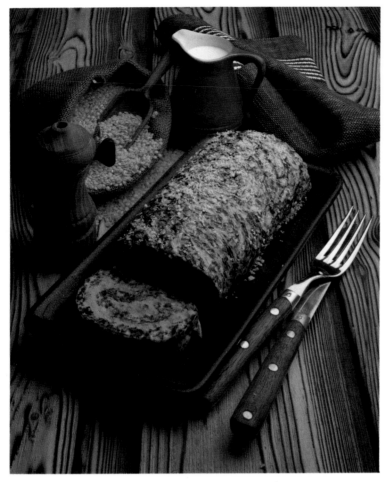

Above:
SPINACH AND LENTIL
ROULADE
This very pretty pale green and yellow roll is an elegant party dish, as well as a firm family favourite.

Opposite:
LEEK AND MACARONI GRATIN
Like parsnips, leeks are one of our most neglected vegetables. They have a mild but distinctive flavour and make wonderful soups and pies. Combined with Cotswold cheese and macaroni in this gratin, they are ideal for a warming family meal.

SPINACH AND LENTIL ROULADE

175 g (6 oz) red lentils

1 small onion, skinned and finely chopped

30 ml (2 level tbsp) tomato ketchup

15 ml (1 level tbsp) creamed horseradish

125 g (4 oz) English butter

salt and freshly ground pepper

450 g (1 lb) spinach, cleaned and trimmed

50 g (2 oz) flour

300 ml (½ pint) milk

2 eggs, separated

dry breadcrumbs

1. Butter and line a 28-cm (11-inch) Swiss-roll tin.
2. Cook the lentils with the onion in a large saucepan of boiling salted water until tender. Drain well, then return to the pan and heat to evaporate excess moisture. Add the tomato ketchup, horseradish and 50 g (2 oz) butter. Rub through a sieve or purée in a blender. Season and set aside.
3. In a pan, gently cook spinach, sprinkled with salt (do not add any liquid), for 3–4 minutes. Turn into a colander, press with a potato masher, and chop finely.
4. To make the sauce, melt the remaining butter in a pan, stir in the flour and cook gently for 1 minute, stirring. Remove pan

from the heat and gradually stir in the milk. Bring to the boil and continue to cook, stirring, until the sauce thickens. Remove from the heat. Stir in spinach and egg yolks. Season.
5. Whisk egg whites until stiff and gently fold into spinach mixture. Spoon into prepared tin. Level surface. Bake in the oven at 200°C (400°F) mark 6 for 20 minutes, until well risen and golden.
6. Turn out on to greaseproof paper sprinkled with dried breadcrumbs. Peel off greaseproof lining. Spread lentil purée over surface. Roll up Swiss-roll style and return to oven for 5 minutes.
Serves 4

BRUSSELS SPROUT AND BACON SOUFFLÉ

700 g (1½ lb) trimmed brussels sprouts

125 g (4 oz) smoked bacon rashers, chopped

50 g (2 oz) English butter

50 g (2 oz) flour

pinch of grated nutmeg

300 ml (½ pint) milk

3 eggs, separated

salt and freshly ground pepper

1. Butter a 1.4-litre (2½-pint) soufflé dish. Preheat the oven at 200°C (400°F) mark 6.
2. Cook the brussels sprouts in a saucepan of boiling salted water until tender. Drain well.
3. Meanwhile, in a small saucepan, sauté the bacon in its own fat for about 2 minutes. Stir in the butter, flour and nutmeg and cook gently for 1 minute, stirring. Remove pan from the heat and gradually stir in the milk. Bring to the boil and continue to cook, stirring, until the sauce thickens. Simmer for 2 minutes.
4. Chop half the sprouts. In a blender, purée the remaining sprouts with the egg yolks and a little sauce. Fold the purée and the chopped sprouts into the sauce. Season well.
5. Whisk the egg whites until stiff and gently fold into the brussels sprout mixture. Turn into the soufflé dish and bake in the oven for 30–35 minutes. Serve immediately accompanied by a salad.
Serves 4

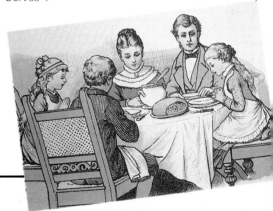

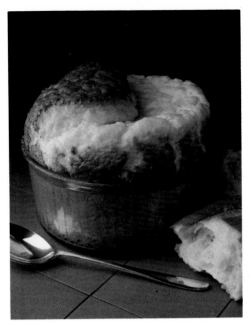

CHEESE SOUFFLÉ

40 g (1½ oz) English butter

200 ml (7 fl oz) milk

1 onion, skinned and sliced

1 carrot, peeled and sliced

bay leaf

6 peppercorns

30 ml (2 level tbsp) flour

10 ml (2 level tsp) French mustard

salt and freshly ground pepper

4 eggs, separated, plus 1 egg white

150 g (5 oz) Double Gloucester cheese, grated

1. Rub the inside of a 1.4-litre (2½-pint) soufflé dish with 15 g (½ oz) butter.
2. Place the milk, onion, carrot, bay leaf and peppercorns in a saucepan, bring to the boil and remove from the heat. Leave to infuse for 15 minutes. Strain, reserving milk.
3. To make the sauce, melt the remaining butter in a pan, stir in the flour and cook gently for 1 minute, stirring. Remove pan from the heat and gradually stir in the reserved milk. Bring to the boil and continue to cook, stirring, until the sauce thickens, then add mustard, salt and freshly ground pepper to taste. Cool a little.
4. Beat the egg yolks into the sauce, one at a time. Add the cheese, reserving 15 ml (1 tbsp). Stir until well blended.
5. Whisk the egg whites until stiff. Mix in one spoonful of sauce, then pour the remaining sauce over the egg whites and cut and fold the ingredients together.
6. Put the mixture gently into the prepared dish. Smooth the top and sprinkle over the remaining cheese. Place on a baking sheet and bake in the centre of the oven at 180°C (350°F) mark 4 for 30 minutes. Serve at once with crusty bread and a green salad.

Serves 4

LEEK AND MACARONI GRATIN

125 g (4 oz) shortcut macaroni

50 g (2 oz) English butter

275 g (10 oz) leeks, cleaned, trimmed and roughly chopped

25 g (1 oz) flour

568 ml (1 pint) milk

175 g (6 oz) Cotswold cheese with chives, grated

salt and freshly ground pepper

25 g (1 oz) fresh breadcrumbs

30 ml (2 tbsp) chopped fresh chives

1. Cook the macaroni in a saucepan of fast boiling salted water, until tender, but not soft; about 8–10 minutes. Drain well.
2. Melt the butter in a pan, and sauté the leeks for 2 minutes. Stir in the flour and cook gently for 1 minute, stirring. Remove pan from the heat and gradually stir in the milk. Bring to the boil and continue to cook, stirring, for 2 minutes. Off the heat, stir in the macaroni and all but 30 ml (2 tbsp) cheese. Season to taste.
3. Spoon the mixture into a buttered 1.1-litre (2-pint) shallow ovenproof dish. Mix together the breadcrumbs, chives and remaining cheese, and sprinkle in lines evenly across the dish.
4. Bake in the oven at 190°C (375°F) mark 5 for 30–35 minutes, until golden. Serve immediately.

Serves 4

Left:
CHEESE SOUFFLÉ
Success in making a soufflé depends largely on the adequate whisking of the egg whites and their very light but thorough incorporation into the other mixture.

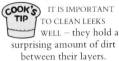

IT IS IMPORTANT TO CLEAN LEEKS WELL – they hold a surprising amount of dirt between their layers. Remove the coarse outer leaves and cut off the tops and roots. Slit the leeks down to within 2.5 cm (1 inch) or so of the bottom, to ensure that all the grit is removed, and if necessary cut them through completely. Wash thoroughly under cold running water.
To use whole, slit the outer leaves down a few inches, as these harbour the most grit.
Pack them tightly, leaf downwards, in a deep container full of cold water. Leave for 30 minutes. You will be astonished at what remains when you lift out what you thought were clean leeks!

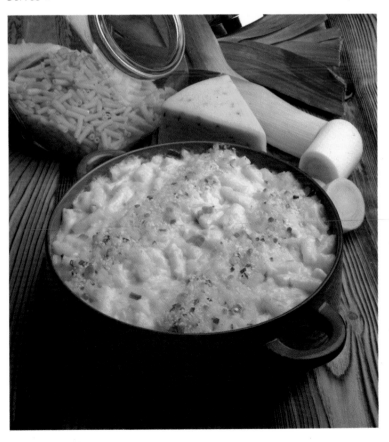

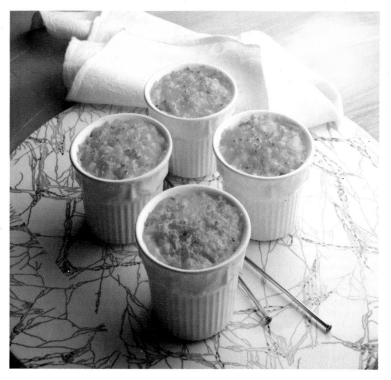

Above:
HADDOCK AU GRATIN
A considerable amount of haddock is smoked, especially in Scotland, and Findon, a small fishing village near Aberdeen, has given its name to the very delicious creamy-yellow 'Finnan haddies' which are smoked there over oak chips. This gratin of haddock looks very tempting served in individual soufflé dishes.

HADDOCK AU GRATIN

175 g (6 oz) fresh haddock fillet

175 g (6 oz) smoked haddock fillet

60 ml (4 tbsp) dry white wine

6 peppercorns

bay leaf

1 small onion, skinned and sliced

125 g (4 oz) button mushrooms, wiped and sliced

50 g (2 oz) English butter

30 ml (2 level tbsp) flour

freshly ground black pepper

50 g (2 oz) Red Leicester cheese, grated

25 g (1 oz) fresh breadcrumbs

1. Place the fresh and smoked fish in a saucepan with 300 ml ($\frac{1}{2}$ pint) water and the wine. Add peppercorns, bay leaf and onion and bring to the boil. Cover and poach gently for about 15 minutes.
2. Strain off liquid and reserve. Flake the fish, discarding skin and bone. Also discard flavouring ingredients.
3. Sauté the mushrooms in the butter for 2 minutes, stir in the flour and cook gently for 1 minute, stirring. Remove pan from the heat and gradually stir in the strained cooking liquid. Bring to boil, and continue to cook, stirring, until the sauce thickens, then add the fish, half the grated cheese and seasoning to taste.
4. Spoon the mixture into six individual soufflé dishes. Top with remaining cheese and crumbs.
5. Bake in the oven at 220°C (425°F) mark 7 for about 15 minutes, until golden brown. Serve hot.
Serves 6

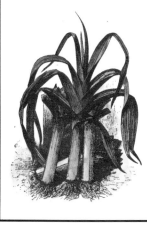

LEEK AND RICE AU GRATIN

450 g (1 lb) leeks

75 g (3 oz) long grain rice

75 g (3 oz) English butter

45 ml (3 level tbsp) flour

300 ml ($\frac{1}{2}$ pint) chicken stock

45 ml (3 tbsp) dry white wine

salt and freshly ground pepper

100 g (4 oz) ham, shredded

4 large tomatoes, skinned and sliced

125 g (4 oz) English Cheddar cheese, grated

40 g (1$\frac{1}{2}$ oz) walnuts, chopped

1. Slice the leeks crosswise into 1-cm ($\frac{1}{2}$-inch) pieces, wash thoroughly and drain. Boil the rice in a saucepan of fast boiling salted water until tender, but not soft, then drain and set aside.
2. Melt 50 g (2 oz) butter in a frying pan and sauté the leeks until golden.
3. Remove from the heat and stir in the flour, stock, wine and seasoning. Boil for 3–4 minutes, stirring, then add the ham to the sauce.
4. Use the tomato slices to line the sides of four individual ramekin dishes; spoon the leek mixture into the centre of each.
5. In a bowl, mix the cheese, rice and walnuts together and spoon over the leeks. Dot with remaining butter.
6. Bake in the oven at 180°C (350°F) mark 4 for 25–30 minutes, until golden. Serve immediately.
Serves 4

BUTTER BEAN AND TUNA GRATIN

225 g (8 oz) dried butter beans

400 ml ($\frac{3}{4}$ pint) milk

small piece of onion

small piece of carrot

bay leaf

6 peppercorns

blade of mace

450 g (1 lb) fresh or frozen broccoli

198-g (7-oz) can tuna, drained

salt and freshly ground pepper

40 g (1$\frac{1}{2}$ oz) English butter

60 ml (4 level tbsp) flour

50g (2 oz) English Cheddar cheese, grated

1. Soak beans overnight in cold water.
2. Put the milk, vegetables, bay leaf and spices in a saucepan, bring slowly to the boil. Remove from the heat and leave, covered, to infuse.
3. Drain the beans and cook in a pan of

gently boiling water until tender, about 1¼ hours. Drain.

4. Meanwhile, break the broccoli into florets and cook in a little boiling salted water until just tender. Drain and arrange in a buttered shallow ovenproof dish.

5. Flake the tuna and combine with the cooked beans and seasoning. Pile in the centre of the dish.

6. To make the sauce, melt the butter in a pan, stir in the flour and cook gently for 1 minute, stirring. Remove pan from the heat and gradually stir in the strained milk. Bring to the boil and continue to cook, stirring, until the sauce thickens, then add seasoning to taste. Pour over the tuna and broccoli mixture.

7. Sprinkle with the cheese and bake in the oven at 200°C (400°F) mark 6 for 15–20 minutes, until golden and bubbling.

Serves 4

LAMB AND SPINACH AU GRATIN

900 g (2 lb) spinach, cleaned and trimmed
100 g (4 oz) English butter
1.4 kg (3 lb) fillet end leg of lamb, boned and minced
1 garlic clove, skinned and crushed
700 g (1½ lb) tomatoes, skinned and chopped
40 g (1½ oz) flour, plus 45 ml (3 level tbsp)
10 ml (2 tsp) dried oregano
10 ml (2 tsp) dried rosemary
300 ml (½ pint) dry white wine
salt and freshly ground pepper
275 g (10 oz) lasagne
900 ml (1½ pints) milk
225 g (8 oz) Lancashire cheese, grated

1. In a pan, gently cook the spinach, sprinkled with salt (do not add any liquid), for 3–4 minutes. Turn into colander, press with potato masher and chop.

2. In a large saucepan, melt half the butter and brown the lamb well. Stir in the garlic, spinach, tomatoes, 45 ml (3 level tbsp) flour and herbs. Cook for 1–2 minutes, then add the wine. Season. Bring to boil and simmer for about 30 minutes, uncovered. Cool.

3. Meanwhile, cook lasagne in a saucepan of fast boiling salted water, until tender, but not soft. Drain, being careful not to break lasagne sheets, and lay each sheet flat on a work surface.

4. Spread lamb mixture over the sheets and roll each up from the short side. Cut rolls into three, stand upright and pack tightly together in one large or two small 5-cm (2-inch) deep, straight-sided ovenproof dishes.

5. To make the sauce, melt the remaining butter in a pan, stir in the remaining flour and cook gently for 1 minute, stirring.

Remove pan from the heat and gradually stir in the milk. Bring to the boil and continue to cook, stirring, until the sauce thickens, then add seasoning to taste. Pour sauce over pasta and cover with foil.

6. Bake in the oven at 200°C (400°F) mark 6 for about 40 minutes, then uncover, sprinkle with cheese and grill until golden.

Serves 10

CIDER AND CHEESE CHOPS

100 g (4 oz) mushrooms, wiped and sliced
2 cooking apples, peeled, cored and sliced
1 onion, skinned and sliced
salt and freshly ground pepper
4 pork chops
300 ml (½ pint) dry cider
50 g (2 oz) dry breadcrumbs
100 g (4 oz) English Cheddar cheese, grated

1. Butter a 1.7-litre (3-pint) shallow ovenproof dish. Place the mushrooms, apples and onions in the base of the dish and season to taste.

2. Place pork chops on top and cover with cider. Mix breadcrumbs and cheese together and sprinkle over chops.

3. Bake in the oven at 200°C (400°F) mark 6 for 1¼–1½ hours, until chops are cooked.

Serves 4

Below:
BUTTER BEAN AND TUNA GRATIN
In this recipe the tuna loses its strong tangy flavour and acquires a very delicate taste. It combines deliciously with the butter beans and broccoli in the cheesy sauce.

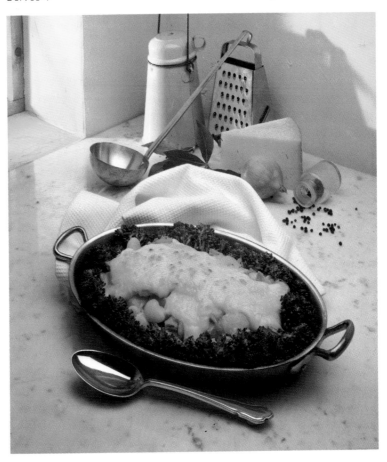

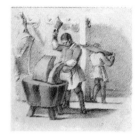

GOULASHES AND STEWS

DEVILLED KIDNEYS

8 sheep's kidneys

15 ml (1 tbsp) mustard powder

10 ml (2 tsp) Worcestershire sauce

50 g (2 oz) English butter

salt and freshly ground pepper

4 pieces of hot toast

1. Skin the kidneys, cut in half and core. Mix the mustard with the Worcestershire sauce.
2. Heat the butter in a saucepan, add the kidneys, salt and freshly ground pepper; brown quickly for 2 minutes, lower the heat and cook very gently for 6 minutes with the pan covered.
3. Add the mustard mixture to the kidneys, stir well and cook slowly for 2 minutes. Stir and serve on the hot toast.

Serves 4

COOK'S TIP WHEN CHOOSING MEAT a good butcher will usually advise on your selection. The general rules are to choose meat which does not have an undue amount of fat; what fat there is should be firm and free from dark marks or discolouration.
Lean meat should be finely grained with a marbling of fat, firm and slightly elastic. The muscles in the hind part of an animal work less and therefore these cuts of meat are generally more tender.
Meat with a coarser grain and a lot of gristle or connective tissue should be cooked slowly; in a casserole, for example, or as a pot roast.

ITALIAN LIVER

350 g (12 oz) lamb's liver

25 g (1 oz) flour

salt and freshly ground pepper

40 g (1½ oz) English butter

450 g (1 lb) onions, skinned and thinly sliced

150 ml (¼ pint) beef stock

300 ml (½ pint) milk

30 ml (2 level tbsp) tomato purée

1 garlic clove, skinned and finely chopped

1.25 ml (¼ tsp) mixed dried herbs

30 ml (2 tbsp) fresh double cream

chopped fresh parsley

1. Cut the liver into small pieces and coat in seasoned flour.
2. Melt the butter in a frying pan and add the liver. Brown on all sides, then remove from pan and set aside.
3. In the butter remaining in the pan, fry the onions slowly until tender. Gradually stir in the stock, milk, tomato purée, garlic and herbs. Bring the sauce to the boil, stirring continuously.
4. Add the liver to the sauce. Cover pan and cook gently for 10–15 minutes, until the liver is tender. Adjust seasoning to taste.
5. Place liver and sauce on a hot serving dish. Trickle the fresh cream over the sauce and sprinkle with chopped parsley.

Serves 4

Opposite:
ITALIAN LIVER
The Italians are very fond of all types of offal. This classic dish, using small pieces of liver served in a tasty sauce, comes from the canal city of Venice.

YORKSHIRE CUTLETS

4 lamb cutlets, trimmed

30 ml (2 level tbsp) fresh breadcrumbs

salt and freshly ground pepper

50 g (2 oz) English Cheddar cheese, finely grated

50 g (2 oz) English butter

4 onions, skinned and sliced

300 ml (½ pint) milk

25 g (1 oz) flour

30 ml (2 tbsp) fresh cream

1. Wash and dry the cutlets. Grill in ovenproof dish, on one side.
2. Meanwhile, mix together breadcrumbs, seasoning and grated cheese.
3. Turn cutlets and top with crumb mixture, dot with 25 g (1 oz) butter and continue to grill until thoroughly cooked.
4. While the cutlets are cooking, boil the onions in the milk. Melt the remaining butter in a pan, stir in the flour and cook gently for 1 minute. Remove the pan from the heat and gradually stir in the onions and milk. Bring to the boil and continue to cook, stirring, until the sauce thickens, then stir in the fresh cream and season to taste.
5. Pour the sauce over the cutlets, or serve separately.

Serves 4

GOULASH

700 g (1½ lb) stewing steak, cut into 1-cm (½-inch) cubes

50 g (2 oz) flour, plus 45 ml (3 level tbsp)

salt and freshly ground pepper

2 medium onions, skinned and sliced

1 green pepper, seeded and chopped

30 ml (2 tbsp) oil

10 ml (2 level tsp) paprika

45 ml (3 level tbsp) tomato purée

pinch of grated nutmeg

300 ml (½ pint) beef stock

2 large tomatoes, skinned and quartered

bouquet garni

150 ml (¼ pint) beer

142 ml (5 fl oz) soured cream

1. Coat the meat with 50 g (2 oz) seasoned flour. In a flameproof casserole dish fry the onions and pepper lightly in the oil for 3–4 minutes.
2. Add the meat and fry gently for about 5 minutes, until golden brown, then add the paprika and fry for 1 minute. Stir in the tomato purée, nutmeg, seasoning and remaining flour.
3. Add the stock, tomatoes and bouquet garni, cover, and cook in the oven at 170°C (325°F) mark 3 for 1½–2 hours, until meat is tender. Add the beer, cook for a few minutes longer and remove the bouquet garni.
4. Before serving stir in the soured cream.

Serves 4

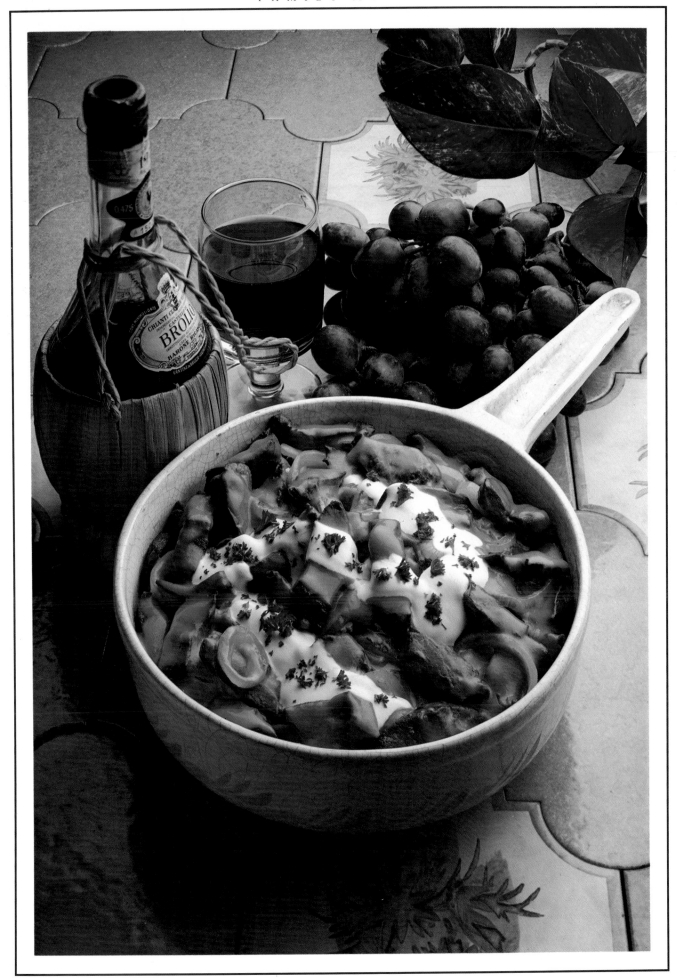

KIDNEYS IN YOGURT

450 g (1 lb) calf's kidneys

15 ml (1 level tbsp) flour

2.5 ml (½ level tsp) paprika

salt and freshly ground pepper

30 ml (2 tbsp) vegetable oil

1 small onion, skinned and finely chopped

10 ml (2 tsp) fresh rosemary or 5 ml (1 tsp) dried rosemary

142 g (5 oz) natural yogurt

chopped fresh parsley

1. Skin the kidneys and slice thinly, removing any core with scissors. Toss in the flour, seasoned with the paprika, salt and freshly ground pepper.
2. Heat the oil in a frying pan, add the onion and fry until soft and golden.
3. Add the flour-coated kidneys and rosemary. Fry over a high heat for about 5 minutes, until the kidneys are tender, but still juicy.
4. Stir the yogurt and add to the pan. Reheat without boiling, season, then skim and serve, sprinkled with chopped parsley.

Serves 4

LIVER IN STROGANOFF SAUCE

450 g (1 lb) lamb's liver

30 ml (2 level tbsp) flour

salt and freshly ground pepper

225 g (8 oz) onions, skinned and thinly sliced

75 g (3 oz) English butter

450 g (1 lb) tomatoes, skinned and quartered, or 396-g (14-oz) can tomatoes, drained

10 ml (2 tsp) dried sage

142 ml (5 fl oz) soured cream

1. Thinly slice the lamb's liver into strips. Toss in seasoned flour.
2. In a frying pan, lightly brown the onions in the butter. Add the tomatoes, push to the side of the pan, then add the liver and cook over a high heat for about 5 minutes.
3. Sprinkle over the sage. Reduce the heat and spoon in the stirred soured cream.
4. Combine pan ingredients, adjust seasoning and heat, but do not boil. Serve hot.

Serves 4

Below:
LIVER IN STROGANOFF SAUCE
The food value of liver is high – it contains protein, vitamin A, vitamin B complex and iron in appreciable amounts. In fact, liver eaten once a week supplies a good portion of the iron we require. This dish is a quick and sophisticated way of serving a very nourishing food.

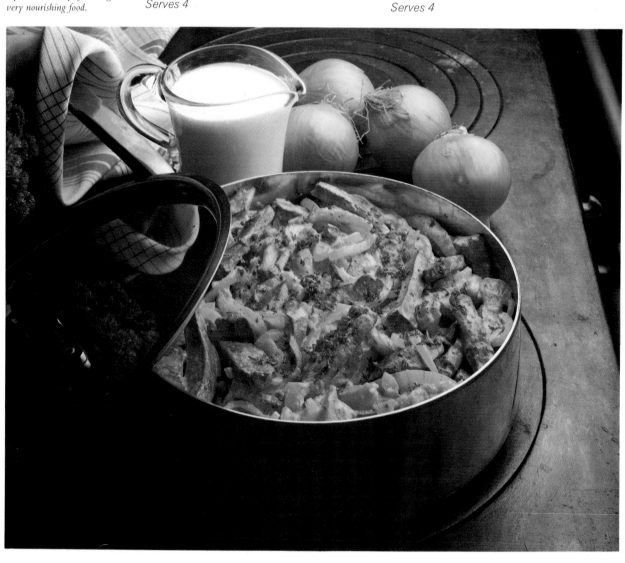

PARCELLED PORK

4 medium pork chops
25 g (1 oz) English butter
1 medium onion, skinned and finely chopped
225 g (8 oz) mushrooms, wiped and sliced
90 ml (6 tbsp) dry cider
30 ml (2 tbsp) lemon juice
142 ml (5 fl oz) soured cream
salt and freshly ground pepper

1. Trim the chops of any rind and excess fat. Melt the butter in a large frying pan and brown the chops well. Remove the chops from the pan and place on pieces of foil about 20 cm (8 inches) square.
2. Add the onion and mushrooms to the butter remaining in the pan and cook for 5 minutes.
3. Stir in the cider and lemon juice and bring to the boil. Reduce the liquid over a high heat until reduced by half, then remove from the heat and stir in the soured cream. Season well.
4. Place a quarter of the mushroom mixture on top of each chop, then shape the foil into neat parcels and seal well.
5. Place the parcels in a small ovenproof dish and bake in the oven at 180°C (350°F) mark 4 for about 50 minutes, until the chops are tender.
6. To serve, place each parcel on a plate and open carefully so that no juices escape. Serve with small new potatoes, boiled in their jackets, and green beans.
Serves 4

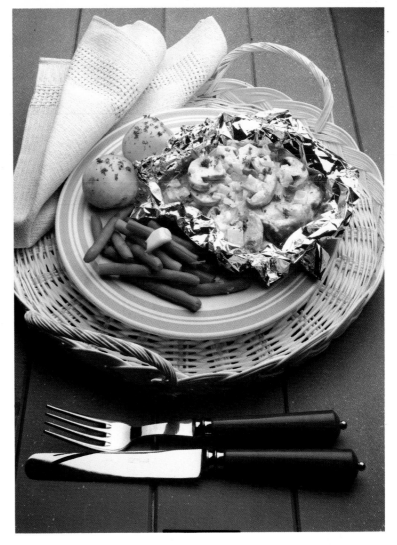

Above:
PARCELLED PORK
Foil-wrapped food cooks in its own steam and is wonderfully tender and tasty. This tempting dish is very quick to prepare and is more interesting to eat than plain grilled chops.

VEAL GOULASH WITH CARAWAY DUMPLINGS

1.4 kg (3 lb) stewing veal
75 g (3 oz) English butter
700 g (1½ lb) onions, skinned and thinly sliced
450 g (1 lb) carrots, peeled and thinly sliced
60 ml (4 level tbsp) paprika
30 ml (2 level tbsp) plain flour
900 ml (1½ pints) chicken stock
60 ml (4 tbsp) dry white wine
salt and freshly ground pepper
225 g (8 oz) self-raising flour
125 g (4 oz) shredded suet
10 ml (2 level tsp) caraway seeds
142 ml (5 fl oz) soured cream

1. Cut the veal into 4-cm (1½-inch) pieces. In a frying pan, heat the butter and brown the veal, a little at a time. Drain and place in a shallow ovenproof dish.
2. Fry the onions and carrots in the butter remaining in the pan until lightly browned. Add the paprika and plain flour and fry for 2 minutes. Gradually stir in the stock, wine and seasoning, bring to boil and pour over the veal.
3. Cover tightly, cook in the oven at 150°C (300°F) mark 2 for 2 hours.
4. Mix the remaining four ingredients together with 75 ml (5 tbsp) of water, seasoning well. Divide into 16 dumplings, place on top of the goulash and sprinkle with extra caraway seeds. Return to the oven, covered, for a further 45 minutes.
Serves 8

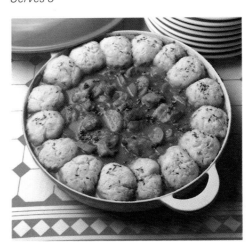

Left:
VEAL GOULASH WITH CARAWAY DUMPLINGS
Hungary claims goulash as a traditional dish. It features paprika – a fine subtle spice made from pimentoes which ranges from sweet to hot and from rose to scarlet – and caraway seeds (which have a spicy, slightly liquorice-like, sharp taste and are one of the oldest spices known to Europe).

FISH PIES AND BAKES

HARVEST MACKEREL

1 mackerel
1 apple, peeled, cored and grated
25 g (1 oz) fresh breadcrumbs
50 g (2 oz) English Cheddar cheese, grated
75 ml (2½ fl oz) fresh single cream
75 g (3 oz) natural yogurt
salt and freshly ground pepper
lemon wedges and chopped fresh parsley to garnish

1. Wash and dry the mackerel thoroughly. Place in a shallow ovenproof dish.
2. Place the apple, breadcrumbs, cheese, fresh cream and yogurt in a bowl and mix well. Season to taste. Spoon the mixture over the mackerel and cover the dish with foil.
3. Bake in the oven at 180°C (350°F) mark 4 for about 25 minutes, until the fish is cooked through. Serve hot garnished with lemon wedges and sprinkled with parsley.
Serves 4

COOK'S TIP FRESH FISH rapidly becomes stale and should be cooked as soon as possible after it is caught. When it is really fresh, fish should have no unpleasant odour, the flesh should be firm, the body stiff, the gills red, the eyes bright and not sunken, and the scales plentiful and sparking.

Fish of a medium size have better flavour than over-large ones; a thick slice cut from a smaller fish is preferable to a thin slice cut from a large one.

PLAICE WITH STILTON SAUCE

4 large plaice fillets, each about 175 g (6 oz)
75 ml (5 level tbsp) flour
salt and freshly ground pepper
65 g (2½ oz) English butter
10 ml (2 tsp) olive or corn oil
300 ml (½ pint) milk
75 g (3 oz) Blue Stilton cheese, crumbled
30 ml (2 level tbsp) dry breadcrumbs
watercress to garnish

1. Cut each fillet into four pieces, and coat the fish with 30 ml (2 level tbsp) flour mixed with salt. In a frying pan, fry the fillets briskly in 40 g (1½ oz) butter and the oil, allowing 3 minutes each side, then transfer to a 450-ml (1½-pint) buttered ovenproof dish.
2. To make the sauce, melt the remaining 25 g (1 oz) butter in a pan, stir in the remaining flour and cook gently for 1 minute, stirring. Remove pan from the heat and gradually stir in the milk. Bring to the boil and continue to cook, stirring, until the sauce thickens, then add the cheese and seasoning to taste. Whisk gently until smooth. Pour over the fish.
3. Sprinkle breadcrumbs over the top, heat in the oven at 190°C (375°F) mark 5 for 20 minutes and serve garnished with watercress.
Serves 4

CIDER BAKED MACKEREL

4 mackerel, gutted and cleaned
salt and freshly ground pepper
75 g (3 oz) English butter
2 dessert apples, peeled and grated
1 small onion, skinned and grated
150 g (5 oz) English Cheddar cheese, grated
50 g (2 oz) fresh breadcrumbs
45–60 ml (3–4 tbsp) dry cider
lemon wedges and chopped fresh parsley to garnish

1. Season the mackerel inside and out with salt and pepper.
2. Melt the butter in a small pan over a low heat.
3. Mix the apple, onion, 75 g (3 oz) cheese and the breadcrumbs in a bowl and bind with 15 ml (1 tbsp) melted butter. Stuff the fish with this mixture and secure the opening of each with two or three skewers.
4. Place the mackerel in an ovenproof dish and sprinkle remaining cheese over each. Pour over the remaining melted butter and sufficient cider to cover the base of the dish.
5. Lay a piece of buttered foil or greaseproof paper loosely over the dish. Bake in the oven at 180°C (350°F) mark 4 for·25–35 minutes, until the mackerel are cooked right through and golden brown. Serve straight from the dish and garnish with lemon wedges and parsley.
Serves 4

STUFFED HERRINGS

4 large herrings, with soft roes
75 g (3 oz) fresh breadcrumbs
10 ml (2 tsp) chopped fresh parsley
salt and freshly ground pepper
50 g (2 oz) English butter
1 egg
30 ml (2 tbsp) lemon juice
300 ml (½ pint) milk
lemon slices to garnish

1. Split the fish and remove the roes. In a bowl, mix the roes, breadcrumbs, parsley and seasoning together.
2. Melt half the butter in a saucepan, add the egg and the breadcrumb mixture, stir well together and cook gently until the egg is just cooked. Cool, then stuff the fish with this mixture.
3. Place the stuffed fish in a buttered shallow ovenproof dish, dot with the remaining butter, sprinkle with the lemon juice, salt and freshly ground pepper.
4. Pour the milk in the dish, cover with greaseproof paper and bake in the oven at 180°C (350°F) mark 4 for about 20 minutes until the fish is cooked. Serve garnished with lemon slices.
Serves 4

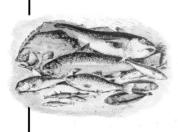

TOMATO FISH BAKE

50 g (2 oz) fresh breadcrumbs

50 g (2 oz) English Cheddar cheese, grated

1 small onion, skinned and finely chopped

2.5 ml ($\frac{1}{2}$ tsp) mixed herbs

salt and freshly ground pepper

300 ml ($\frac{1}{2}$ pint) milk, plus 30–45 ml (2–3 tbsp)

450 g (1 lb) white fish

25 g (1 oz) English butter

50 g (2 oz) mushrooms, wiped and sliced

25 g (1 oz) flour

30 ml (2 level tbsp) tomato purée

5 ml (1 tsp) lemon juice

pinch of sugar

450 g (1 lb) potatoes, peeled

chopped fresh parsley or watercress to garnish

1. To make a stuffing, mix the breadcrumbs, grated cheese, onion, herbs and seasoning with the 30–45 ml (2–3 tbsp) milk.
2. Wash and skin the fish. Place half on the base of a buttered shallow flameproof dish. Spread stuffing over the fish and top with remaining fish.
3. Melt the butter in a saucepan and fry the mushrooms until soft. Add the flour, the remaining 300 ml ($\frac{1}{2}$ pint) milk, tomato purée, lemon juice, sugar and seasoning. Heat, whisking continuously, until the sauce thickens. Pour over fish. Bake in the oven at 190°C (375°F) mark 5 for 20 minutes.
4. Meanwhile, boil the potatoes in a saucepan of fast boiling water until tender. Drain and mash. Remove the fish from the oven and pipe a border of mashed potato around the dish. Return to the oven or place under the grill to brown. Garnish with chopped parsley or watercress.

Serves 4

HADDOCK SAVOURY

450 g (1 lb) smoked haddock

568 ml (1 pint) milk

4 rashers of bacon, cut in half

1 onion, skinned and finely chopped

25 g (1 oz) English butter

25 g (1 oz) flour

100 g (4 oz) English Cheddar cheese, grated

freshly ground pepper

4 tomatoes, skinned and sliced

1. Soak the fish in bowl of cold water for 30 minutes, then drain. Put the fish in a saucepan with the milk, bring to the boil and simmer for 15 minutes.
2. Strain the milk into a basin. Remove skin and bones from the fish and flake the flesh.
3. Fry the bacon in a frying pan with the onion.
4. To make the sauce, melt the butter in a pan, stir in the flour and cook gently for 1 minute. Remove pan from the heat and gradually stir in the reserved milk. Bring to the boil slowly and cook, stirring, until the sauce thickens, then add 75 g (3 oz) cheese and season with pepper.
5. Arrange the fish, bacon, onion and tomatoes in layers in an ovenproof dish. Pour over the sauce and sprinkle with the remaining cheese. Bake in the oven at 190°C (350°F) mark 5 for 20 minutes until hot.

Serves 4–6

Below:
TOMATO FISH BAKE
This is one of those comforting dishes which is easy to make and a little different from the usual. Choose a firm fish such as cod, haddock or whiting.

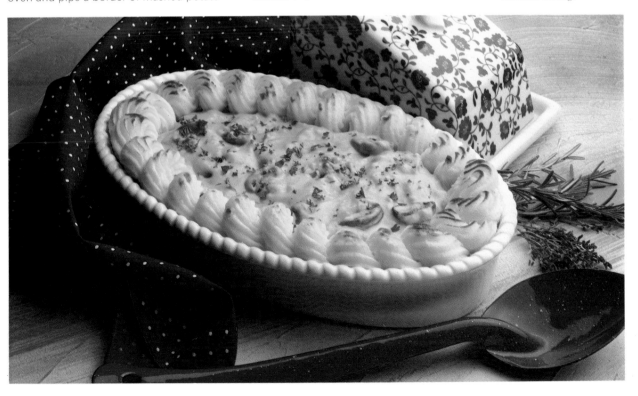

Right, top:
FISHERMAN'S HOT POT
Dishes of cod cooked with sliced
potatoes are found in seaports
around Europe, although each
town has its own version.
Layers of onions and mushrooms
and the delicious cheese sauce
give this hot pot its own unique
character.

SPECIAL FISH PIE

450 g (1 lb) haddock fillet

300 ml (½ pint) milk, plus 90 ml (6 tbsp)

bay leaf

6 peppercorns

1 onion, skinned and sliced

salt and freshly ground pepper

65 g (2½ oz) English butter

45 ml (3 level tbsp) flour

2 eggs, hard-boiled and roughly chopped

150 ml (5 fl oz) fresh single cream

30 ml (2 tbsp) chopped fresh parsley

125 g (4 oz) cooked prawns

900 g (2 lb) potatoes, peeled

1 egg, beaten, to glaze

1. Rinse and drain the fish. Place in a pan and pour over 300 ml (½ pint) of milk; add the bay leaf, peppercorns, onion and a pinch of salt. Bring to the boil and simmer for 10 minutes.
2. Lift from the pan using a slotted spoon and remove the skin and bones. Strain the cooking liquid and reserve.
3. Melt 40 g (1½ oz) of the butter in a pan, stir in the flour and cook gently for 1 minute, stirring. Remove the pan from the heat and gradually stir in the reserved cooking liquid. Bring to the boil and continue to cook, stirring, until the sauce thickens, then cook for a further 2–3 minutes. Season. Add the eggs to the sauce with the fresh cream, fish, parsley and prawns. Check the seasoning, and spoon the mixture into a 1.1-litre (2-pint) pie dish.

Below:
SPECIAL FISH PIE
Haddock is somewhat similar in
appearance and colour to cod,
but it has a more pronounced
flavour; it may be identified by a
black streak down the back and
two black spots, one at each side
above the gills. At its best from
September to February, haddock
is an excellent fish to use in fish
pies.

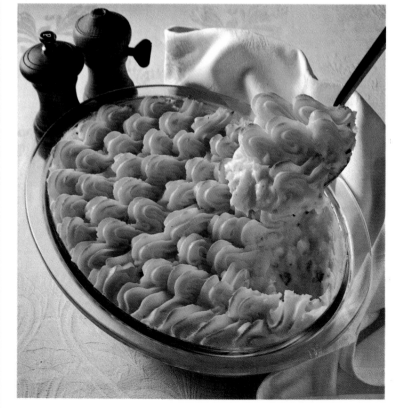

4. Meanwhile, boil the potatoes, drain and mash without any liquid. Heat the remaining 90 ml (6 tbsp) of milk and remaining 25 g (1 oz) butter and beat into the potatoes and season. Spoon into a piping bag and pipe across the fish mixture. Alternatively, spoon the potato over the fish and roughen the surface with a fork.
5. Bake in the oven at 200°C (400°F) mark 6 for 10–15 minutes, until the potato is set. Brush the beaten egg over the pie. Return to oven for a further 15 minutes, until golden brown.
Serves 4

HERRING PIE

4 herrings, boned and filleted

50 g (2 oz) English butter

4 medium potatoes, peeled and thinly sliced

2 medium cooking apples, peeled and finely chopped

salt and freshly ground pepper

1. Leave the fish to soak in salted water for 1 hour. Drain
2. Rub half the butter over the sides and bottom of an ovenproof dish. Line sides and bottom with some of the potato slices.
3. Arrange the fillets and chopped apple in alternate layers in the dish, season each layer with salt and freshly ground pepper, finish with a layer of potatoes.
4. Dot with remaining butter, cover and bake in the oven at 180°C (350°F) mark 4 for 30 minutes. Remove the cover, and return the dish to the oven for a further 15 minutes, until the top is browned.
Serves 4

FISHERMAN'S HOT POT

450 g (1 lb) cod fillet

40 g (1½ oz) flour

700 g (1½ lb) potatoes, peeled

15–30 ml (1–2 tbsp) lemon juice

salt and freshly ground pepper

1 medium onion, skinned and thinly sliced

225 g (8 oz) mushrooms, wiped and sliced

15 g (½ oz) English butter

150 ml (¼ pint) milk

100 g (4 oz) English Cheddar cheese, grated

1. Skin the cod, cut into 2-cm (¾-inch) squares and toss in 25 g (1 oz) flour.
2. Boil the potatoes until tender, but not soft, then slice them thinly. Arrange one-third on the bottom of a buttered ovenproof casserole. Cover with half the cod, sprinkle with lemon juice, season well.
3. Combine the onion and mushrooms and arrange half the mixture over the fish. Cover with the remaining cod, lemon juice,

one-third of the potatoes and the remaining onions and mushrooms.

4. Melt the butter in a pan, stir in the remaining 15 g ($\frac{1}{2}$ oz) flour and cook gently for 1 minute, stirring. Remove pan from the heat and gradually stir in the milk. Bring to the boil and continue to cook, stirring, until the sauce thickens, then add half the cheese and seasoning to taste.

5. Pour the sauce over the ingredients in the casserole, put the remaining potato slices on top, and sprinkle with the remaining cheese.

6. Bake in the oven, uncovered, at 200°C (400°F) mark 6 for about 40 minutes, until golden.

Serves 4

PERFECT PASTA

PASTA BAKE

450 g (1 lb) minced beef

1 red pepper, seeded and sliced

1 onion, skinned and chopped

100 g (4 oz) button mushrooms, wiped and sliced

396-g (14-oz) can tomatoes, with juice

5 ml (1 tsp) Tabasco sauce

salt and freshly ground pepper

100 g (4 oz) wholewheat spaghetti rings

300 g (10 oz) natural yogurt

1 egg, beaten

50 g (2 oz) flour

2 tomatoes, sliced, and chopped fresh parsley to garnish

1. In a saucepan, gently fry the mince in its own fat, until turning brown. Drain off any fat. Add the pepper, onion, mushrooms, the can of tomatoes and juice, Tabasco sauce and seasoning; simmer gently for 10 minutes.

2. Meanwhile, cook the pasta in a pan of fast boiling water for about 10 minutes, until tender, but not soft. Drain. Place in a 1.4-litre (2$\frac{1}{2}$-pint) ovenproof dish. Top with the mince mixture.

3. Beat together the yogurt, egg and flour until smooth, pour over the mince. Bake in the oven at 180°C (350°F) mark 4 for 40 minutes. Serve hot, garnished with tomatoes and chopped parsley.

Serves 4

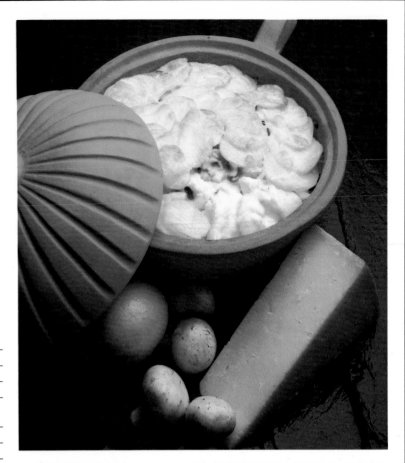

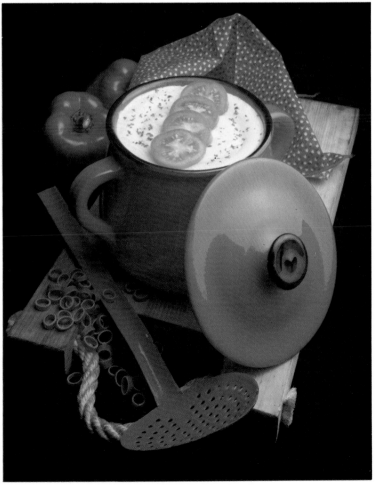

Right:
PASTA BAKE
Pasta is a godsend for family meals as it is quick to prepare and very versatile when combined with a wide range of mouthwatering sauces. This excellent Pasta Bake comes straight from the oven to table as the warming centre of a family meal.

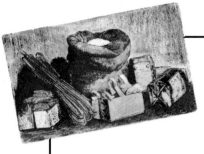

TUNA RIGATONI BAKE

150 g (5 oz) rigatoni pasta
198-g (7-oz) can tuna, drained
225 g (8 oz) cottage cheese
225 g (8 oz) courgettes, thinly sliced
salt and freshly ground pepper
396-g (14-oz) can tomatoes, with juice
25 g (1 oz) English Cheddar cheese, grated

1. Cook the rigatoni in a saucepan of fast boiling salted water for about 8 minutes until tender, but not soft. Drain and set aside.
2. In a bowl flake the tuna into large pieces and gently mix with cottage cheese. Line the bottom of an ovenproof casserole with sliced courgettes, then add a layer of tuna, cottage cheese, then pasta. Continue to layer, finishing with courgettes, and season well.
3. Pour over the can of tomatoes with the juice, spreading the tomatoes evenly over the top of the dish. Sprinkle with the cheese.
4. Bake in the oven at 190°C (375°F) mark 5 for about 30 minutes. Serve hot.
Serves 4

PASTA WITH PEAS AND HAM IN CREAM SAUCE

275–350 g (10–12 oz) tagliatelle or
  spaghetti
100 g (4 oz) English butter
1 large onion, skinned and sliced
100 g (4 oz) ham, cut into thin strips
100 g (4 oz) frozen peas, cooked
60 ml (4 tbsp) fresh single cream
100 g (4 oz) English Cheddar cheese, grated
salt and freshly ground pepper

1. Cook the pasta in a saucepan of fast boiling salted water for about 10 minutes until tender, but not soft. Drain.
2. Meanwhile, heat the butter in a pan, add the onion and cook for about 3 minutes until the onion is soft. Add the ham and peas and cook for a further 5 minutes.
3. Add the drained pasta, stir well and then add the fresh cream and most of the cheese. Toss gently, add seasoning and serve at once, sprinkled with the remaining cheese.
Serves 4

COOK'S TIP TO COOK PASTA WELL try these tips. For 450 g (1 lb) of bought pasta, boil at least 4 litres (7 pints) of water in a very large saucepan and add 45 ml (3 level tbsp) salt. A knob of English butter or 15 ml (1 tbsp) oil added to the water stops the water boiling over and keeps the pasta from sticking.
When the water is boiling very rapidly, drop in the pasta all at once. Turn up the heat and quickly return the water to the boil.
Cook until the pasta is *al dente* – literally 'to the tooth' – just firm to the bite and not completely soft. The cooking time varies from about 8 minutes according to the size and thickness of the pasta. Experiment with pasta shapes as there are many to choose from. There are stars, shells, twists and even pasta in the shape of little bows. In Italy it has been estimated that pasta is made in well over 500 different shapes.

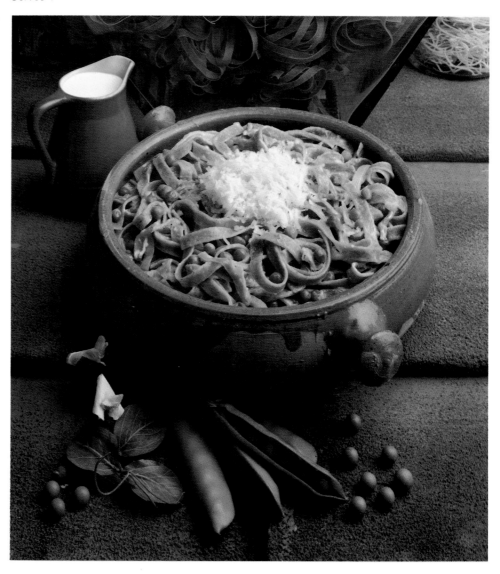

Right:
PASTA WITH PEAS AND HAM IN CREAM SAUCE
Pasta goes well with many unusual combinations of fresh vegetables and meat, as in this lovely dish which is worthy of the finest Italian restaurant.

SPAGHETTI ALLA CARBONARA

4 eggs
150 ml (5 fl oz) fresh single cream
25 g (1 oz) English butter
225 g (8 oz) streaky bacon, chopped
350 g (12 oz) spaghetti
175 g (6 oz) English Cheddar cheese, grated
salt and freshly ground pepper
30 ml (2 tbsp) chopped fresh parsley

1. In a bowl beat together the eggs and fresh cream. Heat the butter in a frying pan and fry the bacon until crisp.
2. Meanwhile, cook the spaghetti in a saucepan of fast boiling salted water for about 8 minutes until tender, but not soft. Drain and add it to the bacon in the frying pan.
3. Cook for 1 minute, stirring all the time. Remove from the heat and add the egg mixture. Mix well. (The heat of the spaghetti will be enough to cook the eggs.)
4. Stir in 125 g (4 oz) cheese and season with salt and pepper. Transfer to a serving dish and serve immediately, sprinkled with the parsley and remaining cheese.

Serves 4

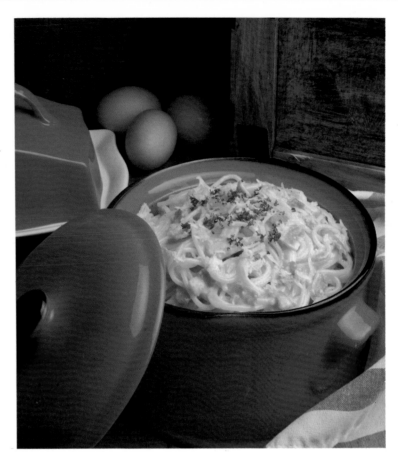

QUICHES AND SAVOURY FLANS

WATERCRESS AND ONION FLAN

175 g (6 oz) shortcrust pastry (see page 230)
2 onions, skinned and sliced
50 g (2 oz) English butter
1 bunch watercress, trimmed and coarsely chopped
salt and freshly ground pepper
2 eggs
150 ml ($\frac{1}{4}$ pint) milk and 150 ml (5 fl oz) fresh single cream, or 300 ml ($\frac{1}{2}$ pint) milk
sliced tomatoes and green olives to garnish

1. Roll out the pastry and use to line a 20.5-cm (8-inch) flan dish or ring placed on a baking sheet. Bake blind in the oven at 200°C (400°F) mark 6 for 10–15 minutes until set.
2. In a frying pan fry onions in butter until soft. Add watercress and cook 3–4 minutes, then season to taste. Place in flan case.
3. Beat together eggs, milk and cream. Pour into flan case.
4. Bake in the oven at 190°C (375°F) mark 5 for 20–30 minutes, until set and golden brown.

5. Serve hot, garnished with sliced tomatoes and green olives.

Variation
Two leeks can be used in place of watercress.

Serves 4–6

ASPARAGUS FLAN

175 g (6 oz) shortcrust pastry (see page 230)
2 eggs
salt and freshly ground pepper
150 ml (5 fl oz) fresh double cream
60 ml (4 tbsp) milk
350-g (12-oz) can asparagus spears, drained, or 350 g (12 oz) fresh asparagus, cooked

1. Roll out the pastry and use to line a 20.5-cm (8-inch) flan dish or ring placed on a baking sheet. Bake blind in the oven at 200°C (400°F) mark 6 for 10–15 minutes until set.
2. In a bowl beat together the eggs, salt, pepper, fresh cream and milk. Pour into the prepared flan case.
3. Arrange the asparagus spears over the top.
4. Bake in the oven at 180°C (350°F) mark 4 for 20–30 minutes, until golden. Serve hot or cold.

Serves 4–6

Above:
SPAGHETTI CARBONARA
The woodcutters who used to go up into the Italian mountains to collect firewood are called carbonari. This nourishing and quickly made dish used to be their staple diet. It became very popular with American servicemen during the Second World War for it combines two of their favourite foods – bacon and eggs!

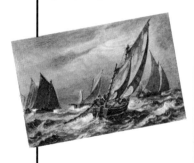

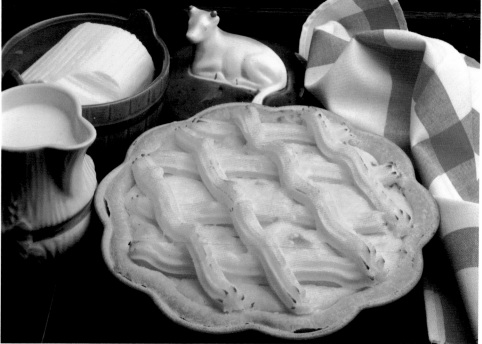

SMOKED HADDOCK FLAN

175 g (6 oz) shortcrust pastry (see page 230)
350 g (12 oz) potato, peeled
350 g (12 oz) smoked haddock
300 ml (½ pint) milk
1 small bunch of spring onions, or shredded green of 1 leek
2 eggs, hard-boiled and quartered
25 g (1 oz) English butter
25 g (1 oz) flour
freshly ground pepper
25 g (1 oz) English Cheddar cheese, grated

1. Roll out the pastry and use to line a 20.5-cm (8-inch) flan dish or ring placed on a baking sheet. Bake blind in the oven at 200°C (400°F) mark 6 for 10–15 minutes until set.
2. Boil the potatoes in a saucepan of boiling salted water until tender, then drain and mash. Set aside. Place the fish in a saucepan with the milk, bring to the boil and simmer for 15 minutes.
3. Strain the milk into a bowl. Remove skin and bones from the fish and flake the flesh. Place in the flan case.
4. Chop the onions and blanch the onions or leek. Place on top of the fish and cover with the eggs.
5. Melt the butter in a pan, stir in the flour and cook gently for 1 minute, stirring. Remove from the heat and gradually stir in the reserved milk. Bring to the boil and cook, stirring, until the sauce thickens. Season with pepper.
6. Spoon the sauce into the flan case and pipe potato across the top in a lattice design.

Sprinkle with cheese and bake in the oven for about 25 minutes until brown. Serve hot.
Serves 4–6

ANCHOVY FLAN

225 g (8 oz) flour
140 g (5½ oz) English butter
175 g (6 oz) English Cheddar cheese, grated
pinch of salt
50-g (2-oz) can anchovy fillets, drained
1 medium onion, skinned and thinly sliced
300 ml (½ pint) milk
pinch of cayenne pepper
pinch of mustard powder
2 eggs, separated

1. In a bowl, lightly work together 200 g (7 oz) flour, 90 g (3½ oz) butter, 75 g (3 oz) cheese and salt to form a manageable pastry dough.
2. Roll out and use to line a 20.5-cm (8-inch) flan dish or ring placed on a baking sheet. Bake blind in the oven at 200°C (400°F) mark 6 for 20 minutes until set.
3. Meanwhile, cook the anchovy fillets and onion in 25 g (1 oz) butter until soft. Place in the pastry case.
4. Melt the remaining 25 g (1 oz) butter in a pan, stir in the remaining 25 g (1 oz) flour and cook gently for 1 minute, stirring. Remove from the heat and gradually stir in the milk. Bring to the boil and cook, stirring, until the sauce thickens. Stir in 50 g (2 oz) cheese and season with cayenne and mustard.
5. Whisk the egg whites until stiff. Beat the egg yolks into the mixture, then fold

in the whisked egg whites.
6. Turn into the flan case, sprinkle with the remaining cheese and bake in the oven at 180°C (350°F) mark 4 for 25–30 minutes.
Serves 4–6

SPINACH AND PRAWN QUICHE

200 g (7 oz) wholemeal flour
salt and freshly ground pepper
100 g (4 oz) English butter
1 egg, beaten
150 ml ($\frac{1}{4}$ pint) milk
125 g (4 oz) peeled prawns
155-g (5$\frac{1}{2}$-oz) packet frozen chopped spinach, thawed

1. In a mixing bowl mix together the flour and pinch of salt, rub in the butter and stir in enough cold water to bind together.
2. Roll out the pastry and use to line a 20.5-cm (8-inch) flan ring placed on a baking sheet. Bake blind in the oven at 200°C (400°F) mark 6 for 20 minutes until set.
3. To the egg, add the milk, prawns and drained spinach. Season well and pour into the flan case.
4. Bake in the oven at 180°C (350°F) mark 4 for about 40 minutes, until just set. Serve hot.
Serves 4–6

CURRIED BACON FLAN

175 g (6 oz) shortcrust pastry (see page 230)
25 g (1 oz) English butter
125 g (4 oz) celery heart, cleaned and sliced
125 g (4 oz) streaky bacon, diced
5 ml (1 level tsp) curry powder
3 eggs, beaten
142 g (5 oz) natural yogurt
salt and freshly ground pepper
225 g (8 oz) tomatoes, skinned and thinly sliced

1. Roll out the pastry and use to line a 21.5-cm (8$\frac{1}{2}$-inch), loose-bottomed French fluted flan tin. Bake blind in the oven at 200°C (400°F) mark 6 for 10–15 minutes until set.
2. Melt the butter in a small frying pan and sauté the celery and bacon until golden brown. Stir in the curry powder and cook for 2 minutes.
3. In a bowl, blend the eggs with the yogurt. Add the pan ingredients and seasoning, and turn into the flan case. Top with tomato slices.
4. Bake in the oven at 190°C (375°F) mark 5 for about 25 minutes until golden brown and set. Serve hot or cold.
Serves 4–6

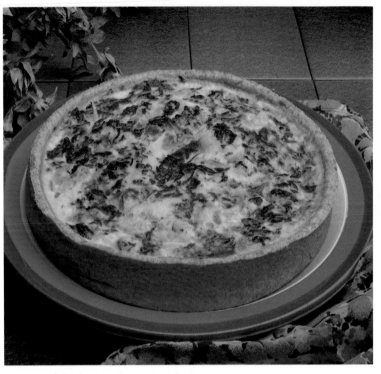

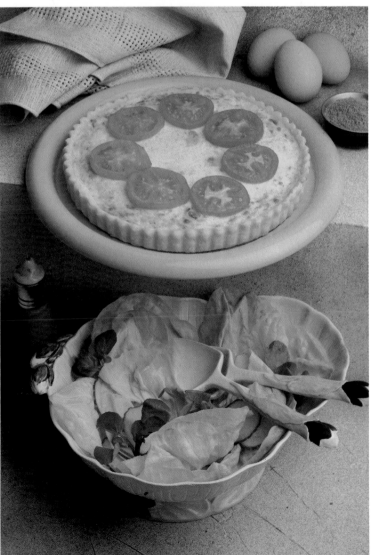

COOK'S TIP BAKING BLIND is the term used to describe the cooking of unfilled pastry cases. Line the pastry with greaseproof paper or foil and fill it with dried beans or rice before baking. This ensures that the case keeps its shape as it cooks.

After baking, carefully lift the lining out of the shell and pour the beans back into a storage jar. The beans may be used again and again for baking blind. Often the pastry is only partially cooked – until it 'sets' – and is then baked for a further period when filled.

MUSHROOM QUICHE

175 g (6 oz) shortcrust pastry (see page 230)

225 g (8 oz) button mushrooms, wiped and thinly sliced

25 g (1 oz) English butter

1 egg, plus 1 egg yolk

150 ml (5 fl oz) fresh single cream

2.5 ml (½ tsp) dried basil, or 5 ml (1 tsp) chopped fresh basil

salt and freshly ground pepper

1. Roll out the pastry and use to line a 21.5-cm (8½-inch) flan dish or ring placed on a baking sheet. Bake blind in the oven at 200°C (400°F) mark 6 for 20 minutes until set.
2. Sauté the mushrooms gently in the butter for 5 minutes. Drain and place in the flan case.
3. Beat together the egg and yolk, add the fresh cream, basil and seasoning and pour over the mushrooms.
4. Bake at 190°C (375°F) mark 5 for about 35 minutes, until just set.
Serves 4–6

BACON AND SPINACH QUICHE

225 g (8 oz) shortcrust pastry (see page 230)

350 g (12 oz) streaky bacon

1 medium onion, skinned and sliced

15 ml (1 tbsp) vegetable oil

2 eggs, beaten

142 g (5 oz) natural yogurt

150 ml (¼ pint) milk

salt and freshly ground pepper

226-g (8-oz) packet chopped spinach, thawed

1. Roll out the pastry and use to line a 24-cm (9½-inch) loose-bottomed flan ring. Bake blind in the oven at 200°C (400°F) mark 6 for 10–15 minutes until set.
2. Dice 125 g (4 oz) bacon. Lightly fry the diced bacon and the onion together in oil until golden.
3. Mix eggs with yogurt, milk and seasoning; stir in the pan ingredients. Lastly, mix in the spinach, well drained. Pour the mixture into the flan case and bake in the oven at 190°C (375°F) mark 5 for about 30 minutes, until just set.
4. Form the rest of the bacon into little rolls and bake (place in the oven 10 minutes after the flan); use as garnish.
Serves 4–6

FLAN PROVENÇAL

300 g (11 oz) flour

5 ml (1 level tsp) cinnamon

150 g (5 oz) English butter

1 egg, beaten

700 g (1½ lb) onions, skinned and thinly sliced

2 garlic cloves, skinned and crushed

90 ml (6 tbsp) olive oil

396-g (14-oz) can tomatoes, drained

30 ml (2 level tbsp) tomato purée

2.5 ml (½ level tsp) dried mixed herbs

salt and freshly ground pepper

56-g (2-oz) can anchovy fillets

12 black olives, stoned

1. Sift the flour and cinnamon into a bowl and rub in the butter. Add enough beaten egg to bind. Roll out and use to line a 25.5-cm (10-inch) flan dish or ring placed on a baking sheet. Bake blind in the oven at 200°C (400°F) mark 6 for 20 minutes until set.
2. Meanwhile, fry the onions and garlic gently in oil in a large pan, until very soft but not coloured.
3. Stir the tomatoes into the onion mixture with the tomato purée, herbs and seasoning. Cook gently for 5 minutes.
4. Turn the mixture into the flan case, decorate with a lattice of anchovies and olives. Brush lightly with olive oil and return to the oven for 20 minutes. Serve hot or cold.
Serves 4–6

POTATO AND BACON FLAN

300 g (11 oz) shortcrust pastry (see page 230)

450 g (1 lb) potatoes, peeled and cut into 1-cm (½-inch) dice

225 g (8 oz) streaky bacon, diced

1 small onion, skinned and sliced

freshly ground pepper

2 eggs

300 ml (½ pint) milk

1. Roll out the pastry and use to line a 25.5-cm (10-inch) flan dish or ring placed on a baking sheet. Bake blind in the oven at 200°C (400°F) mark 6 for 20 minutes until set.
2. Cook the potato dice in a saucepan of boiling salted water until tender, but not soft. Drain.
3. In a frying pan, fry the bacon gently in its own fat for about 2 minutes. Add the sliced onion and cook gently until soft. Place in the

flan case with the potatoes. Season well with pepper.

4. Beat together the eggs and milk; pour over the filling and bake in the oven at 190°C (375°F) mark 5 for about 30 minutes until set. Serve hot.

Serves 4–6

SALAMI AND TOMATO FLAN

175 g (6 oz) rich shortcrust pastry (see page 230)
25 g (1 oz) fresh breadcrumbs
175 g (6 oz) salami, skinned and thinly sliced
225 g (8 oz) tomatoes, skinned and sliced
2 eggs
150 ml ($\frac{1}{4}$ pint) milk
1.25 ml ($\frac{1}{4}$ level tsp) salt and freshly ground pepper
1.25 ml ($\frac{1}{4}$ tsp) Tabasco sauce

1. Roll out the pastry and use to line a 20.5-cm (8-inch) flan dish or ring placed on a baking sheet. Bake blind in the oven at 200°C (400°F) mark 6 for 20 minutes until set.

2. Sprinkle the breadcrumbs over the base of the flan case. Cut the salami slices into strips. Arrange with tomatoes over the breadcrumbs.

3. Beat together the eggs and milk with the salt, pepper and Tabasco. Pour over the filling.

4. Bake in the oven at 190°C (375°F) mark 5 for about 40 minutes, until set.

Serves 4–6

TUNA YOGURT QUICHE

175 g (6 oz) shortcrust pastry (see page 230)
198-g (7-oz) can tuna
15 ml (1 level tbsp) capers
2 eggs, beaten
142 g (5 oz) natural yogurt
salt and freshly ground pepper
30 ml (2 level tbsp) English Cheddar cheese, grated

1. Roll out the pastry and use to line a 20.5-cm (8-inch) flan dish or ring placed on a baking sheet. Bake blind in the oven at 200°C (400°F) mark 6 for 10–15 minutes until set.

2. Flake the tuna into a bowl, then mix in the capers, eggs and yogurt and season to taste.

3. Spoon tuna mixture into flan case, sprinkle with the cheese and bake in the oven at 190°C (375°F) mark 5 for about 30 minutes, until set. Serve hot or cold.

Serves 4–6

CAULIFLOWER AND STILTON FLAN

100 g (4 oz) English butter
175 g (6 oz) flour, plus 30 ml (2 level tbsp)
1.25 ml ($\frac{1}{4}$ level tsp) salt
450 g (1 lb) cauliflower florets
225 g (8 oz) onions, skinned and chopped
200 ml (7 fl oz) milk
freshly ground pepper
125 g (4 oz) Blue Stilton cheese, crumbled
25 g (1 oz) English Cheddar cheese, grated

1. Rub 75 g (3 oz) butter into 175 g (6 oz) flour and salt. Bind to a dough with a little water. Chill in the refrigerator for about 10 minutes.

2. Roll out the pastry and use to line a 23-cm (9-inch) flan dish or ring placed on a baking sheet. Chill again for 10–15 minutes, then bake in the oven at 200°C (400°F) mark 6 for 10–15 minutes until set.

3. Cook the cauliflower florets in a saucepan of boiling salted water for 4–5 minutes until just tender. Drain well and cool.

4. Melt remaining butter in a pan, sauté the onion until soft, then stir in the 30 ml (2 level tbsp) flour and cook gently for 2 minutes, stirring. Remove the pan from the heat and gradually stir in the milk. Bring to the boil and continue to cook, stirring, until the sauce thickens, then add pepper to taste.

5. Sprinkle the Stilton evenly over the base of the flan. Arrange the cauliflower on top. Spoon over the onion sauce and sprinkle with the Cheddar cheese.

6. Bake in the oven at 190°C (375°F) mark 5 for 25–30 minutes until golden and bubbly. Serve hot.

Serves 4–6

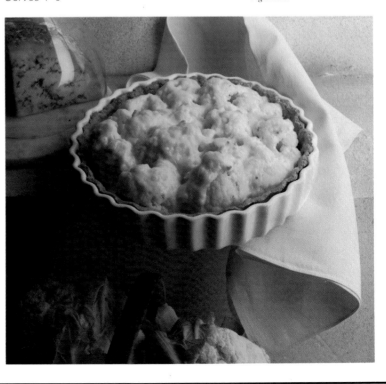

Below:
CAULIFLOWER AND STILTON FLAN
A very sophisticated version of Cauliflower Cheese, this flan uses the 'King of English Cheeses' and the humblest of vegetables.

PREPARING A PASTRY CASE

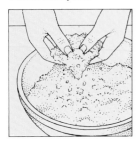

1 Adding the butter to the flour in small pieces

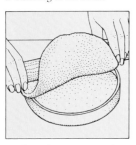

2 Rubbing in the butter

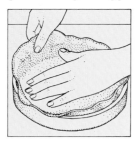

3 Lifting the pastry over the quiche dish using a rolling pin

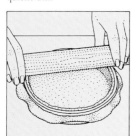

4 Easing the pastry into the quiche dish

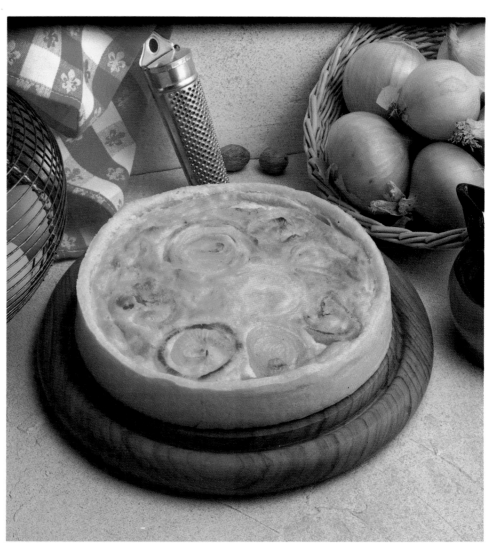

5 Trimming off the excess pastry by pressing the rolling pin over the edges of the dish. The filling can now be poured in

TARTE À L'OIGNON

50 g (2 oz) English butter

700 g (1½ lb) onions, skinned and thinly sliced

175 g (6 oz) shortcrust pastry (see page 230)

2 eggs

50 ml (2 fl oz) milk

150 ml (5 fl oz) fresh single cream

salt and freshly ground pepper

pinch of grated nutmeg

1. Melt the butter in a large frying pan and gently cook the onions, covered, for 20 minutes.
2. Roll out the pastry and use to line a 20.5-cm (8-inch) flan dish or ring placed on a baking sheet.
3. Blend together the eggs, milk, fresh cream and seasonings until smooth.
4. Pour a little of the egg mixture into the pastry case. Add the onions and the remaining egg mixture.
5. Bake in the oven at 200°C (400°F) mark 6 for 30 minutes until golden brown and set.

Serves 4–6

QUICHE LORRAINE

175 g (6 oz) flour

salt and freshly ground pepper

75 g (3 oz) English butter

175 g (6 oz) streaky bacon, chopped

2 eggs, beaten

150 ml (5 fl oz) fresh single cream

175 g (6 oz) English Cheddar cheese, grated

1. Sift together the flour and salt into a bowl. Rub in the butter until the mixture resembles fine breadcrumbs. Add enough water to mix to a firm dough.
2. Roll out the pastry on a lightly floured work surface and use to line a 20.5-cm (8-inch) flan dish or ring placed on a baking sheet.
3. Scatter the bacon over the pastry base. Beat the eggs, fresh cream, seasoning and grated cheese together. Pour the mixture over the bacon. Bake in the oven at 220°C (425°F) mark 7 for 10 minutes.
4. Reduce to 190°C (375°F) mark 5 and cook for a further 20–30 minutes, until set and golden brown. Serve hot or cold.

Serves 4–6

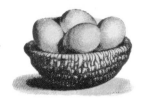

EGG DISHES

SAUSAGE AND SWEET PEPPER OMELETTE

3 eggs

30 ml (2 tbsp) milk

salt and freshly ground pepper

65 g (2½ oz) English butter

225 g (½ lb) pork chipolata sausages

1 small green pepper, seeded and thinly sliced

small bunch of spring onions, trimmed and sliced

50 g (2 oz) haricot beans, cooked

1. Lightly beat together the eggs, milk and seasoning in a bowl.
2. Melt 15 g (½ oz) butter in a frying pan and quickly cook the sausages until golden on all sides. Remove, cut each in half, crosswise, and keep hot.
3. Wipe out the pan with absorbent kitchen paper and melt half the remaining butter. Sauté the pepper, onions and beans for about 2 minutes. Remove from pan and keep hot.
4. Wipe out the pan and melt the remaining butter. Pour in the egg mixture and cook quickly, stirring lightly with the back of a fork until it begins to set.
5. Add sausages and vegetables to the pan.
6. Continue to cook until the egg is just set but still a little runny. Serve immediately.

Serves 2

OMELETTE ARNOLD BENNETT

100 g (4 oz) smoked haddock

50 g (2 oz) English butter

150 ml (¼ pint) fresh double cream

3 eggs, separated

salt and freshly ground pepper

50 g (2 oz) English Cheddar cheese, grated

1. Place the fish in a saucepan and cover with water. Bring to the boil and simmer gently for 10 minutes. Drain and flake the fish, discarding skin and bones.
2. Place the fish in a pan with half the butter and 30 ml (2 tbsp) fresh cream. Toss over a high heat until the butter melts. Leave to cool.
3. Beat the egg yolks in a bowl with 15 ml (1 tbsp) fresh cream and seasoning. Stir in the fish mixture. Stiffly whisk the egg whites and fold in.
4. Heat the remaining butter in an omelette pan. Fry the egg mixture, but make sure it remains fairly fluid. Do not fold over. Slide it on to a flameproof serving dish.

5. Top with the cheese and remaining fresh cream blended together, then quickly bubble under a preheated grill. Slide on to a heatproof serving plate.

Serves 2

NORTH COUNTRY OMELETTE

40 g (1½ oz) English butter

15 g (½ oz) flour

300 ml (½ pint) milk

75 g (3 oz) Lancashire cheese

salt and freshly ground pepper

6 eggs

100 g (4 oz) cooked smoked haddock, flaked into small pieces

1. To make the sauce, melt 15 g (½ oz) butter in a saucepan, stir in the flour and cook gently for 1 minute, stirring. Remove pan from the heat and gradually stir in the milk. Bring to the boil slowly and continue to cook, stirring, until the sauce thickens.
2. Grate 50 g (2 oz) cheese, add to the sauce and stir until melted. Season and keep warm. Cut the remaining cheese into 0.5-cm (¼-inch) cubes.
3. Beat the eggs in a bowl. Add the cubes of cheese and the smoked haddock and season with freshly ground pepper and a very little salt. Beat with a fork.
4. Heat the remaining butter in an omelette pan. Fry half the egg mixture, but make sure it remains fairly fluid. Slide it on to a dish, cover with the cheese sauce and put under a hot grill until the top is nicely browned.
5. Make a second omelette in the same way. Serve immediately.

Serves 4

Opposite:
TARTE À L'OIGNON
A tart which originated in Alsace-Lorraine, on the French-German border, about the sixteenth century. Sometimes cheese is added, but it is also delicious without.

Below:
OMELETTE ARNOLD BENNETT
Arnold Bennett, the author of the 'Five Towns' novels, liked to write about hotels and he immortalised the Savoy Hotel's chef, Jean Baptiste Virlogeux, in his novel Imperial Palace. *In return, Virlogeux created this glorious dish in honour of the novelist.*

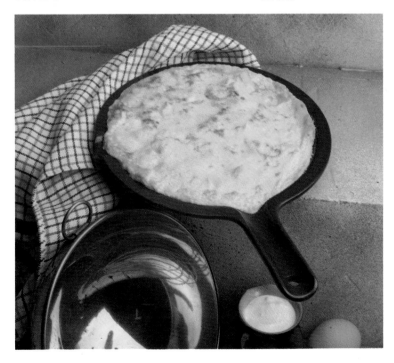

Right:
EGG FRICASSÉE
An excellent way to make the most of fresh eggs – slices of hard-boiled egg in a tarragon-flavoured sauce, accompanied by triangles of light puff pastry.

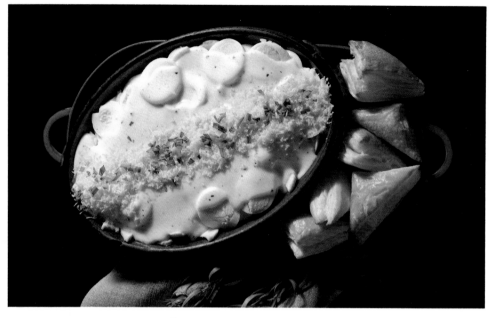

COOK'S TIP

YORKSHIRE PUDDING was originally known as Dripping Pudding and was served with gravy as a first course; it was an ideal way of making the beef go further. In Yorkshire today it is still served separately before the meat, but in much of the rest of the country the pudding is eaten as an accompaniment with the beef.
Those with hearty appetites can follow the old tradition and eat any left over, with jam, for pudding!

EGG FRICASSÉE

200 ml (7 fl oz) milk

small piece of onion

small piece of carrot

bay leaf

6 peppercorns

25 g (1 oz) English butter

30 ml (2 level tbsp) flour

142 ml (5 fl oz) soured cream

2.5 ml ($\frac{1}{2}$ tsp) dried tarragon, or 10 ml (2 tsp) fresh tarragon, snipped

salt and freshly ground pepper

6 eggs, hard-boiled

sprig of fresh tarragon (optional) to garnish

212-g (7$\frac{1}{2}$-oz) packet frozen puff pastry, thawed, for pastry triangles (see below)

1. In a saucepan, bring the milk to the boil with the onion, carrot, bay leaf and peppercorns and leave to infuse for 10 minutes; strain.
2. Melt the butter in a pan and stir in the flour. Remove from the heat and gradually stir in the milk, soured cream, tarragon and seasoning. Return to the heat, bring to boil, stirring all the time until the sauce thickens. Simmer for about 5 minutes.
3. Slice the eggs, reserving the yolk from one. Add the egg slices to the sauce and simmer to warm eggs; adjust seasoning.
4. Sieve the reserved egg yolk and use with the snipped tarragon to garnish the dish. Serve accompanied by pastry triangles.

Pastry triangles:
Roll out the pastry to an oblong 25.5 × 10 cm (10 × 4 inches). Divide into two, lengthwise, and cut each strip into 10 triangles. Bake in the oven at 220°C (425°F) mark 7 for 12–15 minutes until golden brown and well risen.
Serves 4

SAUSAGE YORKSHIRES WITH ONION SAUCE

350 g (12 oz) pork sausagemeat

175 g (6 oz) cooking apple, peeled and cored

5 ml (1 tsp) chopped fresh parsley

salt and freshly ground pepper

125 g (4 oz) flour, plus 15 ml (1 level tbsp)

2 eggs

568 ml (1 pint) milk

lard

175 g (6 oz) onion, skinned and sliced

15 g ($\frac{1}{2}$ oz) English butter

1. Place the sausagemeat in a bowl. Grate the apple into the bowl. Stir in the parsley and seasoning. Work ingredients together and form into 16 small balls.
2. Make a batter from the 125 g (4 oz) flour, the eggs and 300 ml ($\frac{1}{2}$ pint) milk.
3. Preheat the oven to 220°C (425°F) mark 7. Heat a little lard in the bases of four 300-ml ($\frac{1}{2}$-pint) individual ramekin dishes until sizzling hot. Place sausage balls in each and cook in the oven for 10 minutes.
4. Pour the batter over the sausage balls and return to the oven for 35–40 minutes until risen and golden.
5. Meanwhile, cook the onion until soft in the remaining milk. To make the sauce, melt the butter in a pan, stir in the 15 ml (1 level tbsp) flour and cook gently for 1 minute, stirring. Remove pan from the heat and gradually stir in the onions and milk. Bring to the boil and continue to cook, stirring, until the sauce thickens, then add seasoning to taste.
6. When popovers are baked, turn out and pour a little onion sauce into the centre of each.
Serves 4

Opposite:
SAUSAGE YORKSHIRES WITH ONION SAUCE
Crisp, golden popovers filled with tasty sausagemeat balls are served with a delicious onion sauce.

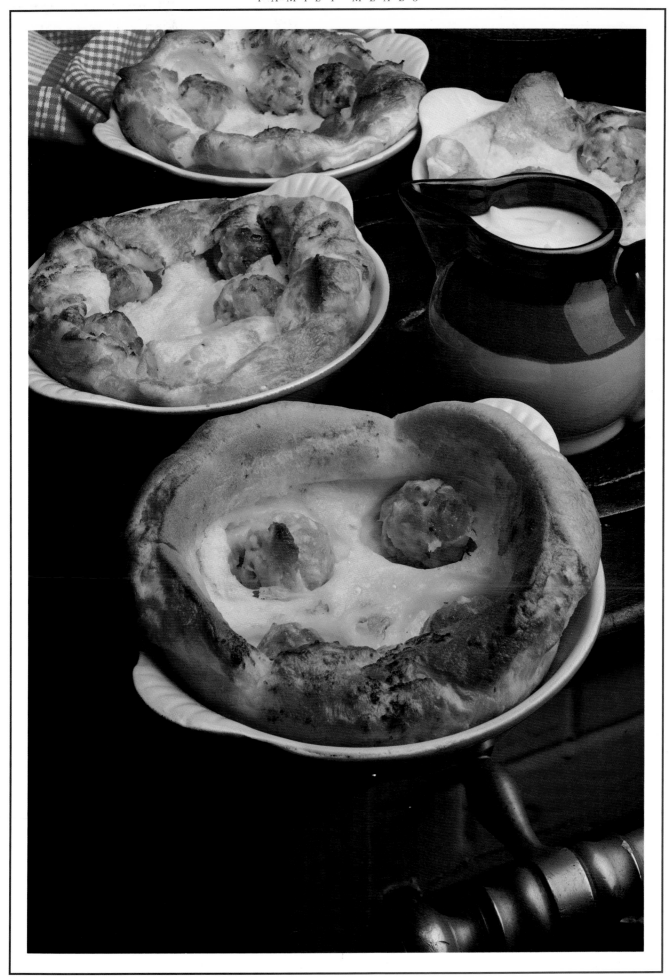

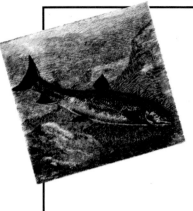

SMOKED FISH PANCAKES

350 g (12 oz) smoked cod fillet
300 ml (½ pint) milk
bay leaf
small pieces of onion
40 g (1½ oz) English butter
30 ml (2 level tbsp) flour
150 ml (5 fl oz) fresh single cream
2 eggs, hard-boiled and chopped
45 ml (3 tbsp) chopped fresh parsley
salt and freshly ground pepper
8 pancakes (see page 276)
fresh chives to garnish

1. Place the fish in a small saucepan, pour over the milk and add the bay leaf and onion. Cover the pan and simmer until the fish begins to flake. Strain off and reserve milk. Flake fish, discard skin and bone.
2. Melt the butter in a saucepan, stir in the flour and cook for 1 minute, stirring. Remove from the heat and gradually stir in the reserved milk and fresh cream. Bring to the boil and cook for 2 minutes, stirring.
3. Remove from the heat, stir in the fish, three-quarters of the chopped egg, parsley and seasoning (add salt with care as the fish may be salty). Cool slightly.
4. Divide the fish mixture between the pancakes, fold over and place in a shallow buttered ovenproof dish.
5. Cover with buttered foil and cook in the oven at 200°C (400°F) mark 6 for 20 minutes.
6. Scatter over remaining egg and snipped chives and serve hot.
Serves 8

EGG AND MUSHROOM SAVOURY

225 g (8 oz) mushrooms, wiped
30 ml (2 tbsp) milk
6 eggs
30 ml (2 tbsp) finely chopped fresh parsley
2.5 ml (½ level tsp) salt
2 large tomatoes, skinned and sliced
75 g (3 oz) Lancashire cheese, crumbled

1. Put the whole mushrooms in a frying pan and pour in the milk. Bring to the boil, and immediately remove from the heat. Transfer the mushrooms to a 600-ml (1-pint) buttered flameproof dish.
2. Beat the eggs into the liquid remaining in the pan, add the parsley and salt, return to the heat and scramble lightly until set. Spoon over the mushrooms, top with slices of tomato and sprinkle thickly with cheese.
3. Brown under a hot grill. Serve with fried potatoes.
Serves 4

SPINACH AND STILTON PANCAKES

900 g (2 lb) fresh spinach, or two 225-g (8-oz) packets frozen chopped spinach
salt and freshly ground pepper
50 g (2 oz) English butter
50 g (2 oz) salted peanuts, chopped
2.5 ml (½ level tsp) paprika
40 ml (8 level tsp) flour
150 ml (5 fl oz) fresh single cream
8 pancakes (see page 276)
300 ml (½ pint) milk
50 g (2 oz) Blue Stilton cheese, grated

1. Tear stalks off the spinach and wash. Place in a saucepan and cook for about 10 minutes, covered, sprinkled with salt (do not add any liquid). Drain well and chop.
2. Heat 25 g (1 oz) butter in a small pan, add the peanuts and paprika and fry gently for 1 minute. Stir in the spinach, 20 ml (4 level tsp) flour, fresh cream, and seasoning. Bring to the boil and cook for 2–3 minutes, stirring. Divide the filling between the pancakes, roll up and place side by side in a buttered ovenproof dish.
3. Melt the remaining butter in a pan, stir in the remaining flour and cook for 1 minute. Remove from the heat and gradually stir in the milk. Bring to the boil, stirring all the time, until the sauce thickens. Stir in the cheese and seasonings. Pour over the pancakes. Cover lightly with foil and bake in the oven at 180°C (350°F) mark 4 for 25–30 minutes.
Serves 8

SAVOURY BAKES
PRAIRIE PIE

4 slices of bread
50 g (2 oz) English butter
350-g (12-oz) can pork luncheon meat
150-g (5-oz) can baked beans
salt and freshly ground pepper
2 eggs, beaten
300 ml (½ pint) milk
50 g (2 oz) English Cheddar cheese, grated

1. Remove crusts from bread, butter thickly on one side and lay two slices, buttered side down, in the base of a 900-ml (1½-pint) ovenproof dish.
2. Chop the luncheon meat, and mix in a bowl with the beans and seasoning. Pour on to the bread base. Top with remaining bread, buttered side up.
3. Mix together the eggs and milk, pour over the bread and sprinkle with grated cheese.
4. Bake in the oven at 190°C (375°F) mark 5 for 30 minutes. Serve hot.
Serves 4

SAVOURY MEAT LOAF

175 g (6 oz) streaky bacon, rinded
225 g (8 oz) cooked meat, minced
40-g (1½-oz) packet bread sauce mix
15 g (½ oz) cornflakes, crumbled
25 g (1 oz) onions, skinned and chopped
2.5 ml (½ tsp) dried mixed herbs
15 ml (1 level tbsp) tomato purée
150 ml (¼ pint) milk
salt and freshly ground pepper
1 egg, beaten

1. Butter a 450-g (1-lb) loaf tin and line with rashers of streaky bacon.
2. In a large bowl, mix together the minced meat, bread sauce mix, cornflake crumbs, onions, herbs and tomato purée.
3. Add the milk and seasoning to the beaten egg and stir into meat mixture. Beat well.
4. Turn into prepared tin, covered with foil. Bake in the oven at 200°C (400°F) mark 6 for 1–1½ hours. Turn out and serve hot or cold.

Serves 4

CHEESE AND NOODLE HOT POT

225 g (8 oz) flat noodles
1 medium onion, skinned and chopped
25 g (1 oz) English butter
300 ml (½ pint) white coating sauce (see page 142)
30 ml (2 level tbsp) tomato purée
50 g (2 oz) hazelnuts, chopped
225 g (8 oz) cottage cheese
salt and freshly ground pepper
50 g (2 oz) Lancashire cheese, crumbled
1 tomato, sliced and chopped fresh parsley to garnish

1. Cook noodles in a saucepan of fast boiling salted water until tender, but not soft. Drain.
2. In a frying pan, fry the onion gently in butter until golden. Stir the noodles and onion into the sauce. Add tomato purée, hazelnuts and cottage cheese. Mix thoroughly. Season to taste.
3. Transfer to a 1.1-litre (2-pint) buttered ovenproof dish and sprinkle with cheese. Bake in the oven at 190°C (375°F) mark 5 for 20–25 minutes, until top is golden.
4. Serve hot garnished with tomato slices and parsley. Serve with a green vegetable.

Serves 4

CHUNKY PORK SUPREME

25 g (1 oz) English butter
2 carrots, peeled and sliced
3 celery stalks, cleaned and chopped
1 small green pepper, seeded and chopped
450 g (1 lb) lean pork, diced
two 34 g (1.2 oz) packets onion sauce mix
568 ml (1 pint) milk
1 bay leaf
salt and freshly ground pepper

1. Melt the butter in a flameproof casserole and fry the carrots, celery and green pepper for 2–3 minutes. Add the pork and cook for 3–4 minutes, stirring frequently.
2. Make up the onion sauce mix with the milk, following the instructions on the packet, then add to the pork with the bay leaf.
3. Mix well, cover and bake in the oven at 180°C (350°F) mark 4 for 1½ hours. Taste and adjust seasoning; remove bay leaf before serving.

Serves 4

Below:
SPINACH AND STILTON PANCAKES
Crisp, light pancakes are as much part of traditional British food as they are French. Served with a delicious sauce combining rich green spinach and tangy Stilton cheese, these pancakes are mouthwatering to look at and delicious to eat.

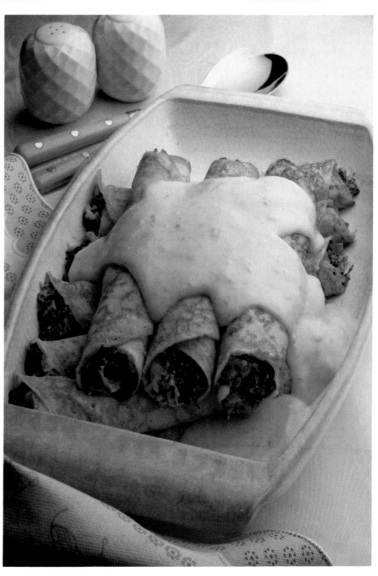

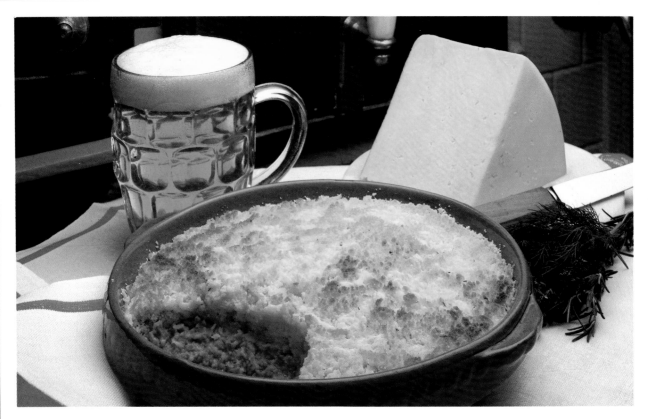

Above:
CHESHIRE LAMB
CRUMBLE
This delicious dish, which can be prepared in advance, is a tasty alternative to Shepherd's Pie. It has a similar minced meat base, with a crisp crumble topping seasoned with cheese and herbs.

BEEF LAYER PIE WITH YOGURT TOPPING

1 medium onion, skinned and chopped

25 g (1 oz) English butter

225 g (8 oz) cooked roast beef, minced

1.25 ml (¼ tsp) dried mixed herbs

30 ml (2 level tbsp) tomato purée

5 ml (1 tsp) Worcestershire sauce

salt and freshly ground pepper

450 g (1 lb) potatoes, peeled

225 g (8 oz) tomatoes, skinned and sliced

1 egg, beaten

25 g (1 oz) flour

142 g (5 oz) natural yogurt

paprika

1. In a saucepan, cook the onion gently in the butter. Add the minced meat, mixed herbs, tomato purée and Worcestershire sauce. Season to taste.
2. Meanwhile, boil the potatoes until tender, but not soft, then slice them thinly. In a 1.1-litre (2-pint) ovenproof casserole, arrange layers of potato slices, then the meat mixture, then tomatoes, finishing with a layer of potatoes. Cover and bake in the oven at 190°C (375°F) mark 5 for 30 minutes.
3. To the egg, blend in the flour and the yogurt. Season to taste and spoon over the pie after it has cooked for 30 minutes.
4. Return dish to the oven and cook for a further 30 minutes. Dust with paprika before serving.

Serves 4

CHESHIRE LAMB CRUMBLE

350 g (12 oz) cooked roast lamb

1 medium onion, skinned

115 g (4½ oz) flour

15 ml (1 level tbsp) tomato purée

300 ml (½ pint) beef stock

salt and freshly ground pepper

50 g (2 oz) English butter

50 g (2 oz) English Cheshire cheese, grated

2.5 ml (½ tsp) dried mixed herbs

1. Mince together the meat and onion. Mix in 15 g (½ oz) flour, the tomato purée, stock and seasoning. Turn into a shallow ovenproof dish.
2. In a bowl, rub the butter into the remaining flour until it resembles fine breadcrumbs, then stir in the grated cheese, herbs and seasoning. Spoon the crumble over the meat.
3. Bake in the oven at 190°C (375°F) mark 5 for 45 minutes–1 hour. Serve immediately.

Serves 4

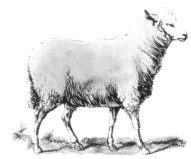

LANCASHIRE GAMMON

25 g (1 oz) English butter

4 gammon steaks

25 g (1 oz) flour

300 ml (½ pint) milk

100 g (4 oz) Lancashire cheese, crumbled

salt and freshly ground pepper

2 eggs, hard-boiled and sliced

watercress or chopped fresh parsley to
    garnish

1. Melt butter in a large pan and fry gammon steaks on both sides. Transfer to a shallow flameproof dish.
2. Stir the flour into the butter remaining in the pan and cook gently for 1 minute, stirring. Remove pan from the heat and gradually stir in the milk. Bring to the boil and continue to cook, stirring, until the sauce thickens, then add 75 g (3 oz) cheese and seasoning to taste.
3. Arrange hard-boiled eggs over gammon and coat with cheese sauce. Sprinkle with remaining cheese.
4. Bake in the oven at 200°C (400°F) mark 6 for 15 minutes. Garnish with watercress or parsley and serve with buttered noodles and peas.
Serves 4

LANCASHIRE HOT POT

900 g (2 lb) neck of mutton

225 g (8 oz) mushrooms, wiped

3 sheep's kidneys

3 large onions, skinned and thinly sliced

12 oysters (optional)

salt and freshly ground pepper

900 g (2 lb) potatoes, peeled and thickly
    sliced

600 ml (1 pint) beef stock

50 g (2 oz) English butter, melted

1. Cut the mutton into cutlets and remove excess fat.
2. Cut the mushrooms in half. Skin and core the kidneys and cut in halves.
3. In a deep ovenproof casserole, place mutton, mushrooms, kidneys, onions and oysters (if used), seasoning each layer. Finish with a layer of potatoes. Pour over the stock. Brush the potatoes with the melted butter.
4. Cover the casserole and cook in the oven at 170°C (325°F) mark 3 for 2 hours, until meat and potatoes are tender.
5. Uncover. Continue to cook at 220°C (425°F) mark 7 for a further 30 minutes, until potatoes are golden brown. Serve hot.
Serves 4

BACON CAKES

7 rashers streaky bacon, rinded

225 g (8 oz) self-raising flour

pinch of salt

25 g (1 oz) English butter

75 g (3 oz) English Cheddar cheese, grated

150 ml (¼ pint) milk

15 ml (1 level tbsp) tomato ketchup

dash of Worcestershire sauce

milk to glaze

1. Grill three rashers of bacon until crisp, then cut into small pieces.
2. Sieve together the flour and salt into a bowl, rub in the butter until it resembles fine breadcrumbs. Add all but 15 g (½ oz) of the cheese and the crumbled bacon.
3. Mix the milk, tomato ketchup and Worcestershire sauce together and add to dry ingredients.
4. Mix to a soft dough and roll out to an 18-cm (7-inch) circle, brush with milk and cut into eight wedges. Arrange on a buttered, floured baking tray in a circle with edges overlapping. Sprinkle with the remaining cheese.
5. Bake in the oven at 200°C (400°F) mark 6 for 30 minutes. Cut the remaining bacon in half and roll up. Place rolls on skewer and grill till crisp. Use as garnish.
Makes 8

Below:
BACON CAKES
Children love these tasty bacon and cheese flavoured cakes, which are spiced with tomato ketchup and a dash of Worcestershire sauce. Serve them piping hot as a welcoming supper dish on a chilly winter's evening.

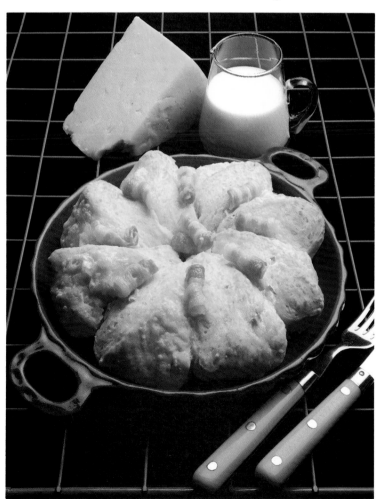

LAMB AND AUBERGINE MOUSSAKA

900 g (2 lb) aubergines, thinly sliced
salt and freshly ground pepper
vegetable oil
350 g (12 oz) lean lamb, minced
2 medium onions, skinned and chopped
45 ml (3 level tbsp) tomato purée
150 ml ($\frac{1}{4}$ pint) dry white wine
226-g (8-oz) can tomatoes, with juice
2.5 ml ($\frac{1}{2}$ level tsp) dried oregano
2.5 ml ($\frac{1}{2}$ level tsp) dried basil
30 ml (2 level tbsp) flour
75 g (3 oz) fresh breadcrumbs
15 g ($\frac{1}{2}$ oz) English butter
300 ml ($\frac{1}{2}$ pint) milk
75 g (3 oz) English Cheddar cheese, grated
1 egg yolk

Below:
LAMB AND AUBERGINE MOUSSAKA
Moussaka is really the Shepherd's Pie of Greece and all the Greek cooks have their own favourite recipes for it. Some will cover it with a cheese sauce, as we do here, others with batter or yogurt. Sometimes potatoes or courgettes are used for the layers instead of aubergines. For a traditional touch serve this delicious moussaka with a crisp green salad and a bottle of retsina, a traditional Greek wine flavoured with pine resin.

1. Sprinkle the aubergines generously with salt. Leave in a colander to drain for 30 minutes.
2. In a saucepan heat 15 ml (1 tbsp) oil. Brown the lamb well. Stir in the onion, tomato purée, wine, tomatoes and herbs with 15 ml (1 tbsp) flour. Bring to the boil, cover and simmer for 30 minutes. Season.

3. Rinse aubergines, squeeze and pat dry. In a frying pan, fry them a few at a time in hot oil, until brown. Drain well on absorbent kitchen paper.
4. Layer the aubergines in a 1.4-litre (2$\frac{1}{2}$-pint) shallow ovenproof dish, with the lamb and 50 g (2 oz) breadcrumbs.
5. To make the sauce, melt the butter in a pan, stir in the remaining flour and cook gently for 1 minute, stirring. Remove pan from the heat and gradually stir in the milk. Bring to the boil and continue to cook, stirring, until the sauce thickens. Remove from the heat, then stir in 50 g (2 oz) cheese and the egg yolk.
6. Spoon the sauce over the moussaka, sprinkle with cheese and the remaining breadcrumbs. Bake in the oven at 180°C (350°F) mark 4 for 45 minutes, until golden. Serve immediately.
Serves 4

VEGETABLE LASAGNE

225 g (8 oz) carrots, peeled and thinly sliced
225 g (8 oz) courgettes, trimmed and thinly sliced
1 onion, skinned and thinly sliced
100 g (4 oz) green pepper, seeded and thinly sliced
100 g (4 oz) celery, cleaned and thinly sliced
1 chicken stock cube
25 g (1 oz) English butter
30 ml (2 level tbsp) flour
300 ml ($\frac{1}{2}$ pint) milk
salt and freshly ground pepper
175 g (6 oz) lasagne
175 g (6 oz) English Cheddar cheese, grated

1. Place the vegetables in a saucepan with the stock cube and 150 ml ($\frac{1}{4}$ pint) boiling water. Bring to boil, cover and simmer for 10 minutes.
2. Melt the butter in a pan, stir in the flour and cook gently for 1 minute, stirring. Remove pan from the heat and gradually stir in the milk. Bring to the boil and continue to cook, stirring, until the sauce thickens, then add seasoning to taste. If the sauce is too thick, add a little stock from the vegetables.
3. Meanwhile, cook lasagne in a saucepan of fast boiling salted water, until tender, but not soft. Drain, being careful not to break lasagne sheets.
4. Make alternate layers of lasagne, vegetables and cheese (use 100 g (4 oz)) in a 1.7-litre (3-pint) shallow ovenproof dish finishing with a layer of lasagne. Top with the sauce, then sprinkle over remaining cheese.
5. Bake in the oven at 190°C (375°F) mark 5 for about 30 minutes.
Serves 4

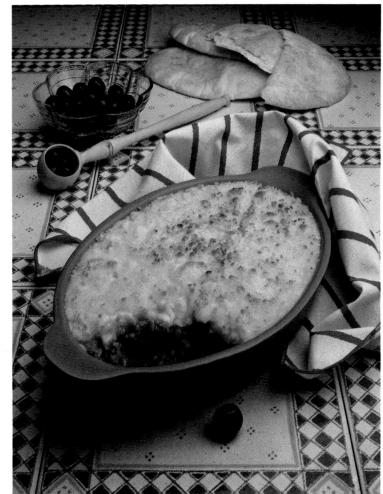

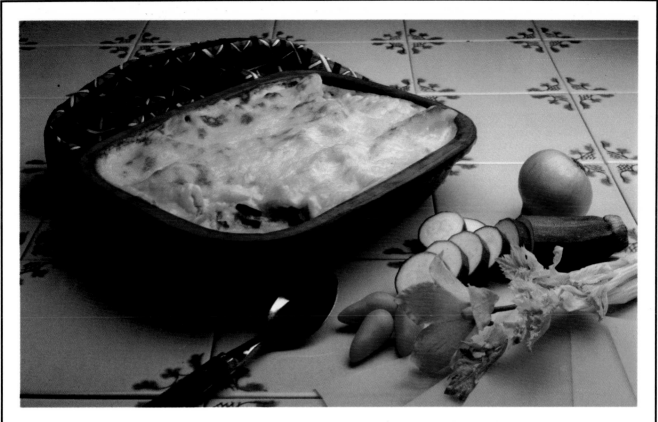

HIDDEN GREENS WITH SAUSAGE

450 g (1 lb) spring greens, washed and trimmed

450 g (1 lb) pork sausagemeat

50 g (2 oz) fresh breadcrumbs

salt and freshly ground pepper

25 g (1 oz) lard

40 g (1½ oz) English butter

40 g (1½ oz) flour

568 ml (1 pint) milk

15 ml (1 level tbsp) French mustard

100 g (4 oz) mature English Cheddar cheese, grated

1. Cook the spring greens with 45 ml (3 tbsp) salted water in a tightly covered pan. Drain well and finely chop. Return to a clean pan and cook, stirring over a moderate heat for 3–5 minutes to evaporate excess moisture.
2. Mix together the sausagemeat, chopped greens, breadcrumbs and seasoning. Shape into 12 small balls.
3. In a frying pan, melt the lard and brown the balls well on all sides. Drain and place in a shallow ovenproof dish.
4. Melt the butter in a pan, stir in the flour and cook gently for 1 minute, stirring. Remove from the heat and gradually stir in the milk. Bring to the boil and continue to cook, stirring, until the sauce thickens. Remove from the heat and stir in the mustard and cheese. Spoon the sauce evenly over the sausage balls.
5. Bake in the oven at 200°C (400°F) mark 6 for about 35 minutes, until golden. Skim well before serving.

Serves 4

VEGETABLE BAKE

25 g (1 oz) English butter

25 g (1 oz) flour

568 ml (1 pint) milk

salt and freshly ground pepper

pinch of grated nutmeg

450 g (1 lb) onions, skinned and thinly sliced

900 g (2 lb) potatoes, peeled and thinly sliced

175 g (6 oz) mushrooms, sliced

1 stick of celery, cleaned and chopped

150 ml (5 fl oz) fresh single cream

50 g (2 oz) English cheese, grated

1. Melt the butter in a pan, stir in the flour and cook gently for 1 minute, stirring. Remove pan from the heat and gradually stir in the milk. Bring to the boil and continue to cook, stirring, until the sauce thickens, then add seasoning to taste.
2. Combine the onions, potatoes, mushrooms and celery with the sauce and turn into 1.1-litre (2-pint) ovenproof casserole. Pour over the fresh cream and bake in the oven at 180°C (350°F) mark 4 for about 1¼ hours then remove pie from oven. Scatter top with grated cheese and return dish to oven for about 15 minutes until the vegetables are cooked.

Serves 6

Above:
VEGETABLE LASAGNE
Italy produces pasta in a huge variety of shapes and sizes and lasagne can be recognised by the fact it is made in flat sheets, each roughly the size of a postcard.

Before being layered in this recipe with vegetables and delicious grated English Cheddar, the lasagne is cooked until tender, but not soft, in rapidly boiling salted water. To avoid breaking it, lift out each sheet on a fish slice.

SPROUT AND MACARONI BAKE

700 g (1½ lb) brussels sprouts, trimmed
salt and freshly ground pepper
175 g (6 oz) wholewheat macaroni
75 g (3 oz) English butter
30 ml (2 level tbsp) flour
568 ml (1 pint) milk
175 g (6 oz) English Cheddar cheese, grated
75 g (3 oz) salted peanuts, roughly chopped

1. Cook the brussels sprouts in boiling salted water until just tender. Drain well. Reserve one-third of the sprouts. Roughly chop the remainder.
2. Meanwhile, cook macaroni in a saucepan of fast boiling salted water until tender, but not soft. Drain well.
3. Melt 25 g (1 oz) butter in a pan, stir in the flour and cook gently for 1 minute, stirring. Remove pan from the heat and gradually stir in the milk. Bring to the boil, and continue to cook, stirring, until the sauce thickens, then add 75 g (3 oz) grated cheese and seasoning to taste.
4. Stir chopped sprouts and macaroni into sauce. Season and spoon into a 1.4-litre (2½-pint) shallow ovenproof dish.
5. Melt remaining butter in a pan, stir in peanuts and remove from heat. Cut the reserved sprouts in half and arrange over sauce in the dish. Top with the remaining cheese and spoon over peanut mixture.
6. Bake in the oven at 190°C (375°F) mark 5 for about 35 minutes. Cover if the top is becoming too brown.
Serves 4

LETTUCE DOLMAS

225 g (8 oz) smoked mackerel fillet
125 g (4 oz) brown rice
1 large cos lettuce
50 g (2 oz) English butter
1 medium onion, skinned and finely chopped
45 ml (3 level tbsp) flour
150 ml (¼ pint) milk
142 ml (5 fl oz) soured cream
salt and freshly ground pepper
30 ml (2 tbsp) lemon juice
2 eggs, hard-boiled and chopped
100 ml (4 fl oz) chicken stock
fresh herb butter (see page 28)

1. Flake the fish and set aside. Discard skin and any bones. Boil the rice in a saucepan of boiling salted water for 40–45 minutes until tender. Drain. Set aside.
2. Ease off 12 lettuce leaves and cut out tough stalk from core end. Blanch a few leaves at a time in a saucepan of boiling salted water for 1 minute. Drain.

3. Finely chop a further four lettuce leaves. Melt the butter in a pan and soften chopped lettuce and onion. Stir in the flour, milk, soured cream and seasoning. Bring to boil and cook gently for 2 minutes, stirring. Add lemon juice.
4. Stir flaked fish, rice and egg into the sauce, and cool. Adjust seasoning.
5. Divide filling among the blanched lettuce leaves and fold each leaf into a parcel.
6. Pack in a single layer into ovenproof dish, pour over stock and cover tightly.
7. Bake in the oven at 200°C (400°F) mark 6 for about 20 minutes. Top with herb butter and serve.
Serves 6

CHEESE AND ASPARAGUS CHARLOTTE

5 slices of brown bread
English butter
298-g (10½-oz) can asparagus spears, drained
175 g (6 oz) English Cheddar cheese, grated
3 eggs
568 ml (1 pint) milk
salt and freshly ground pepper
pinch of mustard powder

1. Cut the crusts from the bread and butter one side of each slice. Place a layer of bread slices, butter side up and cut to fit, in a buttered ovenproof dish. Layer with the asparagus spears and half the grated cheese. Cover with the remaining bread, butter side down.
2. In a bowl, lightly beat together the eggs, milk and seasoning. Pour over the bread in the dish and leave to stand for 15 minutes.
3. Bake in the oven at 190°C (375°F) mark 5 for about 50 minutes, until set and lightly browned. Serve immediately.
Serves 4

HOT VEGETABLE LAYER

450 g (1 lb) potatoes, peeled and thinly sliced
175 g (6 oz) streaky bacon, chopped
225 g (8 oz) carrots, peeled and sliced
50 g (2 oz) mushrooms, wiped and sliced
100 g (4 oz) frozen sliced green beans
100 g (4 oz) English Cheddar cheese, finely grated
2 eggs, size 2
300 ml (½ pint) milk
salt and freshly ground pepper
2 tomatoes, sliced to garnish

1. Butter a 1.1-litre (2-pint) ovenproof dish. Place layers of potato, bacon, carrots, mushrooms, beans and grated cheese in the

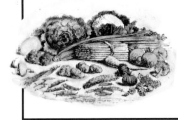

dish. Repeat until all ingredients are used, finishing with a layer of cheese.

2. In a bowl, beat together the eggs, milk and seasoning. Pour over the ingredients in the dish.

3. Bake in the oven at 180°C (350°F) mark 4 for 1–1½ hours, until set and golden in colour. Serve hot, garnished with tomato slices.

Serves 4

CHICKEN DISHES

CHICKEN JULIENNE

175 g (6 oz) long grain rice
40 g (1½ oz) English butter
40 g (1½ oz) flour
300 ml (½ pint) chicken stock
300 ml (½ pint) milk
350 g (12 oz) cooked chicken, cut into long narrow strips
30 ml (2 tbsp) lemon juice
100 g (4 oz) green beans, cooked
pinch of dried thyme
salt and freshly ground pepper
15 ml (1 tbsp) chopped fresh parsley
100 g (4 oz) carrot, peeled, cut into julienne strips and blanched
25 g (1 oz) flaked almonds, toasted

1. Cook the rice in a saucepan of boiling salted water until tender, but not soft. Set aside and keep hot.

2. Melt the butter in a pan, stir in the flour and cook gently for 1 minute, stirring. Remove pan from the heat and gradually stir in the stock and milk. Bring to the boil and continue to cook, stirring until the sauce thickens.

3. Gently stir in the chicken, lemon juice, green beans, thyme and seasoning and cook for 5–10 minutes until heated through.

4. Add the parsley to the cooked rice and toss lightly. Make a border of rice on a serving dish and spoon the chicken into the centre. Decorate with carrot and almonds.

Serves 4

DEVILLED DRUMSTICKS

50 g (2 oz) English butter
15 ml (1 level tbsp) demerara sugar
10 ml (2 level tsp) French mustard
2.5 ml (½ level tsp) salt
12 chicken drumsticks

1. Melt the butter in a saucepan and add it to the sugar, mustard and salt.

2. Place the drumsticks in a mixing bowl and pour over the butter mixture, turning the drumsticks to coat evenly.

3. When butter glaze has set, wrap each drumstick separately in foil.

4. Place on a baking sheet and cook in the oven at 190°C (375°F) mark 5 for 1 hour. Open up foil for last 20 minutes to brown.

Serves 6

Below:
CHICKEN JULIENNE
This elegant chicken dish is simple to make and is a delicious way of using meat left over from another meal. The term 'Julienne' refers to the technique of cutting the cooked chicken, or any other food such as raw vegetables, into long thin strips.

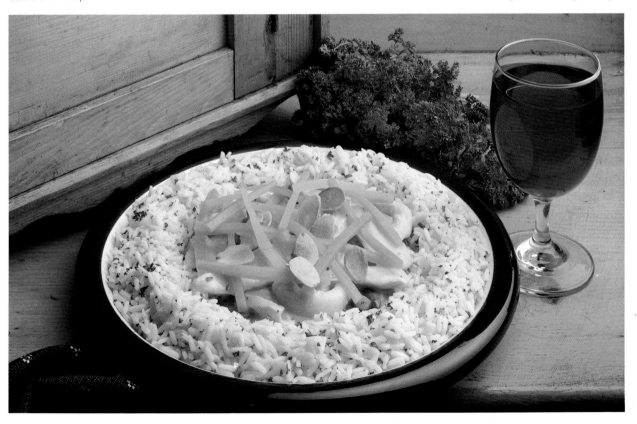

COOK'S TIP WHEN CHOOSING FRESH CHICKEN look for a bird which is plump, with a well rounded breast and thin, moist, tender skin. To test the age of a fresh chicken, hold the breastbone between finger and thumb. The younger the bird, the softer and more flexible the breastbone will be. Frozen chicken must be thawed completely before cooking. Thaw it at room temperature and not in the refrigerator. Thaw the bird in its wrappings and remove the giblets and neck as soon as they are free. A 1.4 kg (3 lb) oven-ready chicken takes 9 hours to thaw. Chicken joints need 3–6 hours to thaw.

HONEY BARBECUED CHICKEN

50 g (2 oz) English butter

100 g (4 oz) onions, skinned and finely chopped

1 garlic clove, skinned and finely chopped (optional)

396-g (14-oz) can tomatoes, with juice

30 ml (2 tbsp) Worcestershire sauce

15 ml (1 tbsp) honey

salt and freshly ground pepper

100 g (4 oz) long grain rice

4 chicken drumsticks

mushrooms, tomatoes and watercress to garnish

1. To make the barbecue sauce, combine the butter, onions, garlic (if used), tomatoes, Worcestershire sauce, honey and plenty of salt and freshly ground pepper in a saucepan. Gently cook for 30 minutes.
2. Meanwhile, cook the rice in a saucepan of fast boiling salted water until tender, but not soft. Set aside and keep hot.
3. Place the chicken drumsticks in the grill pan and brush liberally with the barbecue sauce. Grill for 10 minutes on each side, brushing frequently with more sauce.
4. Serve on a bed of rice garnished with grilled mushrooms and tomatoes and sprigs of watercress. Serve remaining sauce separately.
Serves 4

SPECIAL CURRIED CHICKEN

3 medium onions, skinned and sliced

25 g (1 oz) English butter

15 ml (1 level tbsp) curry powder

450 g (1 lb) cauliflower florets

225 g (8 oz) carrots, peeled and sliced

1 medium green pepper, seeded and chopped

2 sticks of celery, cleaned and chopped

450 g (1 lb) cooked chicken, chopped

150 ml (¼ pint) milk

30 ml (2 level tbsp) mango chutney

salt and freshly ground pepper

1. Fry the onion in butter in a large pan until soft. Stir in the curry powder and cook for another 2 minutes. Add the rest of the vegetables, the chicken and milk.
2. Cover and simmer for 30 minutes. Stir in the mango chutney and season to taste.
3. Serve hot with a side dish of yogurt mixed with chopped cucumber.
Serves 4

CHICKEN CURRY

50 g (2 oz) English butter

2 onions, skinned and sliced

1 cooking apple, peeled and chopped

25 g (1 oz) flour

15 ml (1 level tbsp) curry powder

2.5 ml (½ level tsp) ground ginger

2.5 ml (½ level tsp) cinnamon

300 ml (½ pint) milk

150 ml (¼ pint) chicken stock

15 ml (1 level tbsp) mango chutney

salt and freshly ground pepper

350 g (12 oz) cooked chicken, chopped

1. Melt the butter in a large saucepan and fry the onion and apple until soft.
2. Add the flour, curry powder, ginger and cinnamon. Cook gently for a few seconds before blending in the milk and stock.
3. Stir in the chutney, salt, freshly ground pepper and chicken. Bring to the boil and simmer gently for 20 minutes. Serve with plain boiled rice and a dish of yogurt and chopped cucumber.
Serves 4

SPICED CHICKEN

25 g (1 oz) English butter

1 onion, skinned and chopped

50 g (2 oz) mushrooms, wiped and sliced

25 g (1 oz) flour

300 ml (½ pint) milk

salt and freshly ground pepper

350 g (12 oz) cooked chicken, chopped

1.25 ml (¼ level tsp) grated nutmeg

1.25 ml (¼ level tsp) ground ginger

142 g (5 oz) natural yogurt

2 egg yolks

lemon slices and chopped fresh parsley to garnish

1. Melt the butter in a saucepan and fry the onion and mushrooms. Remove vegetables from pan and set aside. Stir in the flour and cook gently for 1 minute, stirring. Remove pan from the heat and gradually stir in the milk. Bring to the boil and continue to cook, stirring, until the sauce thickens, then add seasoning to taste.
2. Remove from the heat and add the chicken, nutmeg, ginger, mushrooms and onions.
3. Blend the yogurt with the egg yolks, then add to the chicken mixture. Heat gently without boiling, until mixture thickens.
4. Serve garnished with lemon and parsley.

Variation
Substitute lamb or veal which is lean and tender for chicken.
Serves 4

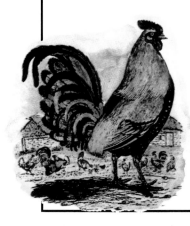

CHICKEN IN CELERY SAUCE

100 g (4 oz) English butter

4 chicken portions

1 small head of celery, cleaned and diced

25 g (1 oz) flour

450 ml (¾ pint) milk

¼ cucumber, sliced

15 ml (1 level tbsp) capers

salt and freshly ground pepper

1. Heat 75 g (3 oz) of butter in a pan and gently fry the chicken until tender. Keep hot. Cook the celery in salted water until tender, then rub through a sieve or purée in a blender.
2. Melt the remaining butter in a pan, stir in the flour and cook gently for 1 minute, stirring. Remove pan from the heat and gradually stir in the milk. Bring to the boil, add the celery, and continue to cook, stirring, for 5 minutes, then add the cucumber, capers and seasoning to taste.
3. Put the chicken on a hot serving dish and pour the sauce over.

Serves 4

Below:
HONEY BARBECUED CHICKEN
Tender moist chicken and sweet delicately scented honey are two foods which naturally complement each other. Traditional dishes combining these two ingredients are found throughout the world, especially in the Middle East and China. Try this mouthwatering recipe with its shiny barbecue glaze for an exciting new way of serving chicken.

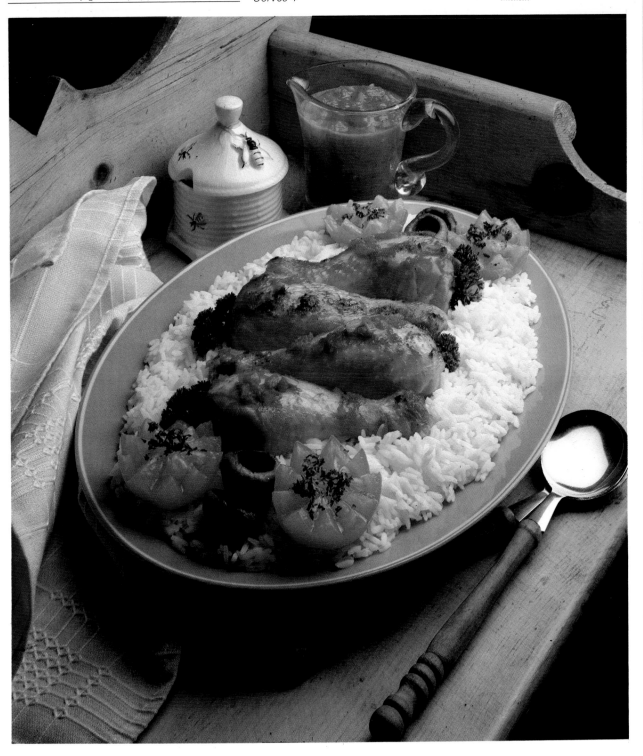

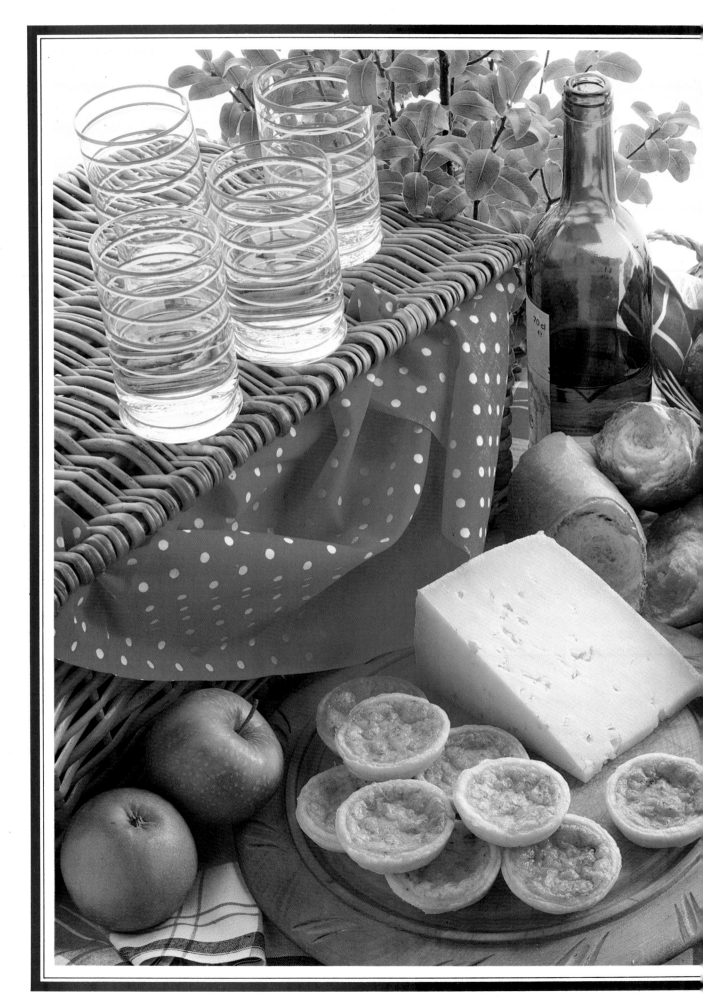

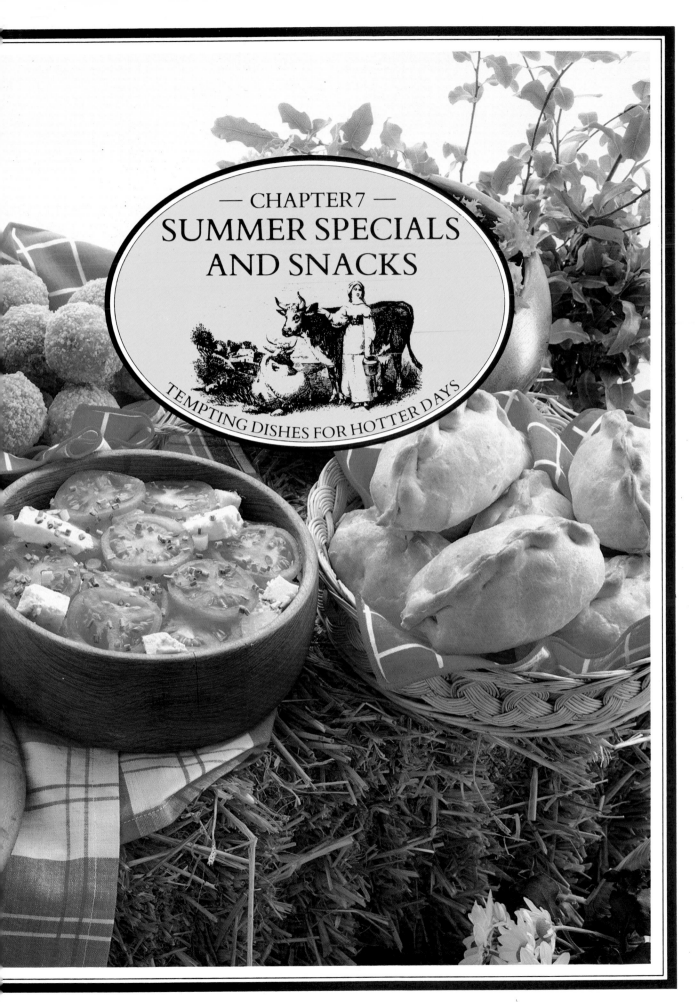

— CHAPTER 7 —
SUMMER SPECIALS AND SNACKS

TEMPTING DISHES FOR HOTTER DAYS

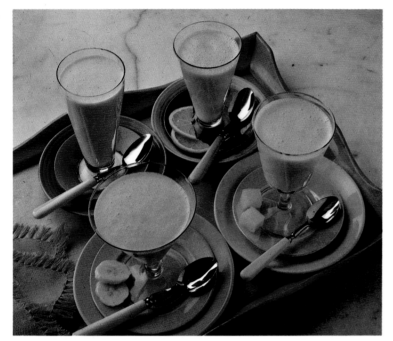

Above: clockwise from top
*HONEY AND YOGURT
COOLER, ORANGE
FRESHER, HAWAIIAN
QUENCHER, AND
NUTTY BANANA
WHIRL*
*A meal in a glass is a delicious
and time-saving way of keeping
your energy level high during
hot summer days. Using a
blender you can quickly whizz
up these four cooling and
nourishing ideas for leisurely
summer living.*

MEALS IN A GLASS

ORANGE FRESHENER

142 g (5 oz) natural yogurt
150 ml (¼ pint) fresh orange juice
slice of orange

1. Whisk the yogurt and orange juice together – a blender is useful here.
2. Pour into a serving glass and add a slice of orange.
Serves 1

NUTTY BANANA WHIRL

568 ml (1 pint) cool, fresh milk
1 banana, peeled and thinly sliced
5 ml (1 tsp) honey
dash of lemon juice
50 g (2 oz) almonds, chopped

1. Put all the ingredients into a blender and blend for about 1 minute until frothy.
2. Pour into tall glasses and serve immediately.
Serves 2

HAWAIIAN QUENCHER

142 g (5 oz) natural yogurt
150 ml (¼ pint) pineapple juice
5 ml (1 tsp) clear honey
fresh pineapple, cubed

1. Whisk the yogurt, pineapple juice and honey together until blended.
2. Serve in tumblers with pineapple cubes.
Serves 2

HONEY AND YOGURT COOLER

1 egg
15 ml (1 tbsp) honey
300 g (10 oz) natural yogurt
juice of 1 orange

1. Put all the ingredients into a blender and blend for 1 minute.
2. Pour into a tall glass and serve immediately.
Serves 1

The summer should be one long holiday when you can turn your back on the kitchen as often as possible. Summertime cooking should be relaxed and easy as you can make it, with light tempting meals that call for little, if any, cooking and the minimum of heat in the kitchen. These are ideal times for doing cook-ahead meals or for preparing hot dishes which can be finished off or reheated later. You should also take as much advantage as possible of all the lovely summer fruits and vegetables at their best, cheapest and most plentiful.

Cheese and eggs are very versatile and provide lots of inspiration for quick and easy meals and light snacks. Yogurt and soured cream give many dishes a sharp refreshing note that we all appreciate on hot, sticky days.

Summer days are salad days and they should be light, cool and tempting. The lightest and coolest of all hot weather dishes are the cold savoury mousses and soufflés, as delicate as they are delicious.

Summer is also the time for picnics and outings, long days spent swimming, sailing, walking, and generally using up energy. So we've included a section of substantial foods that can be packed up and taken with you, and also ones you can cook yourself over a fire out in the open, in the garden, on a camp site, picnic spot or on the beach.

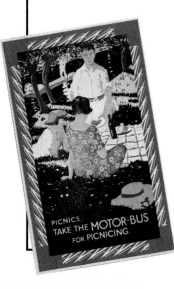

PICNICS.
TAKE THE MOTOR-BUS
FOR PICNICING.

SAVOURY MOUSSES AND SOUFFLÉS

PRAWN AND ASPARAGUS MOUSSE

300 ml (½ pint) milk
slices of carrot and onion
1 bay leaf
6 peppercorns
blade of mace
25 g (1 oz) English butter
30 ml (2 level tbsp) flour
15 ml (3 level tsp) gelatine
425-g (15-oz) can green asparagus
2.5 ml (½ level tsp) salt
freshly ground pepper
75 ml (5 tbsp) fresh double cream
200-g (7-oz) can peeled prawns
2 egg whites

1. For béchamel sauce, bring milk, carrot, onion, bay leaf, peppercorns and mace nearly to the boil. Leave off the heat to infuse for 10 minutes. Melt the butter in a saucepan, stir in the flour and cook gently for 1 minute, stirring. Remove pan from the heat and gradually stir in the strained flavoured milk. Bring to the boil slowly and continue to cook, stirring, until the sauce thickens.
2. Sprinkle gelatine over 45 ml (3 tbsp) water in a small bowl and leave to soak. When swelled up, beat into the hot sauce, stir to dissolve. Turn into a basin, cover closely and allow to cool but not set.
3. Reserve a few pieces of asparagus for garnish. Purée the rest in a blender with the sauce. Season.
4. Lightly whip the fresh cream. Fold into the puréed mixture with the prawns (reserving 6 to garnish) and whisked egg white. Turn into individual dishes and refrigerate to set. Garnish with the reserved prawns and asparagus.

Serves 6

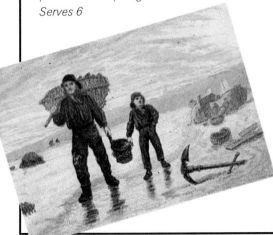

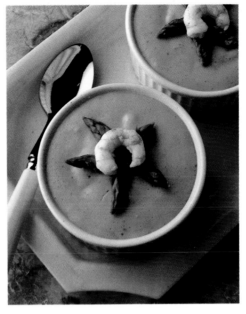

Left:
PRAWN AND ASPARAGUS MOUSSE
Prawns and asparagus are foods with delicate and complementary flavours which are particularly appealing in hot weather. Serve this pretty mousse in your palest china for a cool and elegant start to a summer dinner party.

PARTY MOUSSE

1 egg, hard-boiled and chopped
chopped fresh parsley
600 ml (1 pint) aspic jelly
568 ml (1 pint) milk
2 bay leaves
20 ml (4 level tsp) gelatine
75 g (3 oz) English butter
90 ml (6 level tbsp) flour
900 g (2 lb) boiled bacon, roughly chopped
1 onion, skinned and roughly chopped
30 ml (2 tbsp) creamed horseradish
120 ml (8 tbsp) fresh double cream
30 ml (2 tbsp) sherry
salt and freshly ground pepper

1. Set the egg with the parsley and a little liquid aspic in the base of eighteen oval ramekin dishes each holding about 100 ml (4 fl oz).
2. Infuse the milk with the bay leaves. Sprinkle gelatine over 60 ml (4 tbsp) water in a small bowl and leave to soak.
3. Melt the butter in a saucepan, stir in the flour and cook gently for 1 minute, stirring. Remove pan from the heat and gradually stir in the strained flavoured milk. Bring to the boil slowly and continue to cook, stirring, until the sauce thickens. While still hot stir in the soaked gelatine until dissolved.
4. Place the bacon and onion in a food processor or powerful blender with the cool sauce and horseradish; blend until smooth. This will need to be done in several lots. Turn out into a bowl and stir in the fresh cream, sherry and seasoning to taste.
5. Spoon into dishes and refrigerate to set.
6. Run a warm knife around the mousses and dip the bases of the dishes in warm water for about 10 seconds to loosen the aspic. Turn out on to a serving platter.

Serves 18

PRAWNS can be obtained all the year round; they are at their best from February to October.

Fresh prawns are usually sold boiled in the shell and before using them, you pull off the tail and head and shell them. Uncooked prawns should be boiled for approximately 10 minutes in lightly salted water before being shelled. Ready-shelled frozen prawns are a good buy, but they often have less flavour than prawns which are bought whole.

COOK'S TIP WHEN PACKING PICNICS If you don't have a picnic basket, pack everything in a sturdy cardboard box.
Don't forget a corkscrew. Salt, pepper, sugar and milk are also essentials. A pocket knife is another useful item to pack.
Test your liquid containers to make sure they are leak-proof.
Take a kitchen roll to use as napkins and to wipe up spills.
Take a packet of straws as they make drinking from cans easier and less sticky.
Pack dressings separately from salads and add them just before eating. Prepare salads the night before and leave them to chill in the fridge. Pack them last thing before leaving so they're fresh and crisp.
Stick the tips of any sharp knives in a cork for safety.
Slice and butter rolls before leaving and seal them in plastic bags.
Carry a flan or quiche in the tin it was cooked in and cover it with foil.
Don't forget to take something to sit on.
Keep the countryside tidy by taking a spare plastic bag to carry all litter home.

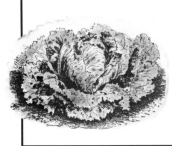

CHILLED HAM AND MUSHROOM SOUFFLÉ

175 g (6 oz) onion, skinned and chopped
100 g (4 oz) tomato, skinned and chopped
175 g (6 oz) button mushrooms, wiped and sliced
2 garlic cloves, skinned and crushed
65 g (2½ oz) English butter
40 g (1½ oz) flour
450 ml (¾ pint) milk
salt and freshly ground pepper
3 eggs, separated
175 g (6 oz) ham
15 ml (1 level tbsp) tomato purée
20 ml (4 level tsp) gelatine
300 ml (½ pint) aspic jelly to garnish

1. Sauté the prepared chopped onion and tomato, mushrooms (reserving a few for garnish) and garlic together in 25 g (1 oz) butter for 8 minutes – do not brown.
2. To make a sauce, melt the remaining butter in a pan, stir in the flour and cook gently for 1 minute, stirring. Remove pan from the heat and gradually stir in the milk. Bring to the boil slowly and continue to cook, stirring until the sauce thickens then simmer for 5 minutes. Season and beat in egg yolks.
3. Purée the vegetables, white sauce, diced ham and tomato purée together in a blender. Turn into a large bowl.
4. Sprinkle gelatine over 45 ml (3 tbsp) water in a small bowl. Place the bowl over a pan of hot water and stir until dissolved. Cool then add to the ham purée. Season well.
5. Stiffly whisk the egg whites and fold into the purée. Turn into a 1.6-litre (3-pint) soufflé dish and chill until set.
6. Garnish with the mushrooms and aspic jelly.
Serves 6–8

CHILLED SMOKED MACKEREL AND TOMATO SOUFFLÉ

300 ml (½ pint) mayonnaise
142 ml (5 fl oz) soured cream
30 ml (2 tbsp) horseradish sauce
15 ml (1 level tbsp) tomato purée
10 ml (2 tsp) anchovy essence
350 g (12 oz) tomatoes, skinned, quartered and seeded
350 g (12 oz) smoked mackerel fillets
salt and freshly ground pepper
15 ml (3 level tsp) gelatine
2 egg whites

1. Place the mayonnaise in a large bowl and stir in the soured cream, horseradish, tomato purée and anchovy essence.
2. Thinly slice the tomato quarters and flake the fish. Stir into the mayonnaise base; check seasoning.
3. Sprinkle gelatine over 45 ml (3 tbsp) water in a small bowl. Place the bowl over a pan of hot water and stir until dissolved. Cool then stir into the mayonnaise.
4. Stiffly whisk the egg whites and fold in. Turn into a 1.4-litre (2½-pint) soufflé dish and chill to set.
Serves 8

MAIN-COURSE SALADS

PRAWN AND PINEAPPLE SALAD

1 Webb or Cos lettuce
425-g (15-oz) can pineapple cubes, well drained
175 g (6 oz) fresh or frozen peeled prawns
175 g (6 oz) Derby cheese, diced
142 ml (5 fl oz) soured cream
paprika and cucumber slices to garnish

1. Wash the lettuce and shake leaves dry. Tear into bite-size pieces and use to cover four individual plates.
2. Mix the pineapple cubes well together with the prawns and cheese. Pile equal amounts on top of the lettuce.
3. Spoon over the soured cream. Garnish lightly with paprika and cucumber slices.
Serves 4

CRUNCHY SALAD

175 g (6 oz) Caerphilly cheese, grated
25 g (1 oz) walnuts, chopped
50 g (2 oz) sultanas
3 medium sticks celery, cleaned and chopped
1 small green pepper, seeded and chopped
2 red dessert apples, cored and diced
45 ml (3 tbsp) olive oil
25 ml (1½ tbsp) lemon juice
salt and freshly ground pepper
175 g (6 oz) ham, roughly chopped

1. Mix together the cheese, walnuts, sultanas, celery, pepper and apples, and toss together thoroughly.
2. Whisk the oil, lemon juice and seasonings together. Add to the salad and mix well.
3. Arrange the ham and salad mixture alternately on serving dish.
Serves 4

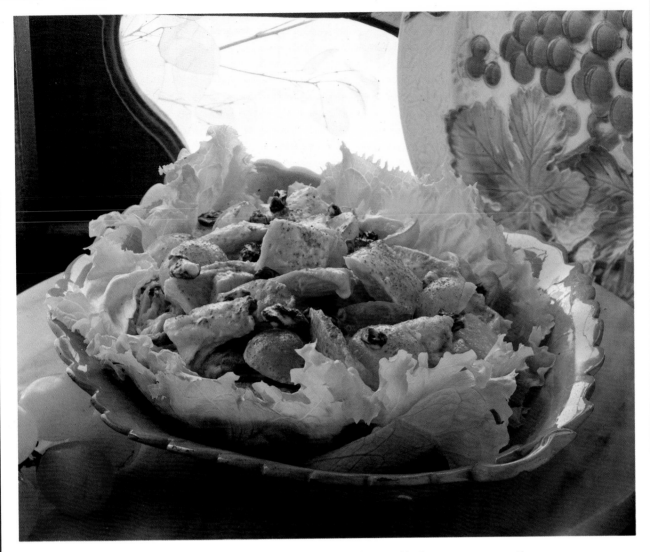

CHICKEN AND GRAPE SALAD

1.4 kg (3 lb) roasting chicken

1 onion, skinned

1 carrot, peeled

1 bay leaf

6 peppercorns

2 eggs

90 ml (6 tbsp) lemon juice (about 2 lemons)

45 ml (3 tbsp) clear honey

150 ml (5 fl oz) fresh whipping cream

225 g (8 oz) white grapes, halved and seeded

50 g (2 oz) raisins

salt and freshly ground pepper

lettuce and paprika to garnish

1. Poach the chicken with the onion, carrot, bay leaf and peppercorns in enough water to just cover, for about 50 minutes, until tender. Cool in the stock, then divide the flesh into bite-size pieces. Reserve the stock for soups, sauces or freezing.

2. Beat the eggs with 60 ml (4 tbsp) lemon juice and honey. Cook in a double boiler or in a basin standing over a saucepan of hot water until thick. Cover with damp greaseproof paper and cool.

3. Whip the fresh cream until softly stiff; fold into the cold lemon mixture.

4. To the grapes add the remaining lemon juice, then combine with the chicken, raisins, sauce and seasoning.

5. Serve garnished with lettuce and paprika, and accompanied by cold cooked rice.

Serves 4–6

Above:
CHICKEN AND GRAPE SALAD
White grapes, tender chicken and cream are a cool classic combination of foods which originated in French cookery under the name Chicken Véronique. Crisp and sharply sweet, the grapes provide an excellent contrast to the blandness of the chicken. Try this lovely recipe, accompanied by cold cooked rice, for a spectacular main course at a summer dinner party.

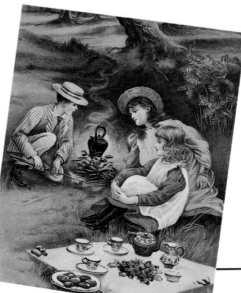

COOK'S TIP SOURED CREAM adds a delicious tangy note to many savoury dishes and can be bought ready for use. To make your own soured cream, stir 5 ml (1 tsp) lemon juice into 150 ml (¼ pint) fresh single cream and leave it to stand for 30 minutes.

COLD BEEF IN SOURED CREAM

30 ml (2 tbsp) corn oil
450 g (1 lb) lean rump steak in a thin slice, cut into thin strips
salt and freshly ground pepper
1 medium onion, skinned and finely chopped
225 g (8 oz) button mushrooms, wiped and thinly sliced
5 ml (1 level tsp) French mustard
10 ml (2 tsp) chopped fresh thyme or 2.5 ml (½ tsp) dried
1 green dessert apple, thinly sliced
142 ml (5 fl oz) soured cream
15 ml (1 tbsp) lemon juice

1. Heat the oil in a large frying pan. When hot quickly brown steak in a shallow layer, turning occasionally. Don't crowd the pan, the meat should remain pink in the centre.
2. Transfer the beef to a bowl using a slotted spoon. Season with salt and pepper.
3. Reheat residual fat; fry the onion until golden brown. Add the mushrooms, mustard and thyme. Fry over high heat for 1 minute. Add to the beef, cover and leave to cool.
4. Combine the apple with the soured cream and lemon juice in a bowl.
5. To serve, line a shallow dish with crisp lettuce. Combine contents of bowls. Check seasoning and pile into centre of lettuce. Tuck in slices of freshly toasted bread.
Serves 4

Below:
COLD BEEF IN SOURED CREAM
Combining thin strips of freshly cooked steak with a piquant soured cream sauce, this salad is an unusual summery version of Beef Stroganoff. Seasoned with mustard and thyme and combined with apple slices, it should be piled on a bed of crisp, green lettuce.

CHEDDAR CHEESE AND APPLE SALAD

½ round lettuce
142 ml (5 fl oz) soured cream
45 ml (3 tbsp) milk
5 ml (1 tsp) lemon juice
5 ml (1 level tsp) icing or caster sugar
1.25 ml (¼ level tsp) salt
2 dessert apples, peeled, cored and diced
225 g (8 oz) English Cheddar cheese, diced
2 canned pineapple rings, coarsely chopped
4 slices of orange, unpeeled, to garnish
8 black olives to garnish

1. Wash the lettuce and shake leaves dry. Tear into bite-size pieces and use to cover the base of a serving dish.
2. Combine the soured cream with the milk, lemon juice, sugar and salt.
3. Add the apples, cheese and pineapple to the soured cream mixture and toss lightly together. Pile over the lettuce and garnish with orange slices and olives.
Serves 4

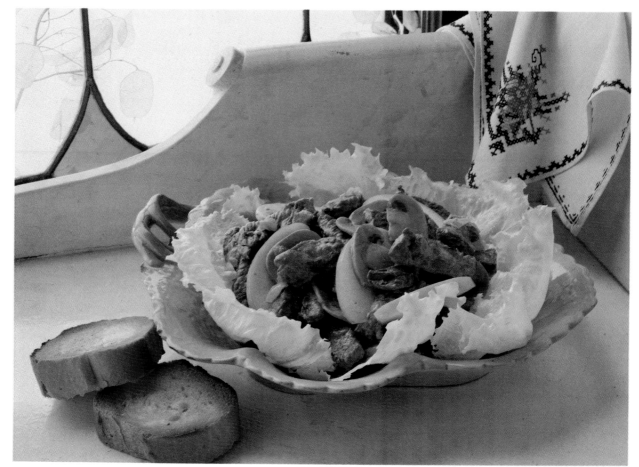

TURKEY PINEAPPLE AND PASTA SALAD

700 g (1½ lb) cooked turkey meat

45 ml (3 tbsp) oil

30 ml (2 tbsp) lemon juice

about 5 ml (1 level tsp) paprika

salt and freshly ground pepper

225 g (8 oz) wholemeal shortcut macaroni

300 ml (10 fl oz) soured cream

30 ml (2 level tbsp) horseradish sauce

30 ml (2 level tbsp) tomato ketchup

225 g (8 oz) celery, wiped and sliced

340-g (12-oz) can pineapple cubes, drained

25 g (1 oz) peanuts to garnish

1. Cut the turkey into bite-size pieces. Mix the oil, lemon juice, 2.5 ml (½ level tsp) paprika and seasoning and stir in the turkey. Leave in a cool place for about 1 hour.
2. Cook the macaroni in a saucepan of boiling salted water until tender, drain well.
3. Stir together in a large bowl the soured cream, horseradish and ketchup. Fold in the macaroni, celery and drained pineapple. Season well.
4. Stir the turkey into the macaroni mixture, cover and chill well. Adjust seasoning. Serve with lettuce garnished with peanuts and paprika pepper.
Serves 6

CHEESE AND CHICORY SALAD

2 large heads of chicory, wiped and trimmed

100 g (4 oz) Cotswold or English Cheddar cheese, cubed

1 green pepper, seeded and chopped

2 sticks of celery, cleaned and chopped

100 g (4 oz) radishes, trimmed and sliced

30 ml (2 tbsp) beef stock

salt and freshly ground pepper

90 ml (6 tbsp) vegetable oil

45 ml (3 tbsp) white wine vinegar

5–10 ml (1–2 level tsp) soft brown sugar

1 small garlic clove, skinned and crushed

100 g (4 oz) walnut halves

1. Chop the chicory coarsely. Place the cheese cubes in a salad bowl with the chicory. Add the pepper, celery and sliced radish and mix together.
2. Place the stock, salt, pepper, oil, vinegar, sugar and garlic in a screw-top jar and shake well to combine. Pour over the salad and stir in the walnuts.
Serves 4

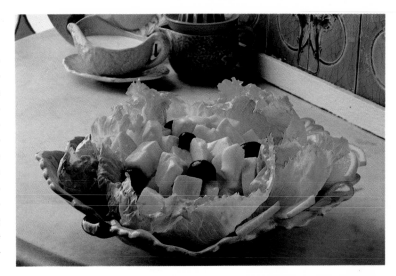

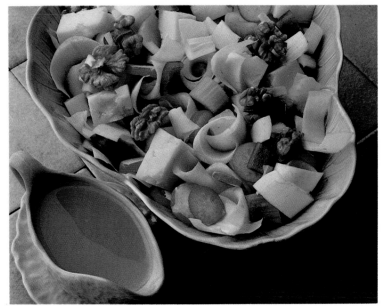

SIDE SALADS

COLESLAW

450 g (1 lb) white cabbage, finely shredded

4 stalks celery, cleaned and chopped

1 small onion, skinned and finely chopped

2 dessert apples, peeled and coarsely grated

30 ml (2 tbsp) vegetable oil

15 ml (1 tbsp) vinegar

5 ml (1 level tsp) sugar

salt and freshly ground pepper

15 ml (1 tbsp) mayonnaise

150 ml (5 fl oz) fresh single cream

1. Mix the finely shredded cabbage in a salad bowl with the chopped celery, onion and grated apple.
2. Stir in the oil, vinegar, sugar, salt and pepper, then the mayonnaise. Stir in the fresh cream just before serving the salad.
Serves 6–8

Above, top:
CHEDDAR CHEESE AND APPLE SALAD
A firm tasty cheese such as Cheddar is perfect with crisp tangy apples for salads. Choose firm apples such as Sturmer, Pippins, Granny Smiths or Blenheim Oranges for this delicious summer dish.

CHEESE AND CHICORY SALAD
Chicory is an unusual salad plant which has an interesting, faintly bitter taste which combines well with a good full-flavoured English cheese.

With the addition of crunchy celery, green pepper, walnuts and a mouthwatering dressing, this lovely recipe is an ideal way to enjoy chicory at its best.

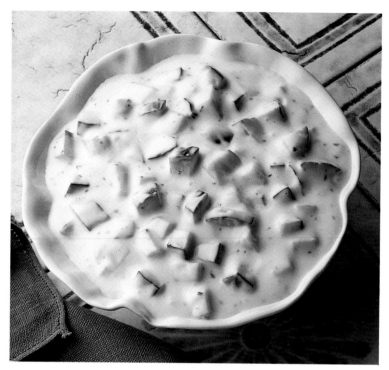

Above:
TZAZIKI
Tangy natural yogurt is widely used in the cookery of the Middle East and it is also the main ingredient of this cool, delicious salad which comes from Greece. For the best result, use fresh chopped mint, as well as the garlic, and chill the mixture well in the refrigerator to allow the flavours to develop. Serve it accompanied by hot pitta bread for the perfect start to a summer meal.

This dish is pronounced 'Zat-zee-kee' and it is usually offered as a starter on the menus of most good Greek restaurants.

STILTON AND TOMATO SALAD

225 g (8 oz) Blue Stilton cheese

450 g (1 lb) tomatoes, skinned and thinly sliced

small bunch of spring onions, trimmed and chopped

150 ml ($\frac{1}{4}$ pint) French dressing (see page 134)

chopped fresh chives to garnish

1. Cut the cheese into sticks; it does not matter if it crumbles.
2. Arrange the tomatoes and cheese in a shallow plate with the onions. Spoon over the French dressing. Cover and chill.
3. Sprinkle with the chives before serving.
Serves 4

TUNA PASTA SALAD

75 g (3 oz) small pasta shells

225 g (8 oz) small courgettes, cut into 0.5-cm ($\frac{1}{4}$-inch) diagonal slices

salt and freshly ground pepper

200-g (7-oz) can tuna fish

142 g (5 oz) natural yogurt

30 ml (2 tbsp) milk

5 ml (1 tsp) anchovy essence

15 ml (1 tbsp) lemon juice

12 small black olives, halved and stoned

paprika to garnish

1. Cook the pasta shells in boiling salted water, until just tender.
2. Add courgettes to the boiling pasta for the last 2 minutes of cooking time. Drain well and rinse under the cold tap.
3. Flake the tuna fish, reserving the oil.
4. In a large bowl whisk together the tuna oil, yogurt, milk, anchovy essence, lemon juice and seasoning.
5. Add the pasta, courgettes, tuna and olives to the dressing; stir gently to mix. Cover the salad and chill well before serving.
6. Spoon into individual dishes and dust with paprika.
Serves 4

TZAZIKI

$\frac{1}{2}$ medium cucumber, skinned and roughly diced

salt and freshly ground pepper

142 g (5 oz) natural yogurt (use a firm set yogurt if possible)

1 garlic clove, skinned and crushed

15 ml (1 tbsp) chopped fresh mint

1. Place the cucumber in a colander, sprinkle with salt and leave to stand for 30 minutes to draw out the juices. Rinse, drain well and dry with absorbent kitchen paper.
2. Place in a serving bowl. Pour over the yogurt, add the garlic, mint, seasoning and mix well. Cover and chill in the refrigerator before serving.
Serves 4

ONION AND OLIVE SALAD

900 g (2 lb) tomatoes, skinned and thinly sliced

175 g (6 oz) onion, skinned and thinly sliced

10 black olives, stoned and thinly sliced

142 ml (5 fl oz) soured cream

15 ml (1 tbsp) tarragon vinegar

10 ml (2 level tsp) French mustard

salt and freshly ground pepper

1. Combine the tomatoes, onions and olives. Whisk the rest of the ingredients together.
2. At serving time, toss all the ingredients gently together.
Serves 8

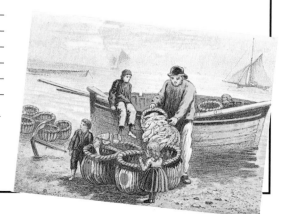

APPLE AND WALNUT SALAD

6 red apples

300 ml (10 fl oz) natural yogurt

30 ml (2 tbsp) lemon juice

salt and freshly ground pepper

125 g (4 oz) walnuts, chopped

1. About 2 hours ahead, core and roughly chop the apples. In a large bowl combine the yogurt, lemon juice and plenty of seasoning. Stir in the apple to coat evenly.
2. Cover with cling film and leave in a cool place. Just before serving stir in the chopped walnuts.
Serves 8

RED CABBAGE AND APPLE SALAD

$\frac{1}{2}$ red cabbage, about 900 g (2 lb), finely shredded

3 dessert apples, peeled, cored and sliced

1 small garlic clove, skinned

300 ml ($\frac{1}{2}$ pint) salad oil

150 ml ($\frac{1}{4}$ pint) cider vinegar

60 ml (4 tbsp) natural yogurt

salt and freshly ground pepper

1. Blanch the cabbage for 2–3 minutes in boiling salted water. Do not overblanch as it will lose its crisp texture. Drain and cool.
2. Combine the apple with the cabbage in a bowl. Put the rest of the ingredients in a screw-top jar, shake well. Pour at once over the cabbage, toss.
3. Refrigerate the salad covered overnight. Toss again to mix well before serving.
Serves 8

ENDIVE, ORANGE AND WALNUT SALAD

2 endive

6 oranges

25 g (1 oz) walnuts, chopped

15 ml (1 level tbsp) caster sugar

142 ml (5 fl oz) soured cream

salt and freshly ground pepper

60 ml (4 tbsp) corn oil

30 ml (2 tbsp) lemon juice

1. Pull the endive apart, wash, dry thoroughly. Tear into pieces. Place in a salad bowl.
2. Grate the rind of one orange into a bowl and squeeze in the juice. Remove the skin and all pith from the remaining oranges and segment free of membrane. Add to the endive. Add the walnuts. Cover and keep refrigerated.

3. Just before serving combine the sugar, soured cream, seasoning, reserved orange juice and rind. Beat in the oil gradually and stir in the lemon juice. Spoon completed dressing over the endive and then toss the mixture lightly with two forks.
Serves 8

DRESSINGS

TOMATO AND YOGURT DRESSING

60 ml (4 tbsp) olive or corn oil

5 ml (1 level tsp) salt

5 ml (1 level tsp) caster sugar

30 ml (2 tbsp) wine vinegar

300 ml ($\frac{1}{2}$ pint) tomato juice

142 g (5 oz) natural yogurt

10 ml (2 level tsp) grated onion

30 ml (2 tbsp) horseradish sauce

freshly ground pepper

1. Place the oil, salt, sugar, vinegar and tomato juice in a bowl and whisk well together.
2. Gradually whisk in the yogurt, followed by the grated onion and horseradish. Season well with pepper.
3. This dressing can be kept for up to 1 week in a screw-topped jar in the refrigerator.
Makes 600 ml (1 pint)

COOK'S TIP YOGURT can be a useful and delicious part of a slimming diet, as it is naturally low in calories. In summer it is ideal for use in tangy salad dressings. For the lowest calorie count, slimmers should choose the fat-free and low-fat natural varieties rather than the fruit flavoured or whole fruit yogurts. To make your own yogurt see page 29.

Below:
RED CABBAGE AND APPLE SALAD
Red cabbage and apples are two crisp, delicious foods which traditionally complement each other. Try this delicious colourful salad with its tangy dressing of natural yogurt, cider vinegar and a hint of garlic.

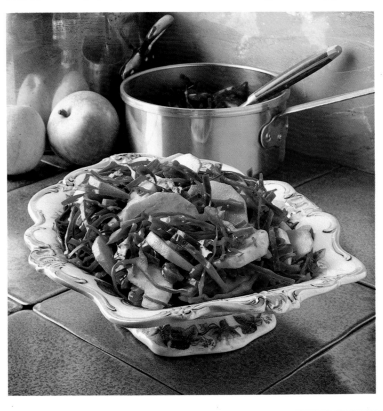

YOGURT DRESSING

142 g (5 oz) natural yogurt
15 ml (1 tbsp) salad oil
5–10 ml (1–2 tsp) cider or wine vinegar
5 ml (1 level tsp) wholegrain mustard

1. Mix all the ingredients well together and chill before serving.
Makes 150 ml ($\frac{1}{4}$ pint)

FRENCH DRESSING

90 ml (6 tbsp) vegetable oil
45 ml (3 tbsp) wine vinegar
pinch of sugar
2.5 ml ($\frac{1}{2}$ level tsp) French mustard
Salt and freshly ground pepper

1. Mix all ingredients well together.
Makes about 150 ml ($\frac{1}{4}$ pint)

Below:
OPEN SANDWICHES
Strictly speaking, these colourful and appetising sandwiches are not really sandwiches at all. In Denmark where they originated, they are called smørrebrød. Rye bread is traditionally used as a base, but other firm-textured types of bread can be substituted. When serving smørrebrød at a party, allow about 3 per person. In Denmark open sandwiches are usually eaten with a knife and fork, rather than fingers.
Left to right, numbers 11, 2, 13, 15 and 20.

OPEN SANDWICHES

1. Ham, cubes of Derby cheese and pineapple rings.

2. Salami, Caerphilly and tomato.
3. Finely grated Leicestershire cheese blended with a little fresh cream topped with dates and shredded lettuce.
4. Finely grated Wensleydale cheese blended with mayonnaise and topped with hard-boiled egg.
5. Finely grated English Cheshire cheese, liver sausage and potato salad.
6. Slices of Ilchester cheese, cold beef and grated carrot.
7. Banana slices (tossed in lemon juice), grilled bacon topped with grated White Stilton cheese.
8. Double Gloucester cheese, pickle and cucumber.
9. Blue Wensleydale cheese, and apple slices.
10. Cold pork, grated Nutwood cheese and apple slices.
11. Lettuce, slices of Blue Stilton cheese and ham rolls.
12. Mild English Cheddar cheese slices, watercress and tomato slices.
13. Crisp lettuce, grated Lancashire cheese and peach slices.
14. Slices of mature English Cheddar cheese topped with peanut butter and salted peanuts.
15. Slices of Lymswold cheese with halved green grapes.
16. Shredded cooked chicken topped with grated Windsor Red cheese.

(continued on p. 135)

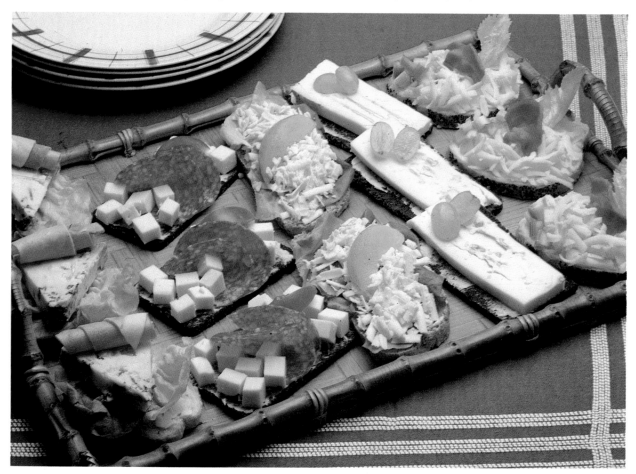

17. Slices of corned beef, grated Sherwood cheese and tomato slices.
18. Cubes of Huntsmen cheese and apple mixed with a little fresh cream or natural yogurt.
19. Chipolata sausages topped with finely grated Cotswold cheese.
20. Finely grated Charnwood or Applewood cheese topped with finely chopped celery and crispy bacon.
21. Slices of Walton cheese topped with pieces of apricot.
22. Crisp lettuce, pear slices, topped with finely grated Blue Cheshire cheese.
23. Chopped hard-boiled egg, mayonnaise and finely grated Cheviot cheese mixed together, topped with shredded lettuce and cress.
24. Finely grated Sage Derby cheese blended with a little mayonnaise topped with shredded turkey and sweetcorn.
25. Cubes of Rutland cheese, chopped celery in a little double cream flavoured with horseradish.

Garnish all sandwiches with sprigs of parsley or watercress. A knife and fork is needed to eat an open sandwich.

PICNICS AND PACKED LUNCHES

SAUSAGE BARS

368-g (13-oz) packet frozen puff pastry, thawed
1 large onion, skinned and finely chopped
225 g (8 oz) sausagemeat
175 g (6 oz) English Cheddar cheese, grated
30 ml (2 tbsp) tomato purée
30 ml (2 tbsp) fresh breadcrumbs
1 egg, beaten
salt and freshly ground pepper
milk to glaze

1. Roll out the pastry into an oblong, approximately 35.5 × 25.5 cm (14 × 10 inches). Place on a dampened baking tray.
2. Combine the onion, sausagemeat, cheese, tomato purée, breadcrumbs, egg, salt and freshly ground pepper, then place in a strip down the centre of the pastry.
3. Dampen edges of pastry and seal together. Turn pastry over so that the join is underneath. Make diagonal cuts in the pastry with a sharp knife; brush with milk.
4. Bake in the oven at 200°C (400°F) mark 6 for 35–40 minutes. Serve the Sausage Bars hot or cold, cut into slices.
Serves 4

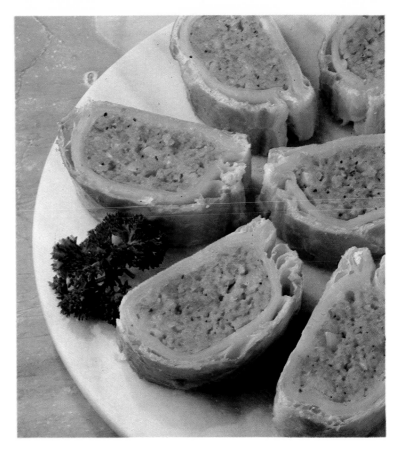

CORNISH PASTIES

225g (8 oz) shortcrust pastry (see page 230)
175 g (6 oz) skirt of beef or chuck steak
2 potatoes, peeled and coarsely grated
1 small turnip, peeled and coarsely grated
1 onion, skinned and finely chopped
salt and freshly ground pepper
40 g (1½ oz) English butter
1 egg to glaze

1. Roll out the pastry on a lightly floured board and, using a large saucer as a guide, cut out four circles.
2. Trim any excess fat from the beef and cut or scrape the meat into paper-thin slices with a sharp knife. Mix the meat with the vegetables.
3. Pile the filling in the centre of each pastry circle. Season with salt and freshly ground pepper and top with a knob of butter.
4. Dampen the pastry edges with cold water and carefully draw up two edges to meet on top of the filling. Pinch and twist the pastry firmly together to form a neat fluted and curve pattern. Cut a small air vent in the side of each.
5. Brush the pasties with the lightly beaten egg and place them on a buttered baking tray.
6. Bake in the oven at 220°C (425°F) mark 7 for 10 minutes. Reduce the heat to 180°C (350°F) mark 4 and bake for a further 30 minutes.
Serves 4

Above:
SAUSAGE BARS
These popular and tasty sausage bars are an ideal snack to take on a picnic. Pack the roll whole, but do remember to include a knife to cut it with.

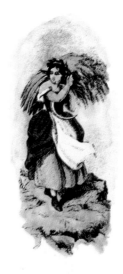

SARDINE TART

175 g (6 oz) shortcrust pastry (see page 230)

110-g (4½-oz) can sardines in oil

1 small onion, skinned and finely sliced

juice of 1 lemon

65 g (2½ oz) natural yogurt

65 ml (2½ fl oz) fresh single cream

50 g (2 oz) cottage cheese

2 eggs, beaten

salt and freshly ground pepper

fresh parsley to garnish

1. Roll out the pastry and use to line an
18-cm (7-inch) flan ring.
2. Drain the oil from the sardines into a small
pan and use to fry the onion until soft.
Remove from the pan and place on the base
of the flan case. Sprinkle with half the lemon
juice.
3. Beat together the yogurt, fresh cream,
cottage cheese, eggs and seasoning. Pour
over the onions. Arrange the sardines on top
like the spokes of a wheel. Sprinkle with the
remaining lemon juice and freshly ground
pepper.
4. Bake in the oven at 220°C (425°F) mark 7
for 15 minutes then reduce the temperature
to 180°C (350°F) mark 4 for a further 25
minutes. Serve hot or cold garnished with
parsley.
Serves 4–6

CHEESE AND BACON BANNOCK

225 g (8 oz) self-raising flour

salt and freshly ground pepper

50 g (2 oz) English butter

1 egg, beaten

120 ml (8 tbsp) milk

100 g (4 oz) streaky bacon, chopped

50 g (2 oz) English butter

100 g (4 oz) English Cheddar cheese, grated

1. Place the flour and a pinch of salt in a
mixing bowl and rub in the butter. Mix in the
egg and 90 ml (6 tbsp) milk to make a soft
dough.
2. Turn on to a floured work surface and
knead lightly into a round. Dust with flour
and mark into six sections. Place on a
buttered baking tray. Bake in the oven at
230°C (450°F) mark 8 for 10–15 minutes,
until well risen and golden brown.
3. To make the filling, fry the bacon lightly.
Beat the butter, grated cheese, seasoning
and remaining milk together to make a
smooth spread. Mix in the cold bacon.
4. Split the bannock in half and fill with the
cheese and bacon mixture. Eat hot or cold.
Serves 6

Below:
*CHEESE AND BACON
BANNOCK*
*The name bannock comes from
the Latin word 'panicum'
meaning 'bread'. It is a large
flattish cake, usually round,
traditionally made in Scotland
and the north of England. In
this recipe the bannock is split in
half and filled with cheese and
bacon for a tasty supper dish.*

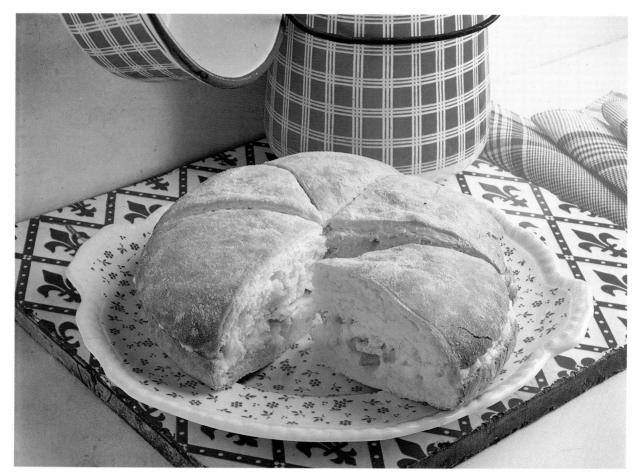

FARMHOUSE TEABREAD

50 g (2 oz) streaky bacon, chopped

1 onion, skinned and chopped

2 sticks of celery, cleaned and chopped

225 g (8 oz) self-raising flour

salt and freshly ground pepper

25 g (1 oz) English butter

1 egg, beaten

150 ml ($\frac{1}{4}$ pint) milk

15 ml (1 tbsp) chopped fresh parsley

2.5 ml ($\frac{1}{2}$ tsp) mixed dried herbs

1. Fry the bacon in its own fat. Add the onion and celery and fry until soft. Allow to cool.
2. Sift the flour and 2.5 ml ($\frac{1}{2}$ level tsp) salt together and rub in the butter until the mixture resembles fine breadcrumbs.
3. Beat the egg and milk together. Season and add parsley and mixed herbs.
4. Add the bacon mixture to the dry ingredients. Stir in the milk and egg and mix to a soft batter consistency. Turn the mixture into a well-buttered 450-g (1-lb) loaf tin or 16-cm (6-inch) cake tin.
5. Bake in the oven at 180°C (350°F) mark 4 for 50–60 minutes, until well risen and golden brown. Turn out and serve hot or cold, sliced and spread with butter. Serve with soup, cheese or cold meats and salad.
Serves 4

SCOTCH CHEESIES

125 g (4 oz) English Cheddar cheese

450 g (1 lb) sausagemeat

15 ml (1 tbsp) French mustard

salt and freshly ground pepper

flour

1 egg, beaten

25 g (1 oz) dry breadcrumbs

1. Divide the cheese into twelve even-sized pieces.
2. Pound the sausagemeat with the mustard and seasoning until well blended.
3. Roll each piece of cheese in sausagemeat, making sure the cheese is completely encased.
4. Coat the balls lightly in flour, beaten egg and breadcrumbs in that order, pressing the crumbs on well.
5. Chill for 30 minutes to set the crumbs, then deep fry at 190°C (375°F) until golden brown. Drain well on kitchen paper. Leave until cold.
Makes 12

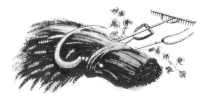

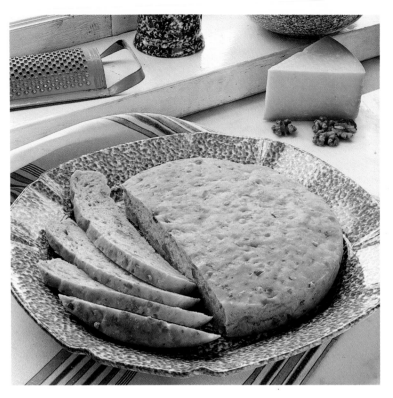

CHEESE AND WALNUT LOAF

15 g ($\frac{1}{2}$ oz) fresh yeast, or 7.5 ml (1$\frac{1}{2}$ level tsp) dried yeast

150 ml ($\frac{1}{4}$ pint) tepid milk

5 ml (1 level tsp) sugar

450 g (1 lb) strong plain flour

7.5 ml (1$\frac{1}{2}$ level tsp) salt

freshly ground pepper

5 ml (1 level tsp) paprika

1.25 ml ($\frac{1}{4}$ level tsp) bicarbonate of soda

50 g (2 oz) walnuts, chopped

75 g (3 oz) English Cheddar cheese, grated

300 ml (10 fl oz) soured cream

1. Butter a 25.5-cm (10-inch) shallow cake tin. Blend the fresh yeast with the milk and sugar. If using dried yeast, sprinkle it into the milk and sugar and leave in a warm place for 15 minutes until frothy.
2. Sift the flour, salt, freshly ground pepper, paprika and bicarbonate of soda into a large bowl. Stir in the walnuts and cheese.
3. Stir the yeast liquid into the flour. Stir in the soured cream and mix to a soft dough.
4. Turn on to a lightly floured work surface and knead for 5 minutes until smooth and no longer sticky. Cover with lightly oiled cling film and leave to rise in a warm place for about 1 hour until doubled in size.
5. Turn on to a floured work surface and knead for 2–3 minutes. Place in the cake tin and cover with lightly oiled cling film. Leave to prove for 30 minutes. Bake in the oven at 220°C (425°F) mark 7 for 35–40 minutes. Cool on a wire rack.
Serves 8–10

Above:
CHEESE AND WALNUT LOAF
Although English walnuts seldom ripen really well owing to the climate, traditional breads flavoured with the nut are common throughout the country. This mouthwatering loaf includes cheese for extra goodness and flavour.

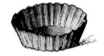

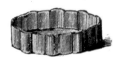

INDIVIDUAL CHEESE TARTS

100 g (4 oz) shortcrust pastry (see page 230)

75 g (3 oz) Red Leicester cheese, grated

150 ml (¼ pint) milk or fresh single cream

1 egg, size 2

10 ml (2 tsp) chopped fresh parsley

salt and freshly ground pepper

1. Roll out the pastry on a floured work surface and use to line twelve 5-cm (2-inch) patty tins.
2. Put the cheese into a bowl, add the milk or fresh cream, egg, parsley and seasoning. Whisk lightly together with a fork.
3. Using a spoon, divide the mixture between the patty tins. Bake in the oven at 180°C (350°F) mark 4 for 20–25 minutes.
Makes 12

SAVOURY SCONE WHEELS

75 g (3 oz) garlic sausage, roughly chopped

50 g (2 oz) salami, roughly chopped

25 g (1 oz) stuffed green olives, roughly chopped

1 medium onion, skinned, finely chopped

50 g (2 oz) English Cheddar cheese, grated

2.5 ml (½ tsp) dried basil

salt and freshly ground pepper

225 g (8 oz) flour

15 ml (3 level tsp) baking powder

40 g (1½ oz) English butter

150 ml (¼ pint) milk

1. Mix the garlic sausage, salami, olives and onion together with the grated cheese, basil and seasoning – go easy on the salt.
2. Sift the flour, baking powder and 2.5 ml (½ level tsp) salt into a mixing bowl and rub in the butter. Bind to a soft dough with the milk.
3. Roll out the scone dough to a rectangle about 30.5×18 cm (12×7 inches) and spread the salami mixture over the surface. Roll up from a narrow edge and cut the roll into eight slices.
4. Place cut side down on a lightly buttered baking sheet. Bake in the oven at 230°C (450°F) mark 8 for about 15 minutes. Cool on a wire rack.
Makes 8

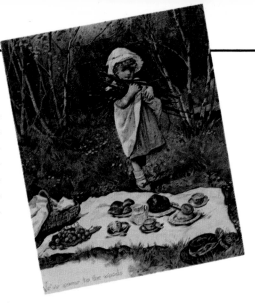

CELERY LUNCH LOAF

225 g (8 oz) self-raising flour

2.5 ml (½ level tsp) salt

1.25 ml (¼ level tsp) cayenne pepper

25 g (1 oz) English butter

125 g (4 oz) celery heart, finely chopped

125 g (4 oz) English Cheddar cheese, grated

15 ml (1 tbsp) chopped fresh parsley

150 ml (¼ pint) milk

1. Sift together the flour, salt and cayenne pepper. Rub in the butter. Stir in the celery, cheese and parsley and mix to a soft dough with the milk.
2. Knead lightly. For a cob-shaped loaf, form into a slightly flattened ball. Slash the top with a knife.
3. Place on a baking sheet, brush with milk and bake in the oven at 190°C (375°F) mark 5 for 45–50 minutes. Cover with foil towards the end of cooking time to prevent over-browning.
Serves 8

WHOLEMEAL TOMATO QUICHES

125 g (4 oz) plain flour

125 g (4 oz) wholemeal flour

150 g (5 oz) English butter

125 g (4 oz) spring onions, trimmed and snipped

8 small firm tomatoes

2 eggs

142 g (5 oz) natural yogurt

45 ml (3 tbsp) fresh single cream

5 ml (1 tsp) dried tarragon

salt and freshly ground pepper

1. Mix the flours together and rub in 125 g (4 oz) of the butter. Bind to a firm dough with about 60 ml (4 tbsp) water and use to line eight 10-cm (4-inch) individual Yorkshire pudding tins. Bake blind in the oven at 200°C (400°F) mark 6 for about 15 minutes.

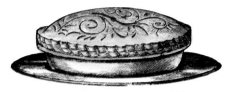

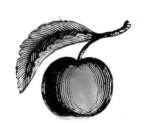

2. Fry the spring onions until golden in the remaining butter.

3. Skin the tomatoes and slice each one thinly into six pieces; arrange in overlapping circles in the pastry cases. Scatter the spring onions over the top.

4. Lightly whisk the eggs with the yogurt, fresh cream, herbs and seasoning and spoon carefully into the pastry cases.

5. Bake in the oven at 180°C (350°F) mark 4 for 20–25 minutes, until just set. Serve warm.

Makes 8

APPLE CAKE

225 g (8 oz) cooking apples, peeled, cored and chopped
225 g (8 oz) sultanas
150 ml (¼ pint) milk
175 g (6 oz) soft brown sugar
350 g (12 oz) self-raising flour
10 ml (2 level tsp) mixed spice
175 g (6 oz) English butter
1 egg, beaten
25 g (1 oz) demerara sugar

1. Mix together the apples, sultanas, milk and sugar. Sieve together the flour and spice, then rub in the butter. Add the fruit mixture and egg; mix well.

2. Place in a buttered and lined 20-cm (8-inch) square cake tin. Sprinkle with demerara sugar and bake in the oven at 170°C (325°F) mark 3 for 1¾ hours, until risen and golden brown.

Serves 6–8

STRAWBERRY FLAN

100 g (4 oz) shortcrust pastry (see page 230)
1 egg yolk
25 g (1 oz) caster sugar
15 g (½ oz) flour
2.5 ml (½ tsp) vanilla flavouring
150 ml (¼ pint) milk
450 g (1 lb) strawberries, hulled
30 ml (2 tbsp) red currant jelly
150 ml (5 fl oz) fresh double cream
15 ml (1 tbsp) milk
15 ml (1 level tbsp) sifted icing sugar
10 ml (2 tsp) orange juice or sherry

1. Roll out the pastry. Use it to line a 15–18-cm (6–7-inch) fluted flan ring resting on a lightly buttered baking tray. Prick well all over. Line with foil and bake blind in the oven at 200°C (400°F) mark 6 for 15 minutes.

2. Remove the foil, return the flan to the oven and bake for a further 15 minutes until crisp and golden. Remove and cool.

3. Beat the egg yolk and sugar together until thick and light. Stir in the flour and vanilla and gradually blend in the milk.

4. Pour into a small saucepan and cook, stirring, until the mixture comes to the boil and thickens. Simmer for 3 minutes. Remove from the heat and cool.

5. When completely cold, spread over the base of the flan case, cover with strawberries and brush with melted red currant jelly.

6. Beat the fresh cream and milk together until thick. Stir in the sugar and either orange juice or sherry.

7. Pipe or spoon the mixture over the fruit filling. Chill for 30 minutes before serving.

Serves 6

COCONUT BROWNIES

75 g (3 oz) English butter, cut into small pieces
50 g (2 oz) plain chocolate
125 g (4 oz) caster sugar
50 g (2 oz) soft brown sugar
2 eggs
100 g (4 oz) self-raising flour
100 g (4 oz) desiccated coconut
2.5 ml (½ tsp) vanilla flavouring
apricot jam to decorate

1. Place the butter in a medium basin. Add broken up chocolate and stand the basin in a pan of simmering water until the butter and chocolate melt. Remove from the heat.

2. Add the sugars, eggs, flour, 25 g (1 oz) desiccated coconut and vanilla flavouring and beat until smooth.

3. Spoon the mixture into a buttered and base-lined 28×18×3-cm (11×7×1¼-inch) oblong cake tin.

4. Bake in the oven at 180°C (350°F) mark 4 for about 35 minutes, until firm; cool in tin.

5. Cut into fingers, ease out of tin.

6. Brush brownies in diagonal strips with warm apricot jam, press reserved coconut on to the jam.

Makes about 16

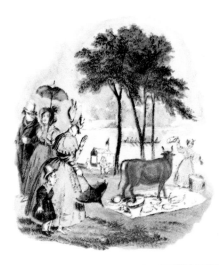

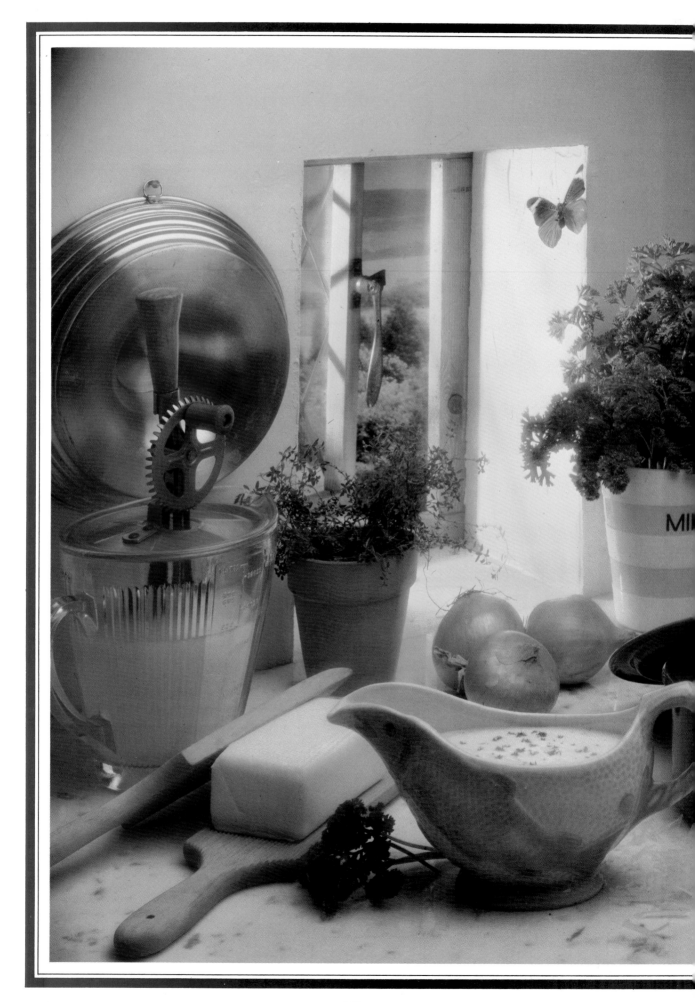

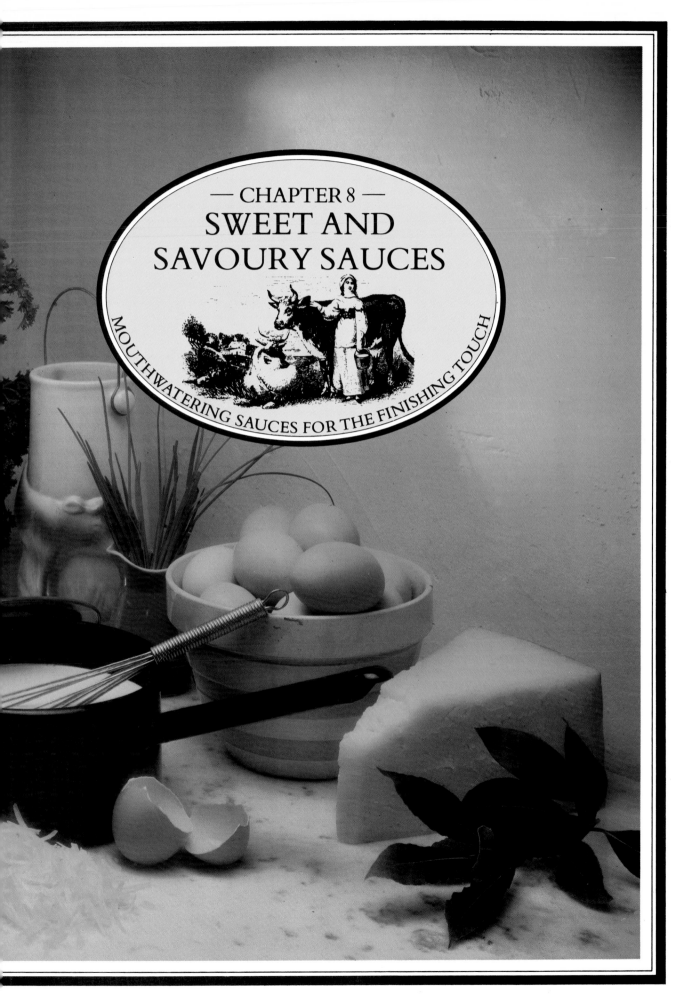

— CHAPTER 8 —
SWEET AND SAVOURY SAUCES

MOUTHWATERING SAUCES FOR THE FINISHING TOUCH

A good sauce can make a dish. It enhances the flavour of the food and can transform the simplest sweet or savoury dish into something special. A sauce is not difficult to make, once the basic principles are mastered – the right amount of flour to liquid and careful regulation of the heat while blending are probably the two factors that have the greatest bearing on the texture of the finished sauce.

Almost all the savoury sauces which we know best have been made in English kitchens for at least six hundred years. Bread sauce has always been served with roast chicken (and sometimes with pheasant or guinea fowl); mint sauce with lamb; horseradish with beef; chestnut sauce or stuffing with turkey; apple sauce with pork, goose or duck; mustard sauce with herrings; and gooseberry sauce with mackerel. All these sauces are traditional British accompaniments to roasts and grills, but there are many others to accompany vegetables and puddings which we also give here.

The secret in making a really smooth sauce lies in giving it your complete attention for the few minutes it takes to prepare it.

If a smooth sauce goes lumpy before boiling, a vigorous beating with a wire sauce whisk should help matters. If it's still lumpy after boiling you'll probably need to strain it through a sieve or blend in an electric blender – provided there are no additives which break down.

When making a basic white sauce in advance it's best to re-heat it in a double boiler to prevent sticking and scorching. To stop a skin forming, dot the surface with tiny flakes of butter which will melt and keep the surface moist. Whisk them in just before serving. Alternatively, keep the surface closely covered with buttered greaseproof.

To give a sauce a glossy finish add a last minute spoonful or two of cream, a knob of butter, or to make the sauce richer, an egg yolk. It's surprising what a difference these additions make as a last minute touch, but once you've added them don't re-boil the sauce or it will curdle. Reheat gently.

SAVOURY SAUCES

BASIC WHITE SAUCES
POURING SAUCE

● **Roux method**

15 g (½ oz) English butter

15 g (½ oz) flour

300 ml (½ pint) milk

5 ml (¼–½ level tsp) salt

salt and freshly ground pepper

1. Melt the butter in a saucepan. Add the flour and cook over low heat, stirring with a wooden spoon, for 2 minutes. Do not allow the mixture (roux) to brown.
2. Remove the pan from the heat and gradually blend in the milk, stirring after each addition to prevent lumps forming. Bring to the boil slowly and continue to cook, stirring all the time, until the sauce comes to the boil and thickens.
3. Simmer very gently for a further 2–3 minutes. Season with salt and pepper.
Makes 300 ml (½ pint)

COATING SAUCE

1. Follow recipe for Pouring Sauce (see above), but increase butter and flour to 25 g (1 oz) each.

● **One-stage method**

1. Use ingredients in same quantities as for Pouring or Coating Sauce (see above).
2. Place butter, flour and milk in a saucepan. Heat, whisking continuously, until the sauce thickens and is cooked.
3. Season to taste with salt and pepper.

● **Blender or food processor method**

1. Use ingredients in same quantities as for Pouring or Coating Sauce (see above).
2. Place the butter, flour, milk and seasonings in the machine and blend until smooth.
3. Pour into a saucepan and bring to the boil, stirring, until the sauce thickens.

Variations
Parsley Sauce

A traditional sauce for bacon, ham and fish dishes.

1. Follow the recipe for the Pouring Sauce or Coating Sauce (see above).
2. After seasoning with salt and pepper, stir in 25–30 ml (1–2 tbsp) finely chopped fresh parsley.

Onion Sauce

For grilled and roast lamb.

1. Follow the recipe for the Pouring Sauce or Coating Sauce (see opposite), but soften 1 large onion, skinned and finely chopped in the butter before adding the flour. Reheat gently before serving.

Cheese Sauce

Delicious with fish, poultry, ham, bacon, egg and vegetable dishes.

1. Follow the recipe for the Pouring Sauce or Coating Sauce (see opposite).
2. Before seasoning with salt and pepper, stir in 50 g (2 oz) finely grated English Cheddar cheese or 50 g (2 oz) crumbled Lancashire cheese, 2.5–5 ml ($\frac{1}{2}$–1 level tsp) prepared mustard and a pinch of cayenne pepper.

Lemon Sauce

For fish, poultry, egg and veal dishes.

1. Follow the recipe for the Pouring Sauce or Coating Sauce (see opposite).
2. Before seasoning with salt and pepper stir in the finely grated rind of 1 small lemon and 15 ml (1 tbsp) of lemon juice. Reheat gently before serving.

BLUE STILTON SAUCE

Use for vegetables such as courgettes, sautéed fennel and cauliflower

25 g (1 oz) English butter
30 ml (2 level tbsp) flour
400 ml ($\frac{3}{4}$ pint) milk
125 g (4 oz) Blue Stilton cheese, crumbled
salt and freshly ground pepper

1. Melt the butter in a saucepan. Add the flour and cook over low heat, stirring, for 2 minutes.
2. Remove from the heat and gradually stir in the milk.
3. Bring to the boil slowly, and continue to cook, stirring, until the sauce thickens. Simmer for a further 2–3 minutes.
4. Stir in the cheese and season well. Reheat but do not boil again.

Makes 400 ml ($\frac{3}{4}$ pint)

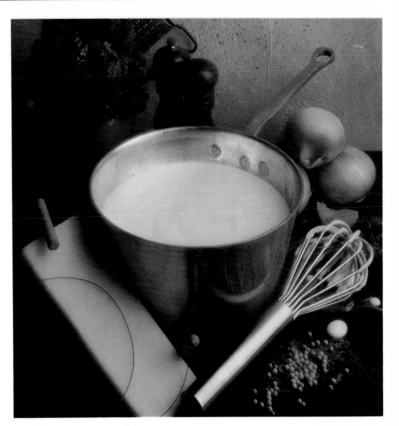

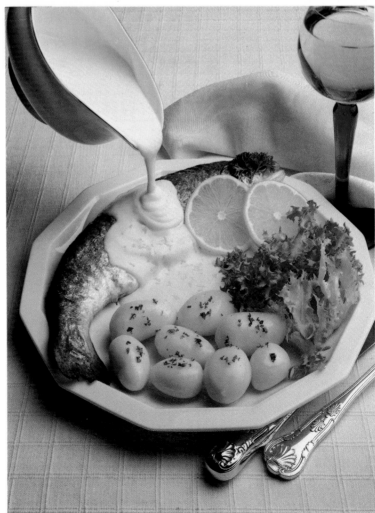

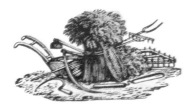

Right:
MUSTARD CREAM
SAUCE
Mustard powder is a mixture of one or more varieties of mustard seed (there are three: white, black and brown) and a cereal added to absorb the myronic oil the seeds contain. The Romans brought mustard to Britain and the plants still flourish in East Anglia, the area which supplies the entire home market. The fresh cream in this sauce is an excellent foil for the mustard's piquancy.

Below:
MILD CURRY SAUCE
A spicy sauce which dates back to the days of the British Raj. It is delicious and can be used to make a quick meat, fish or vegetable curry.

MILD CURRY SAUCE

Use for marrow, cabbage wedges, hard-boiled eggs or combining with pieces of cooked fish, chicken or meat.

1 medium onion, skinned and finely chopped
50 g (2 oz) English butter
15–20 ml (3–4 level tsp) mild curry powder
45 ml (3 level tbsp) flour
400 ml (¾ pint) milk, or half stock and half milk
30 ml (2 level tbsp) mango or apple chutney
salt and freshly ground pepper

1. Sauté the onion in the butter until golden in colour.
2. Stir in the curry powder and cook for 3–4 minutes. Add the flour and cook for 2–3 minutes, stirring.
3. Remove from the heat and gradually stir in the milk.
4. Bring to the boil slowly and continue to cook, stirring, until the sauce thickens. Simmer for a further 2–3 minutes.
5. Add the chutney and season well. Reheat to serving temperature.

Makes 400 ml (¾ pint)

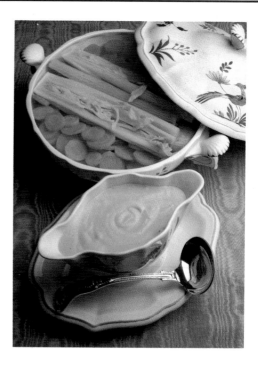

MUSTARD CREAM SAUCE

Use for carrots, celery hearts, herring, mackerel, cheese, ham and bacon dishes.

40 g (1½ oz) English butter
45 ml (3 level tbsp) flour
400 ml (¾ pint) milk
30 ml (2 level tbsp) mustard powder
20 ml (4 tsp) malt vinegar
salt and freshly ground pepper
30 ml (2 tbsp) fresh single cream

1. Melt the butter in a saucepan. Add the flour and cook over low heat stirring, for 2 minutes.
2. Remove from the heat and gradually stir in the milk. Bring to the boil slowly and continue to cook, stirring until the sauce thickens. Simmer for a further 2–3 minutes.
3. Blend the mustard powder with the vinegar and whisk into the sauce, season. Stir in the fresh cream. Reheat but do not boil.

Makes 400 ml (¾ pint)

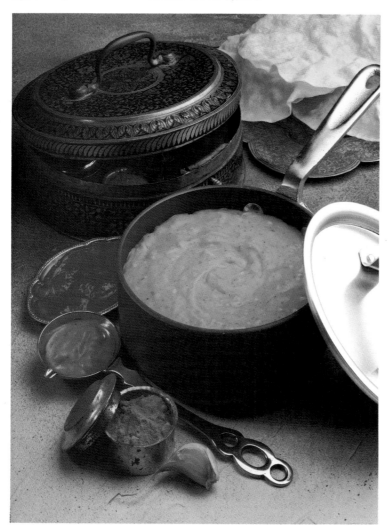

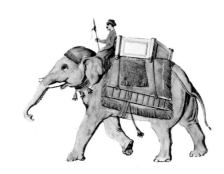

PIMENTO AND PAPRIKA SAUCE

Use for vegetables such as cauliflower, celeriac and marrow.

40 g (1½ oz) English butter

15 ml (1 level tbsp) paprika

45 ml (3 level tbsp) flour

400 ml (¾ pint) milk

salt and freshly ground pepper

5 ml (1 tsp) lemon juice

30 ml (2 tbsp) red wine

115-g (4-oz) can pimento, drained and thinly sliced

1. Melt the butter in a saucepan, stir in the paprika and flour and cook gently for 2 minutes, stirring.
2. Remove the pan from the heat and gradually stir in the milk, beating well after each addition.
3. Bring to the boil and continue to cook, stirring until the sauce thickens. Simmer for about 5 minutes.
4. Season. Add the lemon juice and red wine.
5. Add the pimento to the sauce. Reheat, and check for seasoning.
Makes 400 ml (¾ pint)

EGG SAUCE

Use for poached or steamed fish, or kedgeree.

300 ml (½ pint) Basic White Pouring or Coating Sauce (see page 142)

1 egg, hard-boiled and chopped

5–10 ml (1–2 tsp) chopped fresh chives (optional)

1. Follow the recipe for the Basic White Pouring or Coating Sauce.
2. Add the egg to the sauce with the chives. Season well and reheat for 1–2 minutes.
Makes 300 ml (½ pint)

CAPER SAUCE

Delicious with boiled lamb.

300 ml (½ pint) Basic White Pouring or Coating Sauce (see page 142)

15 ml (1 tbsp) capers

5–10 ml (1–2 tsp) vinegar from the capers, or lemon juice

salt and freshly ground pepper

1. Follow the recipe for the Basic White Pouring or Coating Sauce, using all milk or half milk and half the liquid in which the lamb was boiled.

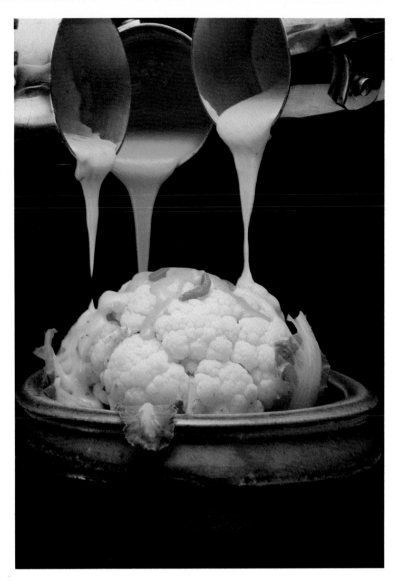

2. When the sauce has thickened, stir in the capers and the vinegar or lemon juice. Season well. Reheat for 1–2 minutes and serve.
Makes 300 ml (½ pint)

ANCHOVY SAUCE

A mouthwatering accompaniment to fish dishes.

300 ml (½ pint) Basic White Pouring or Coating Sauce (see page 142), made with half milk and half fish stock

5–10 ml (1–2 tsp) anchovy essence

squeeze of lemon juice

red colouring, (optional)

1. Follow the recipe for the Basic White Pouring or Coating Sauce. When it has thickened, remove it from the heat and stir in the anchovy essence, then the lemon juice and a few drops of colouring (if used), to tint the sauce a dull pink.
Makes 300 ml (½ pint)

Above:
SAUCY TOUCHES
From left: Prawn Velouté, Pimento and Paprika, and Blue Cheese Sauces. These are just three of the exciting sauces you can use to add variety to your favourite vegetables.

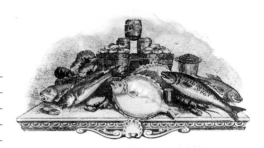

Opposite:
MUSHROOM AND
SHERRY SAUCE
Like many other sauces, this one
employs the same technique as
Basic White Sauce. The roux
(the flour and butter thickening
which is used) was introduced
into England in the seventeenth
century from Italy via French
cooks. Use a dryish sherry such
as fino, manzanilla or
amontillado in this excellent
sauce.

BÉCHAMEL SAUCE

Use for fish, poultry, egg and vegetable dishes.

300 ml (½ pint) milk
1 small onion, skinned and quartered
1 small carrot, peeled and sliced
½ small celery stick, cleaned and sliced
2 cloves
6 white peppercorns
1 blade of mace
1 sprig of parsley
1 sprig of thyme
1 bay leaf
25 g (1 oz) English butter
25 g (1 oz) flour
salt and freshly ground pepper
30 ml (2 tbsp) fresh double cream

1. Put the milk into a saucepan with the onion, carrot, celery, cloves, peppercorns, mace, parsley, thyme and bay leaf. Slowly bring just to the boil, then remove from the heat and cover the pan.
2. Set aside to infuse for 30 minutes. Strain, reserving the milk liquid.
3. Melt the butter in a pan. Stir in the flour and cook gently for 2 minutes, stirring. Do not allow the mixture (roux) to brown. Remove the pan from the heat and gradually stir in the flavoured milk.
4. Bring to the boil and continue to cook, stirring, until the sauce thickens. Simmer very gently for 3 minutes. Remove from the heat and season with salt and pepper. Stir in the fresh cream.

Variations
Cucumber Sauce
Stir in 60 ml (4 level tbsp) of grated, peeled cucumber before the seasoning.

Aurore Sauce
Stir in 30 ml (2 tbsp) tomato purée and 2.5 ml (½ tsp) caster sugar before seasoning.
Makes 300 ml (½ pint)

MUSHROOM AND SHERRY SAUCE

Use for vegetables such as broccoli, new potatoes and cabbage wedges.

400 ml (¾ pint) milk
1 piece of onion
1 piece of carrot
1 piece of celery
1 bay leaf
4 peppercorns
50 g (2 oz) English butter
125 g (4 oz) mushrooms, wiped and finely chopped
45 ml (3 level tbsp) flour
salt and freshly ground pepper
15–30 ml (1–2 tbsp) Madeira or dry sherry

1. Put the milk, vegetables (except the mushrooms), bay leaf and peppercorns in a saucepan and bring to the boil. Remove from the heat, cover the pan and leave to infuse for 15 minutes. Strain and reserve the milk.
2. Melt the butter and gently sauté the mushrooms for about 3 minutes. Stir in the flour and cook for 2 minutes.
3. Remove from the heat and gradually stir in the flavoured milk. Bring to the boil slowly and continue to cook, stirring, until the sauce thickens. Simmer for a further 2–3 minutes. Season and add sherry to taste.
Makes 400 ml (¾ pint)

SUPREME SAUCE

Use for poultry or fish and sometimes for meat and vegetable dishes.

300 ml (½ pint) Velouté Sauce (see page 148)
1–2 egg yolks
30–45 ml (2–3 tbsp) fresh single or double cream
knob of English butter

1. Follow the recipe for Velouté Sauce. Stir in the egg yolks and the additional fresh cream off the heat, and add the butter a little at a time. Reheat if necessary, but don't re-boil, or the sauce will curdle.
Makes 300 ml (½ pint)

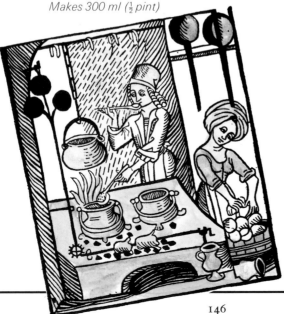

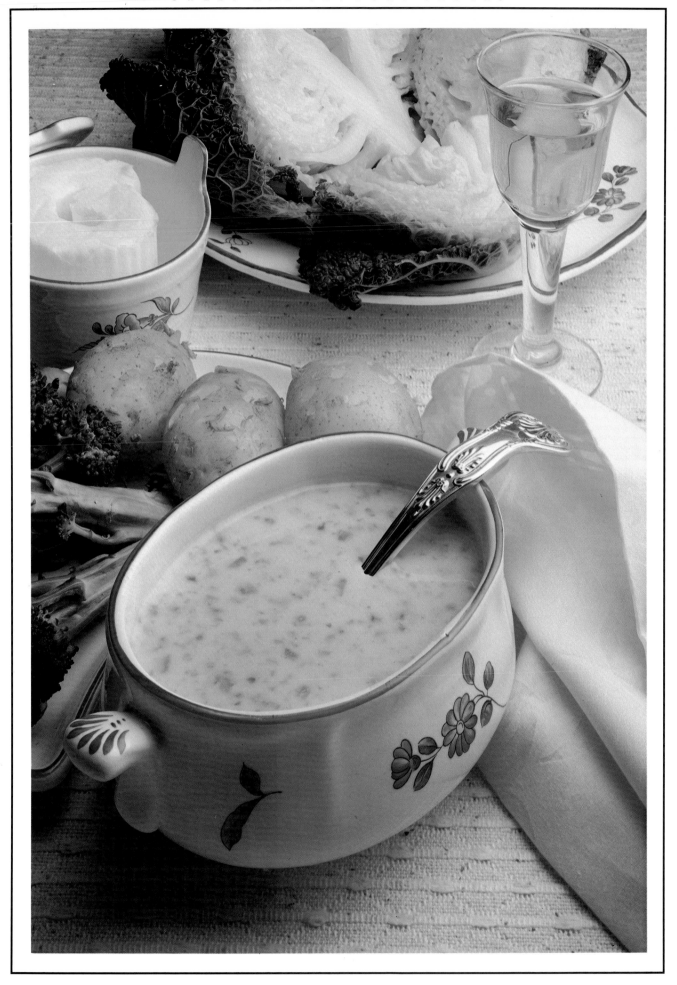

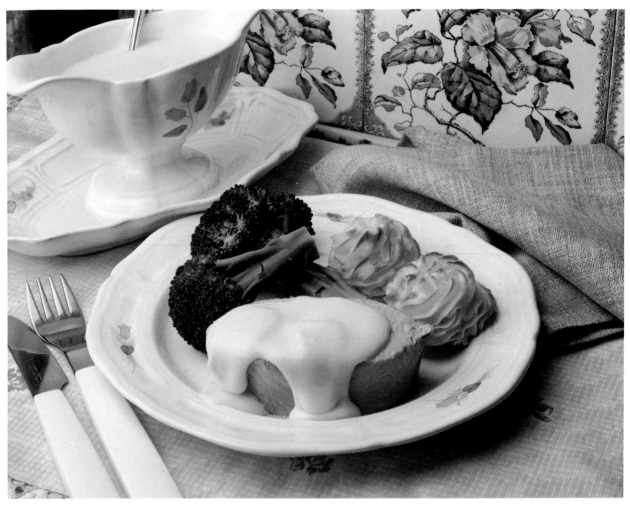

Above:
HOLLANDAISE SAUCE
This delicious sauce is Dutch in origin and is probably the most famous of all. It was one of the five basic sauces which the French chef Escoffier felt no self-respecting cook should be without. Hollandaise is simple to make (see opposite) and transforms the most ordinary dish into a special treat.

PRAWN VELOUTÉ

Use for vegetables such as courgettes, broccoli and cauliflower.

175 g (6 oz) fresh prawns
75 ml (5 tbsp) fresh double cream
40 g (1½ oz) English butter
45 ml (3 level tbsp) flour
300 ml (½ pint) chicken stock
2 egg yolks
15 ml (1 tbsp) lemon juice
30 ml (2 tbsp) chopped fresh parsley
salt and freshly ground pepper

1. Wash the prawns and remove the shells. Put the shells in a small pan with the fresh cream; bring to the boil then leave to infuse for 15 minutes. Divide the prawns into three.
2. Melt the butter in a saucepan, stir in the flour and cook for 2 minutes, stirring. Remove the pan from the heat and gradually stir in the stock. Bring to the boil and continue to cook, stirring until the sauce thickens. Simmer for 2–3 minutes.
3. Remove from the heat and add the egg yolks blended with the strained cream.
4. Add the lemon juice, parsley, prawns and seasoning and reheat gently without boiling.

Makes 300 ml (½ pint)

VELOUTÉ SAUCE

Lovely with poultry, fish or veal.

knob of English butter
30 ml (2 level tbsp) flour
400 ml (¾ pint) chicken or other light stock
30–45 ml (2–3 tbsp) fresh single cream
lemon juice
salt and freshly ground pepper

1. Melt the butter in a saucepan, stir in the flour and cook gently, stirring well, until the mixture is a pale golden colour.
2. Remove the pan from the heat and gradually stir in the stock. Bring to the boil and continue to cook, stirring all the time until the sauce thickens. Simmer until slightly reduced and velvety.
3. Remove from the heat and add the fresh cream, a few drops of lemon juice and seasoning.

Makes about 300 ml (½ pint)

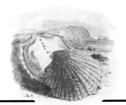

ESPAGNOLE SAUCE

This classic brown sauce is used as a basis for many other savoury sauces.

1 rasher streaky bacon, chopped
25 g (1 oz) English butter
1 shallot, skinned and chopped, or a small piece of onion, chopped
60 ml (4 tbsp) mushroom stalks, wiped and chopped
1 small carrot, peeled and chopped
30–45 ml (2–3 level tbsp) flour
300 ml (½ pint) beef stock
bouquet garni
30 ml (2 level tbsp) tomato purée
salt and freshly ground pepper
15 ml (1 tbsp) sherry (optional)

1. Fry the bacon in the butter for 2–3 minutes, add the vegetables and fry for a further 3–5 minutes, until lightly browned. Stir in the flour, mix well and continue frying until it turns brown.
2. Remove the pan from the heat and gradually add the stock (which can be made from a stock cube), stirring after each addition.
3. Bring to the boil and continue to cook, stirring, until the sauce thickens. Add the bouquet garni, tomato purée, salt and pepper.
4. Reduce the heat and allow to simmer very gently for 1 hour, stirring from time to time to prevent it sticking; alternatively, cook in the oven at 170°C (325°F) mark 3 for 1½–2 hours.
5. Strain the sauce, reheat and skim off any fat, using a metal spoon. Re-season if necessary and add sherry just before the sauce is served.

Makes about 200 ml (⅓ pint)

HOLLANDAISE SAUCE

Delicious with fish, egg, chicken and vegetable dishes.

5 ml (1 tsp) lemon juice
5 ml (1 tsp) wine vinegar
3 white peppercorns
½ small bay leaf
4 egg yolks
225 g (8 oz) English butter, softened
salt and freshly ground pepper

1. Put the lemon juice, vinegar, 15 ml (1 tbsp) water, peppercorns and bay leaf into a saucepan. Boil gently until the liquid is reduced by half. Leave aside until cold and then strain.
2. Put the egg yolks and reduced vinegar liquid into a double saucepan or bowl standing over a pan of gently simmering water. Whisk until the mixture is thick and fluffy.
3. Gradually add the butter, a tiny piece at a time. Continue whisking until each piece has been absorbed by the sauce and sauce itself is the consistency of mayonnaise. Season with salt and pepper, and serve immediately.

Variations
Mousseline Sauce
This is a richer sauce suitable for asparagus and broccoli, poached fish, egg and chicken dishes.
Stir 45 ml (3 tbsp) whipped fresh double cream into the sauce just before serving.
Makes about 300 ml (½ pint)

BÉARNAISE SAUCE

A classic sauce for meat grills and roasts.

30 ml (2 tbsp) tarragon vinegar
45 ml (3 tbsp) wine vinegar
15 ml (1 level tbsp) finely chopped onion
2 egg yolks
100 g (4 oz) English butter, softened
salt and freshly ground pepper

1. Put the vinegars and the onion into a saucepan. Boil gently until the liquid is reduced by about one-third. Leave until cold and then strain.
2. Put the egg yolks, reduced vinegar liquid and 10 ml (2 tsp) cold water into a double saucepan or bowl standing over a pan of simmering water. Whisk until thick and fluffy.
3. Gradually add the butter, a tiny piece at a time. Continue whisking until each piece has been absorbed by the sauce and the sauce itself has thickened. Season with salt and pepper.

Makes about 200 ml (⅓ pint)

MAKING HOLLANDAISE SAUCE

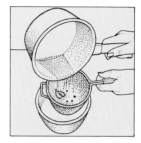

1 Straining the reduced vinegar and lemon juice

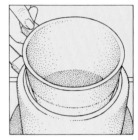

2 Placing the egg yolks and reduced vinegar in a double saucepan. It is now ready to be whisked over hot water until thick

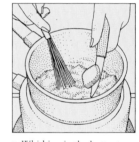

3 Whisking in the butter to the thickened mixture, a little at a time

Below:
BÉARNAISE SAUCE

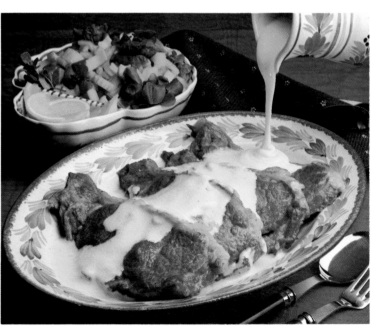

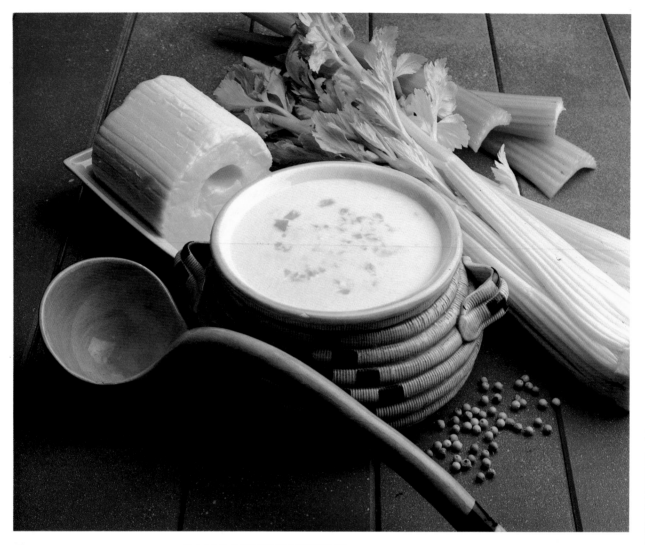

Above:
CELERY BUTTER SAUCE
This sauce is a mouthwatering accompaniment to vegetables, and is also the perfect finishing touch to a delicate-tasting dish such as boiled chicken or poached fish.

SAVOURY BUTTER SAUCES

These consist of melted, clarified butter with one or two simple additions. To keep the butter a good colour during cooking and prevent bitterness and dark speckles, it should be first clarified.

Put the required amount of English butter into a saucepan and melt over a very low heat. Leave aside for a few minutes, then strain through fine muslin into a clean bowl. The butter will now be clear and free of milky solids.

BROWN BUTTER SAUCE

Delicious with hot asparagus and broccoli.

75 g (3 oz) clarified butter

1. Put the butter into a saucepan and cook very slowly until the butter turns a light brown colour.
2. Serve immediately.
Makes enough for 4 servings

BLACK BUTTER SAUCE

A sophisticated sauce for poached and steamed fish, egg and vegetable dishes.

75 g (3 oz) clarified butter
5 ml (1 tsp) vinegar

1. Put the butter into a saucepan and cook very slowly until it turns dark brown.
2. Stir in the vinegar at once and serve immediately.
Makes enough for 4 servings

BLACK BUTTER SAUCE WITH CAPERS

For poached or steamed fish and brain dishes.

75 g (3 oz) clarified butter
5 ml (1 tsp) vinegar
15 ml (1 level tbsp) chopped capers

1. Put the butter into a saucepan and cook very slowly until the butter turns dark brown.
2. Stir in the vinegar and capers at once and serve immediately.
Makes enough for 4 servings

LEMON BUTTER SAUCE

Delicious with poached and steamed fish dishes.

75 g (3 oz) clarified butter
15 ml (1 tbsp) finely chopped fresh parsley
5 ml (1 tsp) lemon juice
freshly ground pepper

1. Put the butter into a saucepan and cook very slowly until it turns a light brown colour.
2. Stir in the remaining ingredients. Serve immediately.

Makes enough for 4 servings

CELERY BUTTER SAUCE

Use with carrots, onions and other vegetables such as Jerusalem artichokes.

3 sticks celery, cleaned and very finely chopped
400 ml (¾ pint) milk
125 g (4 oz) English butter
45 ml (3 level tbsp) flour
salt and freshly ground pepper

1. Put the celery in a saucepan with the milk. Simmer gently, covered, for 12–15 minutes until the celery is tender.
2. Strain, reserving the milk and celery.
3. Melt 40 g (1½ oz) butter in a saucepan, stir in the flour and cook for 2 minutes, stirring.
4. Remove the pan from the heat and gradually stir in the milk. Bring to the boil and continue to cook, stirring until the sauce thickens. Simmer for at least 5 minutes. Add the reserved celery and season with salt and pepper.
5. Add the remaining butter in small knobs, beating in well. Do not boil again.

Makes 400 ml (¾ pint)

BARBECUE SAUCE

A tangy accompaniment to chicken, sausages, hamburgers or chops.

50 g (2 oz) English butter
1 large onion, skinned and chopped
5 ml (1 level tsp) tomato purée
30 ml (2 tbsp) vinegar
30 ml (2 level tbsp) demerara sugar
10 ml (2 level tsp) mustard powder
30 ml (2 tbsp) Worcestershire sauce

1. Melt the butter in a saucepan and fry the onion for 5 minutes, until soft. Stir in the tomato purée and continue cooking for a further 3 minutes.
2. Blend together the remaining ingredients with 150 ml (¼ pint) water until smooth and stir in the onion mixture. Return the sauce to the pan and boil uncovered for a further 10 minutes.

Makes enough for 4 servings

CHESTNUT SAUCE

Rich and satisfying with turkey and other poultry.

225 g (8 oz) chestnuts, peeled
300 ml (½ pint) chicken stock
1 small piece of onion, skinned
1 small piece of carrot, peeled
40 g (1½ oz) English butter
45 ml (3 level tbsp) flour
salt and freshly ground pepper
30–45 ml (2–3 tbsp) fresh single cream

1. Put the peeled nuts into a pan with the stock and vegetables, cover, simmer until soft and mash or sieve.
2. Melt the butter and stir in the flour to form a roux, then add the chestnut purée and bring to the boil, stirring – the sauce should be thick, but it may be necessary at this point to add a little milk or extra stock.
3. Season well with salt and pepper, remove from the heat and stir in the cream. Reheat without boiling and serve at once.

Makes enough for 4 servings

Below:
BARBECUE SAUCE
Sharp velvety sauces like this one are ideal for serving with every barbecue or with plain grills and burgers.

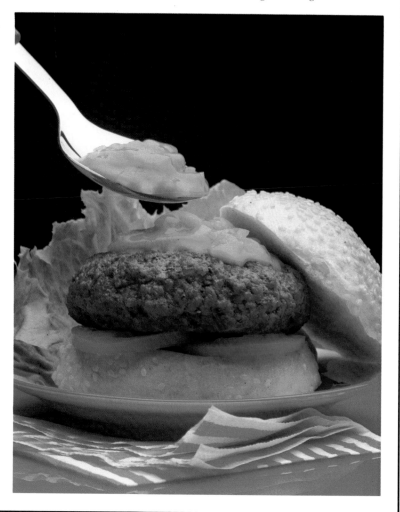

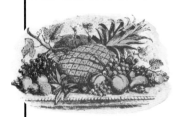

HORSERADISH SAUCE

The traditional touch for roast beef or smoked trout or mackerel.

30 ml (2 level tbsp) finely grated horseradish
10 ml (2 level tsp) caster sugar
salt and freshly ground pepper
1.25 ml (¼ level tsp) prepared mustard
15 ml (1 tbsp) white wine vinegar
150 ml (5 fl oz) fresh double cream

1. Mix together the horseradish, sugar, salt, pepper, mustard and vinegar.
2. Whip the fresh cream until softly stiff and gradually stir into the mixture. Serve chilled.
Makes enough for 4 servings

GOOSEBERRY SAUCE

A lovely eighteenth-century sauce for mackerel and other fish.

350 g (12 oz) gooseberries
25 g (1 oz) English butter
25 g (1 oz) sugar
salt and freshly ground pepper
1.25 ml (¼ level tsp) ground nutmeg

1. Boil the gooseberries in 150 ml (¼ pint) water for 4–5 minutes, until tender and pulped. Then drain and rub through a sieve or purée in a blender.
2. Add the butter, sugar, salt, pepper and the nutmeg. Reheat and serve.
Makes enough for 4 servings

Below:
HORSERADISH SAUCE
The first mention of horseradish in an English publication was in Gerard's Herball, *published in 1597. The plant seems to have arrived here from Germany – it is a native of west and south-east Asia – and en route got its curious name.*

APPLE AND HORSERADISH CREAM

Delicious with smoked mackerel or trout.

142 ml (5 fl oz) soured cream
5 ml (1 level tsp) finely chopped onion
45 ml (3 level tbsp) chopped dessert apple
15 ml (1 level tbsp) creamed horseradish
5 ml (1 level tsp) wholegrain mustard
salt and freshly ground pepper

1. In a bowl, mix together the soured cream, onion, apple, horseradish and mustard.
2. Taste and adjust seasoning with freshly ground pepper and a very little salt.
3. Store in a covered container in the refrigerator for not more than 2 days.
Makes enough for 8 servings

BREAD SAUCE

A welcome accompaniment to roast chicken, turkey or pheasant.

2 cloves
1 medium onion, skinned
1 small bay leaf
400 ml (¾ pint) milk
75 g (3 oz) fresh white breadcrumbs
salt and white pepper
15 g (½ oz) English butter
30 ml (2 tbsp) fresh single cream

1. Stick the cloves into the onion and place in a small heavy-based pan with the bay leaf and the milk to cover.
2. Bring slowly to the boil, remove from the heat, cover and leave to infuse for 10 minutes, then remove the onion and bay leaf.
3. Add the breadcrumbs and seasoning, return to the heat and simmer gently, cover, for 10–15 minutes, stirring occasionally. Stir in the butter and fresh cream.
Makes enough for 6 servings

SWEET SAUCES

SWEET WHITE SAUCE

● Roux method

20 g (¾ oz) English butter
30 ml (2 level tbsp) flour
300 ml (½ pint) milk
25 ml (1½ level tbsp) sugar

1. Melt the butter in a saucepan, stir in the flour and cook gently for 2–3 minutes, stirring.

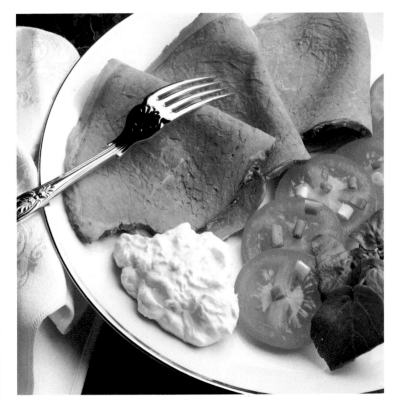

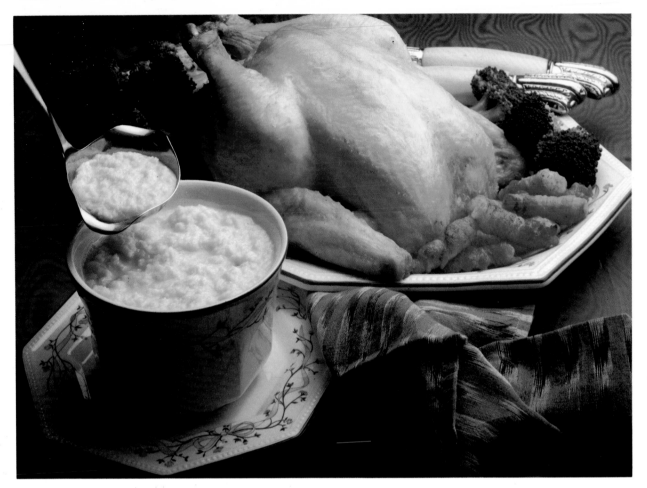

2. Remove the pan from the heat and gradually stir in the milk.

3. Bring to the boil and continue to cook, stirring until the sauce thickens. Add the sugar to taste.

● **Blended method**

25 ml (1½ level tbsp) cornflour
300 ml (½ pint) milk
25 ml (1½ level tbsp) sugar

1. Place the cornflour in a basin and blend with 15–30 ml (1–2 tbsp) milk to a smooth paste.

2. Heat the remaining milk until boiling, pour on to the blended mixture, stirring all the time.

3. Return the mixture to the pan and bring to the boil, stirring continuously. Cook for 1–2 minutes after the mixture has thickened to make a white, glossy sauce. Add sugar to taste.

Note: For those who like a thicker sauce, increase the quantity of cornflour to 30 ml (2 level tbsp). This will be necessary if you add fresh cream, rum or any other form of liquid when the sauce has been made.

Variations

Flavour with any of the following when the sauce has thickened:

5 ml (1 level tsp) mixed spice or ground nutmeg

30 ml (2 level tbsp) jam
Grated rind of ½ orange or lemon
30 ml (2 tbsp) fresh single cream
15–30 ml (1–2 tbsp) rum
1 egg yolk (the sauce must be reheated but not re-boiled)

Makes 300 ml (½ pint)

CUSTARD SAUCE

Use for hot puddings and pies.

25 ml (1½ level tbsp) custard powder
25–30 ml (1½–2 level tbsp) sugar
300 ml (½ pint) milk

1. Blend the custard powder and the sugar with a little of the cold milk, to a smooth paste.

2. Boil the rest of the milk and stir into the blended mixture.

3. Return the sauce to the boil, stirring all the time until it thickens.

Note: Cold thick custard is often used in cold sweets, eg, fruit fool; for this thicker consistency use 30–40 ml (2–2½ level tbsp) custard powder.

Makes 300 ml (½ pint)

Above:
BREAD SAUCE
This recipe can be traced back to medieval times. Sauces then had to be thickened sufficiently not to run off the flat trencher used instead of our plate. Bread was ideal for the purpose. These days, the sauce is usually served only with poultry, but it is also excellent with sweetbreads.

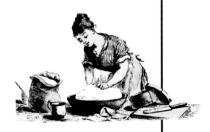

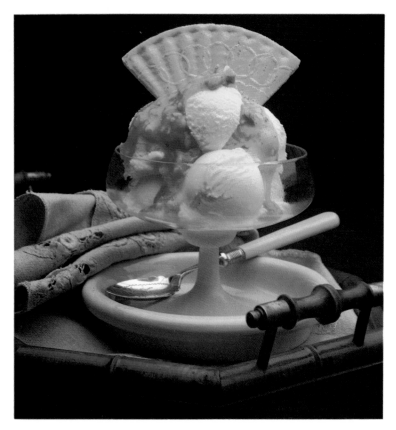

Above:
BUTTERSCOTCH
SAUCE
It is fortunate that children love this delicious sauce so much – it gives us all an excuse to indulge in an old favourite!

BUTTERSCOTCH SAUCE

A scrumptious topping for dairy ice cream.

25 g (1 oz) English butter
30 ml (2 level tbsp) brown sugar
15 ml (1 level tbsp) golden syrup
45 ml (3 level tbsp) chopped nuts
squeeze of lemon juice (optional)

1. Warm the butter, sugar and syrup in a saucepan until well blended.
2. Boil for 1 minute and stir in the nuts and lemon juice. Serve at once.
Makes about 100 ml (4 fl oz)

FUDGE SAUCE

Use with dairy ice cream, steamed and baked puddings.

50 g (2 oz) plain chocolate
25 g (1 oz) English butter
60 ml (4 tbsp) warm milk
225 g (8 oz) soft brown sugar
30 ml (2 level tbsp) golden syrup
5 ml (1 tsp) vanilla flavouring

1. Break up the chocolate and put into a bowl standing over a saucepan of hot water. Add the butter.
2. Leave until the chocolate and butter have melted, stirring once or twice. Blend in the milk and transfer the chocolate mixture to a saucepan. Add the sugar and golden syrup.
3. Stir over a low heat until the sugar has dissolved. Bring to the boil and boil steadily without stirring for 5 minutes.
4. Remove the pan from the heat. Add the vanilla flavouring and mix well. Serve hot.
Makes about 400 ml ($\frac{3}{4}$ pint)

CHOCOLATE SAUCE

Always a family favourite on steamed or baked sponge puddings.

15 ml (1 level tbsp) cornflour
15 ml (1 level tbsp) cocoa powder
30 ml (2 level tbsp) sugar
300 ml ($\frac{1}{2}$ pint) milk
knob of English butter

1. Blend the cornflour, cocoa and the sugar with enough of the milk to give a smooth paste.
2. Heat the remaining milk with the butter until boiling, and pour on to the blended mixture, stirring all the time to prevent lumps forming.
3. Return the mixture to the pan and bring to the boil, stirring until it thickens; cook for a further 1–2 minutes.
Makes 300 ml ($\frac{1}{2}$ pint)

CHOCOLATE FUDGE SAUCE

A luscious sauce for dairy ice cream, profiteroles and other desserts.

75 ml (5 tbsp) fresh single cream
25 g (1 oz) cocoa powder
125 g (4 oz) caster sugar
175 g (6 oz) golden syrup
25 g (1 oz) English butter
pinch of salt
2.5 ml ($\frac{1}{2}$ tsp) vanilla flavouring

1. Combine all the ingredients except the vanilla flavouring in a saucepan and mix well.
2. Slowly bring to the boil, stirring occasionally. Boil for 5 minutes, then add the vanilla flavouring.
3. Cool the sauce slightly before serving.
Makes about 400 ml ($\frac{3}{4}$ pint)

CINNAMON CREAM

A spicy sauce for hot puddings.

150 ml ($\frac{1}{4}$ pint) fresh single cream
5 ml (1 level tsp) caster sugar
1.25 ml ($\frac{1}{4}$ level tsp) ground cinnamon

1. Pour the fresh cream into a bowl, stir in the sugar and cinnamon until evenly blended, then chill.
Makes 150 ml ($\frac{1}{4}$ pint)

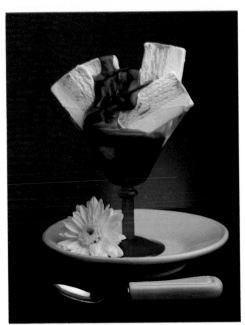

SOURED CREAM SAUCE

Use for hot puddings.

30 ml (2 level tbsp) custard powder
20 ml (4 level tsp) soft light brown sugar
300 ml (½ pint) milk
142 ml (5 fl oz) soured cream

1. In a small basin, mix the custard powder and the sugar to a smooth paste with a little of the milk.
2. Scald the remaining milk and pour on to the custard mixture, stirring well.
3. Return the custard to the pan and bring to the boil, stirring all the time, boil for 2–3 minutes. Lower the heat and carefully stir in the soured cream, then warm through without boiling.
Makes 300 ml (½ pint)

Left:
CHOCOLATE FUDGE SAUCE
A rich luscious chocolate sauce is one of the most tempting finishing touches to dairy ice cream. Chocolate became a popular drink in Britain during the seventeenth century, but it wasn't until the early nineteenth century that powdered cocoa was first made in the Netherlands. This powder is used in this smooth dark sauce which has become a mouthwatering essential to serve with profiteroles and many other desserts.

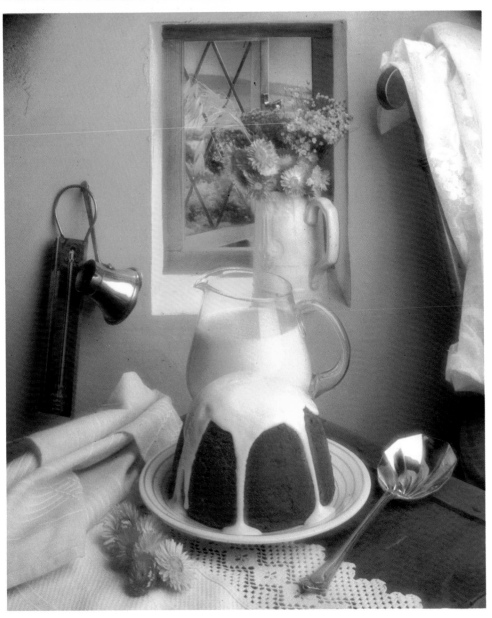

Left:
SOURED CREAM SAUCE
Instead of always serving a custard sauce, try this deliciously different one with a tangy taste.

EGG CUSTARD SAUCE

A traditional sauce for steamed and baked puddings, fruit and mince pies, stewed fruit.

2 eggs
10 ml (2 level tsp) caster sugar
300 ml (½ pint) milk
5 ml (1 tsp) vanilla flavouring (optional)

1. Beat the eggs with the sugar and 45 ml (3 tbsp) milk. Heat the rest of the milk to lukewarm, and beat into the eggs.
2. Pour into a double saucepan or bowl standing over a pan of simmering water. Cook, stirring continuously, until the custard thickens enough to thinly coat the back of a spoon. Do not boil.
3. Pour into a cold jug and stir in the vanilla flavouring. Serve hot or cold. The sauce thickens up slightly on cooling.
Makes 300 ml (½ pint)

SWEET BUTTERS

These traditional English sauces are mouthwatering accompaniments to Christmas Puddings, mince pies, and baked and steamed fruit puddings.

BRANDY BUTTER

100 g (4 oz) English butter, softened
100 g (4 oz) icing sugar, sifted
100 g (4 oz) caster sugar
15 ml (1 tbsp) milk
15 ml (1 tbsp) brandy

1. Beat the butter until pale and light.
2. Gradually beat in the icing and caster sugars, alternately with the milk and brandy. Beat until light and fluffy.
3. Pile into a small dish and leave to harden before serving.
Makes enough for 6–8 servings

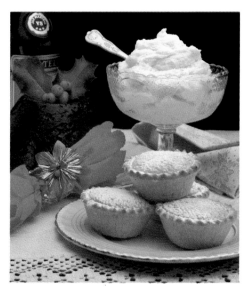

RUM BUTTER

1. Follow the recipe for Brandy Butter, but use soft brown sugar, replace the brandy by 45 ml (3 tbsp) rum and include the grated rind of half a lemon and a squeeze of lemon juice.
Makes enough for 6–8 servings

LEMON OR ORANGE BUTTER

1. Follow the recipe for Brandy Butter, omitting the milk and brandy. Add the grated rind and juice of a lemon or small orange.
Makes enough for 6–8 servings

ALMOND BUTTER

100 g (4 oz) English butter, softened
100 g (4 oz) caster sugar
25 g (1 oz) ground almonds
15 ml (1 tbsp) brandy

1. Cream the butter and sugar together until light and fluffy.
2. Stir in the almonds and brandy.
3. Pile into a small dish and chill well before serving.
Makes enough for 4 servings

SUGAR 'N SPICE

100 g (4 oz) English butter
15 ml (1 level tbsp) brown sugar
15 ml (1 level tbsp) ground cinnamon

1. Whisk the butter and mix in the sugar and cinnamon. Use on waffles or drop scones.
Makes enough for 4 servings

CHOC 'N NUT

100 g (4 oz) English butter
10 ml (2 level tsp) caster sugar
15 ml (1 level tbsp) grated chocolate
30 ml (2 level tbsp) chopped walnuts

1. Whisk the butter and beat in the remaining ingredients. Use to fill cooked pancakes.
Makes enough for 4 servings

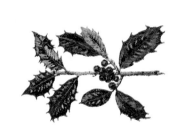

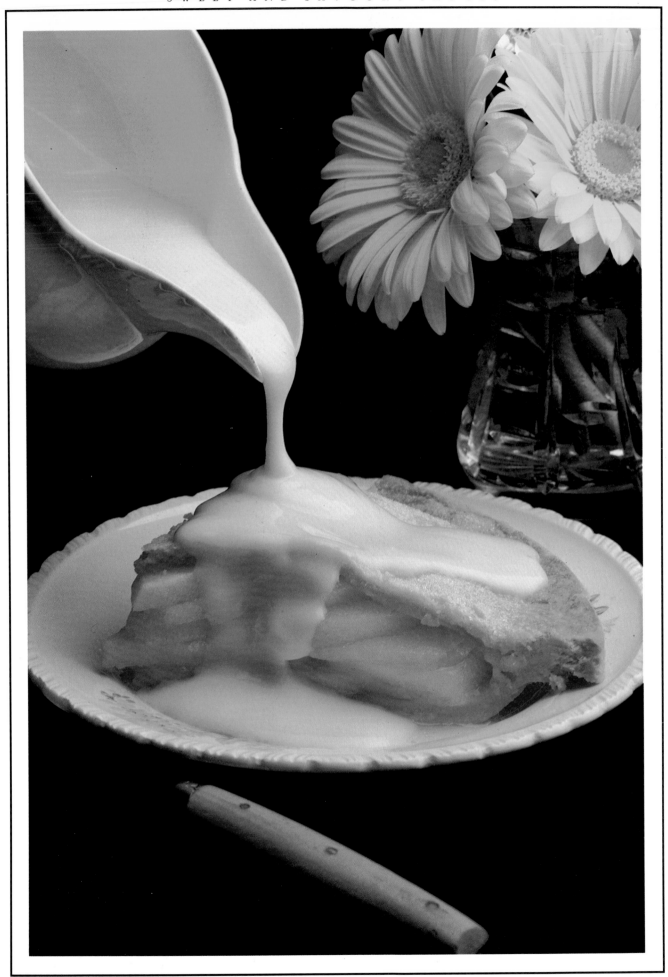

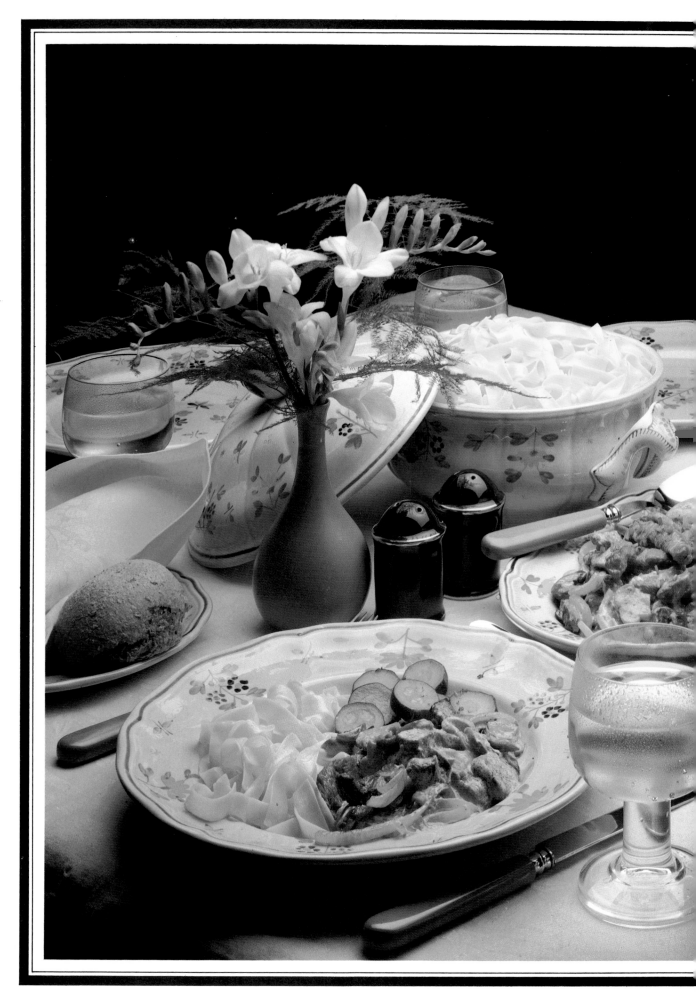

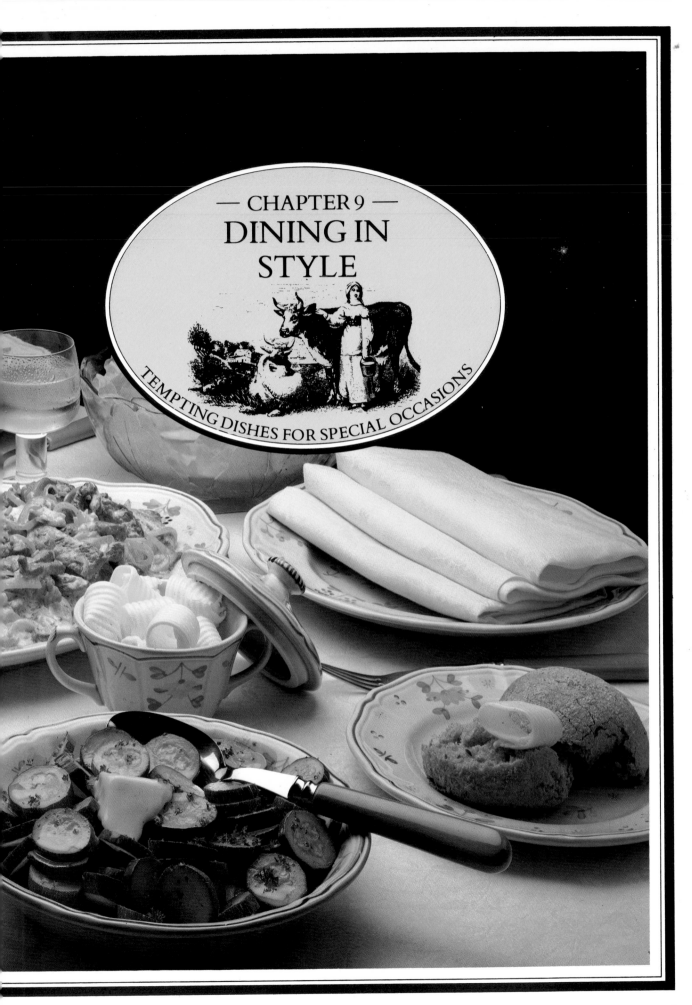

— CHAPTER 9 —
DINING IN STYLE

TEMPTING DISHES FOR SPECIAL OCCASIONS

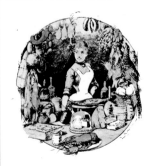

Giving a dinner party is one of the most enjoyable ways of entertaining your friends. It is the time for your best china, soft candlelight, sparkling glasses and delicious food over which that extra bit of care has been taken.

It takes lots of careful planning beforehand to produce an apparently effortless meal in a relaxed and elegant setting. Always try to plan a menu that has plenty of variety and don't be over-ambitious in what you plan to cook. A favourite dish perfectly served is far better than an exotic experiment which flops.

A dinner party is a wonderful opportunity to present food with style and to make each course a joy to look at. The appearance of quite plain food can always be improved with the moderate use of fresh, imaginative garnishes. A plain grill for example, looks much more appetising if set off with watercress, or perhaps a delicious pat of the savoury butters we give on pages 28–9.

Serve dry wines before sweet ones and light before the full-bodied ones, for the good reason that the reverse order turns the dry wine bitter and the light wine insipid. It is also commonsense to serve dry white wine with fish and white meats. Red meats and game, however, need the stronger company of full red wine. Sweet desserts need sweet wine for a partner.

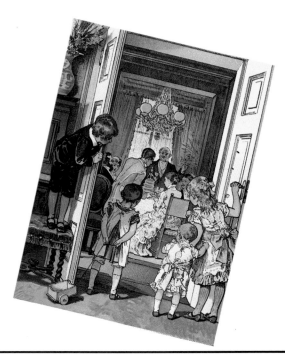

ROASTING IN BUTTER

ROAST TURKEY

Turkey
2.7–3.5 kg (6–8 lb)
  oven-ready serves 6–12
4.5–5.9 kg (10–13 lb)
  oven-ready serves 15–20
6.5–9 kg (14–20 lb)
  oven-ready serves 20–30

English butter for roasting

salt and freshly ground pepper

lemon juice

1 onion, skinned

1 lemon wedge

1. Wash the turkey inside and out, and dry thoroughly. Spread butter over the skin, season with salt, freshly ground pepper and a squeeze of lemon juice. Butter gives a much better taste to turkey than other fats.
2. Place the onion, lemon wedge and a knob of butter inside the body. Stuff the neck end with herb stuffing (see below) before folding the neck skin over.
3. Weigh bird after stuffing. Set oven at 180°C (350°F) mark 4, place bird in roasting tin, cover the breast of large poultry with foil.
Approximate roasting times:
2.3 kg (5 lb) 2 hours
4.5 kg (10 lb) 3 hours
6.8 kg (15 lb) 3¾ hours
9 kg (20 lb) 4¼ hours
Baste occasionally during cooking.
4. To know if the turkey is cooked, pierce the deepest part of the thigh with a skewer. If the juices are colourless the bird is ready; if pink-tinged, cook a little longer. Carving is easier if the bird is left in a warm oven for a while.
5. Serve with gravy and bread sauce. Small sausages, rolls of bacon and watercress may be used to garnish the turkey. Cranberry sauce is also a traditional accompaniment.

HERB STUFFING

3 large onions, skinned and chopped

75 g (3 oz) English butter

175 g (6 oz) fresh breadcrumbs

45 ml (3 tbsp) chopped fresh parsley

salt and freshly ground pepper

1. Fry the onion in the butter until softened. Stir in remaining ingredients and mix well.

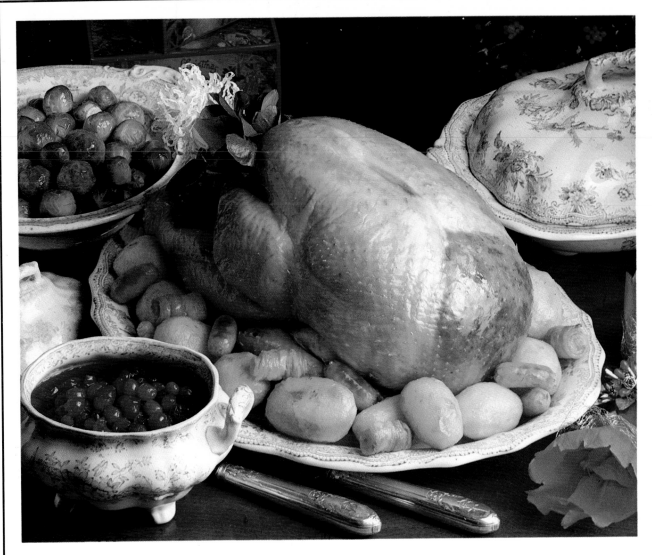

LEMON ROAST CHICKEN

1.8–2.3 kg (4–5 lb) chicken

1 onion, skinned

1 lemon wedge

English butter for roasting

salt and freshly ground pepper

streaky bacon rashers (optional)

1. If the chicken is frozen, allow it to thaw out completely, discarding the bag of giblets. A 1.8 kg (4 lb) bird will take 8–10 hours at room temperature.

2. Wash the bird and dry thoroughly and stuff with half the quantity of herb stuffing (opposite) at the neck end before folding the neck skin over. To add flavour put the onion, lemon wedge and a knob of butter in the body of the bird.

3. Weigh the chicken and place it in a deep roasting tin, brush with melted butter and sprinkle with salt and freshly ground pepper. A few strips of streaky bacon may be laid over the breast to prevent it from becoming dry. Roast in the oven at 200°C (400°F) mark 6, basting from time to time, and allowing 20 minutes per 450 g (1 lb) plus 20 minutes.

4. Put a piece of greaseproof paper over the breast if it shows signs of becoming too brown. Alternatively, wrap the chicken in foil before roasting. Allow the same cooking time, but open the foil for the final 15–20 minutes to allow the bird to brown.

5. Bacon rolls, chipolata sausages, bread sauce and gravy are the usual accompaniments.

Serves 4–6

Above:
ROAST TURKEY
With its generous covering of rich, flavoursome meat, the turkey has become one of the most popular birds to serve not only on Christmas Day but often during the rest of the year as well. Using butter is one of the most simple and delicious ways of roasting poultry. Not only does it bring out the full flavour of the bird, but it keeps the flesh moist and gives a delicious crisp light-golden skin.

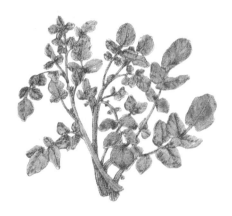

MEAT

STEAK WITH CREAM SAUCE

four 175-g (6-oz) fillet steaks

2 garlic cloves, skinned and crushed or finely chopped (optional)

salt and freshly ground pepper

50 g (2 oz) English butter

125 g (4 oz) button mushrooms, wiped and very thinly sliced

25 g (1 oz) onion, very finely chopped

15 ml (1 tbsp) lemon juice

30 ml (2 tbsp) Worcestershire sauce

15–30 ml (1–2 tbsp) brandy

150 ml (5 fl oz) fresh single cream

15 ml (1 tbsp) finely chopped fresh parsley

fresh parsley to garnish

1. Rub the steaks with the garlic and season well.
2. Heat half the butter in a frying pan and fry the steaks over a high heat for about 2 minutes on each side to brown. If you like your steaks well done, cook longer. Place in a warm serving dish to keep hot.
3. Heat the remaining butter and quickly fry the mushrooms and onion in the pan until tender. Add the lemon juice, Worcestershire sauce and brandy and bring to the boil.
4. Stir in the fresh cream and parsley, bring almost to the boil, check seasoning, then quickly pour over the steaks and serve garnished with a sprig of parsley.

Serves 4

Below:
STEAK WITH CREAM SAUCE
A delicious, quickly-made dish with a delicately piquant sauce.

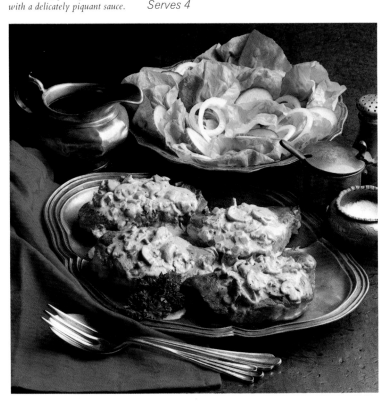

LAMB AND MAÎTRE D'HÔTEL BUTTER

4 large loin lamb chops, trimmed

50 g (2 oz) button mushrooms, wiped and finely chopped

50g (2 oz) English butter

50 g (2 oz) ham, finely chopped

grated rind of 1 small lemon

salt and freshly ground pepper

25 g (1 oz) fresh breadcrumbs

beaten egg

15 ml (1 tbsp) oil

100 g (4 oz) maître d'hôtel butter (see page 28)

1. Using a sharp knife, slit the lean eye of the chop horizontally through the fat edge.
2. Lightly fry the mushrooms in 25 g (1 oz) butter until soft. Add the ham, lemon rind, seasoning and breadcrumbs and bind with a little beaten egg. Allow to cool then stuff the mixture into the incisions in the chops. Secure each chop with string.
3. Heat the oil and remaining butter in a large frying pan and over a high heat, fry well on both sides. Reduce heat and continue to cook for 20 minutes. Remove string before serving.
4. Cut the maître d'hôtel butter into pats and place several on each of the chops to serve.

Serves 4

PIQUANT PORK CHOPS

4 lean loin pork chops

salt and freshly ground pepper

15 ml (1 level tbsp) prepared mustard

30 ml (2 level tbsp) soft brown sugar

450–568 ml ($\frac{3}{4}$–1 pint) milk

25 g (1 oz) cornflour

100 g (4 oz) mushrooms, wiped

25 g (1 oz) English butter

4 peach halves

chopped fresh parsley to garnish

1. Wipe the chops and season, cover evenly with prepared mustard. Place in a flameproof dish and sprinkle with brown sugar.
2. Surround the chops with milk, but do not cover. Bake in the oven at 200°C (400 °F) mark 6 for 15 minutes, then reduce heat to 180°C (350°F) mark 4 and cook for a further 30 minutes until tender.
3. Blend the cornflour with a little water. Place the chops on a warm serving dish and keep warm. Stir the cornflour paste into the cooking juices and heat gently until the sauce thickens. Season to taste.
4. Fry the mushrooms in the butter. Serve the chops garnished with peach halves, fried mushrooms and chopped parsley. Serve sauce in a sauce boat.

Serves 4

PORK MAYONNAISE

6 pork escalopes

45 ml (3 level tbsp) seasoned flour

beaten egg

fine dry breadcrumbs

75 g (3 oz) English butter

60 ml (4 tbsp) oil

150 ml ($\frac{1}{4}$ pint) mayonnaise

142 ml (5 fl oz) soured cream

45 ml (3 level tbsp) grated onion

coarsely grated rind of 2 oranges

30 ml (2 tbsp) chopped fresh mint

1. Dust each escalope lightly with seasoned flour. Dip into beaten egg and then coat with breadcrumbs.

2. Heat half the butter and the oil in a large shallow pan. Add three of the prepared escalopes and cook for 4 minutes on each side. Drain. Cook the remaining escalopes, adding more butter and oil to the pan.

3. For the sauce, mix the remaining ingredients together, adding a little hot water to give a smooth coating consistency.

4. Arrange the escalopes on a serving dish and spoon over the sauce.

Variation

Veal escalopes may be used as an alternative to pork.

Serves 6

BOEUF STROGANOFF

700 g (1$\frac{1}{2}$ lb) rump steak, thinly sliced

45 ml (3 level tbsp) seasoned flour

50 g (2 oz) English butter

1 onion, skinned and thinly sliced

225 g (8 oz) mushrooms, wiped and sliced

150 ml (5 fl oz) soured cream

salt and freshly ground pepper

1. Beat the steak, trim and cut into thin strips.

2. Coat in the seasoned flour. Fry the meat in half the butter for about 5–7 minutes until golden brown.

3. Add the remaining butter, the onion and mushrooms and cook for 3–4 minutes. Stir in the soured cream and season well, using plenty of pepper. Heat to serving temperature and serve at once.

Serves 4

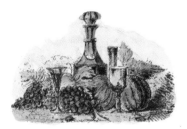

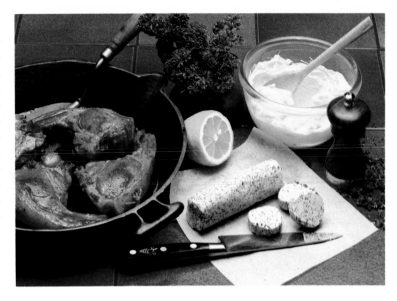

PORK WITH MUSHROOMS

900 g (2 lb) pork fillet, cubed

75 g (3 oz) flour

5 ml (1 level tsp) salt

freshly ground pepper

350 g (12 oz) onions, skinned and sliced

75 g (3 oz) English butter

450 g (1 lb) button mushrooms, wiped and sliced

900 ml (1$\frac{1}{2}$ pints) chicken stock

100 ml (4 fl oz) dry sherry

1. Toss the meat in the flour and seasonings to coat evenly.

2. Fry the onions and meat in butter until lightly browned. Add the mushrooms, stir in any remaining flour and fry gently for 1 minute. Gradually stir in the stock and sherry.

3. Bring to the boil, cover and simmer for 30–40 minutes, until the meat is tender.

Serves 6

Above:
LAMB AND MAÎTRE D'HÔTEL BUTTER
A pat of this delicious savoury butter, flavoured with finely chopped parsley and a piqant dash of lemon juice, is the perfect accompaniment to these unusual stuffed lamb chops. This classic savoury butter adds style to all plain grilled meat and it is also delicious when popped into baked potatoes or stirred into freshly cooked vegetables.

Below:
PORK WITH MUSHROOMS
The best pork comes from young animals and has smooth thin skin with firm flesh and white fat. The fillet, one of the choicest cuts, is used in this delectable stew. Serve it with fennel salad and sauteéd potatoes.

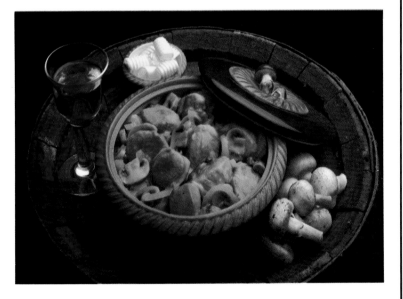

Right:
BLANQUETTE
D'AGNEAU
This delicious, comforting dish,
like many stews, is probably
best made a day ahead and left
to mature. If this is done,
however, the last step – the
addition of the egg yolk and
fresh cream – should be left
until just before serving.
Noddles or boiled potatoes are
an excellent accompaniment.

FRICASSÉE OF VEAL

900 g (2 lb) stewing veal

450 g (1 lb) carrots, peeled

1 medium onion, skinned and sliced

15 ml (1 tbsp) chopped fresh thyme, or
  2.5 ml ($\frac{1}{2}$ level tsp) dried thyme

150 ml ($\frac{1}{4}$ pint) dry white wine

salt and freshly ground pepper

50 g (2 oz) English butter

50 g (2 oz) flour

2 egg yolks

150 ml (5 fl oz) fresh single cream

chopped fresh parsley to garnish

1. Cut the veal into 4-cm (1$\frac{1}{2}$-inch) squares, discarding any skin and fat. Cover the meat with cold water, bring to the boil and bubble for 1 minute. Strain through a colander and rinse under a cold tap to remove all scum. Rinse out the pan thoroughly and replace the meat.
2. Cut the carrots into finger-sized pieces; add to the pan with the onions, herbs, wine, 900 ml (1$\frac{1}{2}$ pints) water and plenty of seasoning. Bring slowly to the boil, cover and simmer gently for about 1$\frac{1}{4}$ hours until the veal is quite tender.
3. Strain off the cooking liquid, make up to 700 ml (1$\frac{1}{4}$ pints) with stock if necessary and reserve; keep the veal and vegetables warm in a covered serving dish.
4. Melt the butter in a pan, stir in the flour and cook gently for 1 minute, stirring. Remove from the heat and gradually stir in the strained cooking liquid and season well. Bring to the boil, stirring all the time. Simmer the sauce for 5 minutes.
5. Mix the egg yolks with the fresh cream; remove the sauce from the heat and stir in the cream mixture. Return to the heat and warm gently – without boiling – until the sauce becomes slightly thicker; adjust seasoning.
6. Pour the sauce over the meat and serve garnished with parsley.
Serves 6

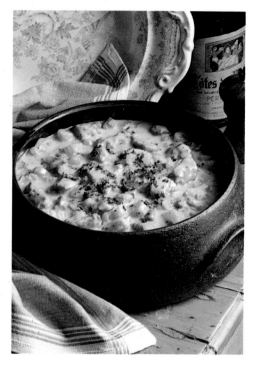

BLANQUETTE D'AGNEAU

700 g (1$\frac{1}{2}$ lb) lean shoulder of lamb, diced

100 g (4 oz) carrots, peeled and sliced

1 onion, skinned and sliced

2 sticks of celery, trimmed and sliced

small bay leaf

5 ml (1 level tsp) dried thyme

salt and freshly ground pepper

300 ml ($\frac{1}{2}$ pint) stock or water

25 g (1 oz) English butter, softened

45 ml (3 level tbsp) flour

1 egg yolk

150 ml (5 fl oz) fresh single cream

chopped fresh parsley to garnish

1. Put the meat, carrots, onion, celery, flavourings and seasonings in a large pan. Cover with stock or water, cover and simmer for 1$\frac{1}{2}$ hours. Remove bay leaf.
2. Blend together the softened butter and flour, and when mixed add to the stew in small knobs and stir until thickened. Simmer for 10 minutes, adding more liquid if necessary.
3. Blend together the egg yolk and fresh cream, add to the stew and reheat without boiling. Garnish with parsley before serving.
Serves 4

Below:
FRICASSÉE OF VEAL
Two cracked veal rib bones added
to the cooking liquid give extra
flavour to this dish. (Remove
them before finishing the sauce.)
Serve with soufflé potatoes and
mushroom stuffed tomatoes.

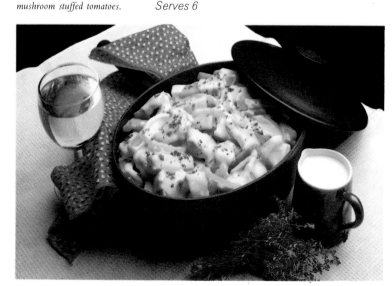

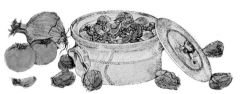

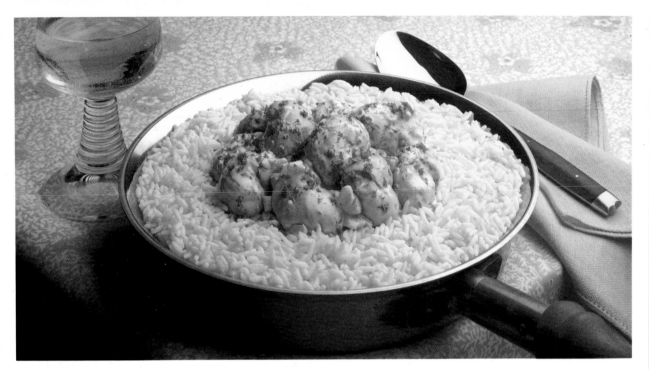

KIDNEYS IN BATTER

225 g (8 oz) flour

pinch of salt

2 eggs

568 ml (1 pint) milk

8 lambs' kidneys, skinned, cored and chopped

1 large onion, skinned and very finely chopped

75 g (3 oz) English butter

350 g (12 oz) mushrooms, wiped and finely chopped

1 garlic clove, skinned and crushed

2 glasses dry sherry

150 ml (5 fl oz) fresh double cream

salt and freshly ground pepper

1. Sieve the flour and salt. Beat in the eggs and milk gradually. Whisk until smooth.
2. Sauté the kidneys and onion in 50 g (2 oz) butter until the onion is transparent; add the mushrooms, crushed garlic and sherry. Cook gently for a few minutes and add the fresh cream.
3. Simmer gently until sauce is reduced and thick, then season.
4. Heat the remaining 25 g (1 oz) butter in a flan dish, add the batter and pour the kidney mixture in the centre. Bake in the oven at 200°C (400°F) mark 6 for 35 minutes, until the pastry is crisp, golden and well risen. Serve at once.

Serves 4

KIDNEYS À LA CRÈME

25 g (1 oz) English butter

8 lambs' kidneys, skinned, cored and halved

1 small onion, skinned and chopped

1 garlic clove, skinned and crushed

30 ml (2 level tbsp) flour

150 ml ($\frac{1}{4}$ pint) beef stock

150 ml (5 fl oz) fresh double cream

salt and freshly ground pepper

1. Melt the butter in a pan, add the kidneys, onions and garlic and cook for 3–4 minutes, until the kidneys are evenly browned.
2. Push the kidneys to one side of the pan, stir in the flour and cook for 2 minutes, gradually adding the stock and fresh cream. Stir gently and reheat without boiling.
3. Season well and serve on a bed of rice.

Serves 4

Above:
KIDNEYS À LA CRÈME
An excellent dish to serve for a light lunch with chilled dry white wine, followed by a simple fruit dessert such as stewed plums.

Below:
KIDNEYS IN BATTER
A crisp golden batter combines marvellously with these kidneys in a fresh cream sauce.

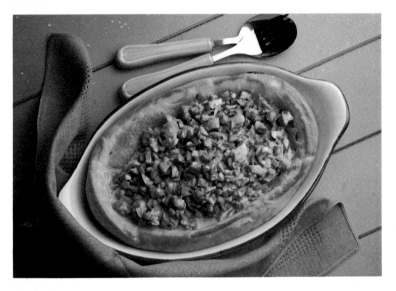

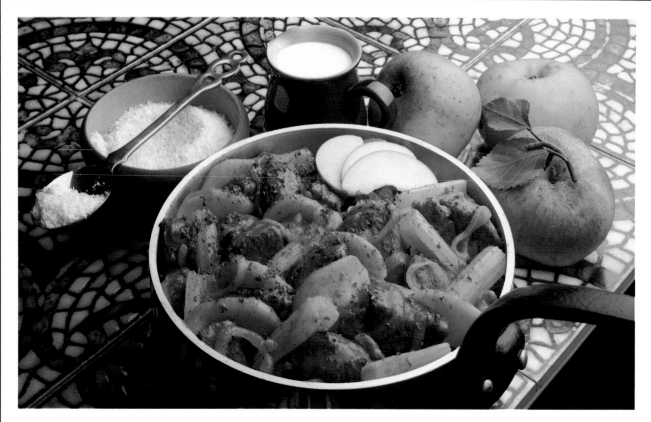

Above:
CHILLI LAMB AND
COCONUT CURRY
An out-of-the-ordinary way to
serve lamb. Browned with celery
and apple, it is spiced with chilli
powder and mellowed with rich
coconut milk for an exotic
Eastern touch.

SWEETBREADS WITH MUSHROOMS AND BRANDY

700 g (1½ lb) lambs' sweetbreads

50 g (2 oz) English butter

1 medium onion, skinned and chopped

225 g (8 oz) button mushrooms, wiped

100 ml (4 fl oz) brandy

170 ml (6 fl oz) fresh single cream

2 egg yolks

salt and freshly ground pepper

chopped fresh parsley to garnish

1. Soak the sweetbreads in cold water for about 4 hours, changing the water several times. Blanch by putting into a pan of cold water then bring to the boil; boil for 2 minutes. Drain and dry sweetbreads on a clean cloth. Snip away any membrane, cut crosswise into slices.
2. Melt half the butter in a frying pan, add the onion and mushrooms; cook until tender. Drain and reserve. Add remaining butter to pan juices, reheat and sauté sweetbreads for 5 minutes.
3. Heat the brandy, ignite and, while flaming, pour over sweetbreads. Cook gently for 10–15 minutes until tender.
4. Combine the fresh cream and egg yolks. Add some hot pan juices to egg mixture, return to pan. Add the onion and mushroom, heat gently to thicken – do not boil. Adjust seasoning to taste. Serve garnished with parsley.

Serves 4–6

CHILLI LAMB AND COCONUT CURRY

50 g (2 oz) desiccated coconut

200 ml (7 fl oz) milk

1.4 kg (3 lb) shoulder of lamb, boned

60 ml (4 tbsp) vegetable oil

4 sticks celery, cleaned and trimmed

1 onion, skinned and sliced

225 g (8 oz) cooking apples, skinned and sliced

2.5 ml (½ level tsp) chilli powder

5 ml (1 level tsp) ground cinnamon

60 ml (4 level tbsp) flour

400 ml (¾ pint) chicken stock

salt and freshly ground pepper

chopped fresh parsley to garnish

1. Bring the coconut to the boil in the milk and 200 ml (7 fl oz) water. Remove from the heat and leave to infuse for 30 minutes. Strain into a jug, pressing the coconut to extract all the juice.
2. Cut up the lamb into 2.5-cm (1-inch) cubes, discarding excess fat. Brown in hot oil in a flameproof casserole, then remove.
3. Cut the celery into 5-cm (2-inch) long pieces and brown with the onion and apple in the residual oil.
4. Stir in the spices and flour. Gradually stir in the stock, coconut milk and seasoning and bring to the boil.
5. Replace meat, cover and cook in the oven at 180°C (350°F) mark 4 for about 1¼ hours. Garnish with parsley.

Serves 4–6

NEPALESE PORK CURRY

700 g (1½ lb) blade of pork

45 ml (3 tbsp) vegetable oil

225 g (8 oz) onion, skinned and sliced

3 dried red chillies

10 ml (2 level tsp) ground cumin

5 ml (1 level tsp) ground cinnamon

15 ml (3 level tsp) ground coriander

2 garlic cloves, skinned and crushed

5 ml (1 level tsp) salt

freshly ground pepper

142 g (5 oz) natural yogurt

1. Cut the pork into 3.5-cm (1½-inch) cubes, discarding skin, bone and excess fat.
2. Brown the meat, a little at a time, in the hot oil in a large sauté pan, then remove.
3. Lightly brown the onion in the residual oil. Halve the chillies, remove the seeds and chop the flesh finely.
4. Add the chillies to the pan with the spices and cook for 1 minute. Stir in 300 ml (½ pint) water with the remaining ingredients and bring to the boil.
5. Replace the meat, cover the pan tightly and simmer for about 1¼ hours, until the pork is tender. Adjust seasoning.
Serves 4

FRICASSÉE OF RABBIT

75 g (3 oz) English butter

100 g (4 oz) bacon rashers, finely chopped

1 young rabbit, jointed

4 medium onions, skinned and chopped

4 cloves

small bunch of mixed herbs (parsley, thyme, marjoram)

1.25 ml (¼ level tsp) grated nutmeg

salt and freshly ground pepper

25 g (1 oz) flour

2 egg yolks

1 sherry glass white wine

grated rind of ½ lemon

1. Melt 25 g (1 oz) butter in a large saucepan, add the bacon and fry gently. Add the rabbit pieces and chopped onions and fry for 3 minutes. Add the cloves, herbs (tied in a muslin bag), nutmeg, salt, pepper and 300 ml (½ pint) water; bring to the boil, cover and simmer for 50 minutes.
2. Mix the flour with 50 g (2 oz) butter, pour on some of the stock from the pan to make a thick gravy, return this to the pan, stir well and simmer for 5 minutes.
3. Beat the yolks, add the wine, the lemon rind and pour over the hot, but not boiling, fricassee. Stir well and serve.
Serves 4

POULTRY

CHICKEN AND COURGETTE EN BROCHETTE

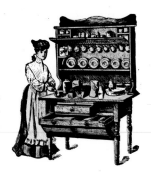

12 dried apricots

four 125-g (4-oz) chicken breasts

30 ml (2 tbsp) lemon juice

75 g (3 oz) English butter

60 ml (4 tbsp) chopped fresh parsley

salt and freshly ground pepper

225 g (8 oz) courgettes, cut into 0.5-cm (¼-inch) slices

1. Soak the apricots overnight in cold water.
2. Skin the chicken breasts and divide each into six even-sized pieces. Place on a flat plate, sprinkle with lemon juice, cover and leave while preparing remaining ingredients.
3. Beat the butter until soft and beat in the parsley with plenty of seasoning.
4. Drain the apricots, halve and pat dry. Stuff the hollow of each apricot with butter.
5. Thread the chicken breasts, stuffed apricots and courgettes alternatively on to flat-bladed kebab skewers. Place in the grill pan without the rack and grill gently for about 25 minutes, turning and basting frequently with pan juices. Serve as soon as possible with juices spooned over.
Serves 4

CHICKEN IN CREAM

4 large chicken joints, skinned and cut in half

40 g (1½ oz) English butter

salt and freshly ground pepper

30 ml (2 tbsp) chopped fresh parsley

30 ml (2 tbsp) chopped fresh mint

150 ml (5 fl oz) fresh double cream

1. Dry the chicken pieces on absorbent kitchen paper.
2. Heat the butter in a large flameproof dish and when bubbling add the chicken pieces.
3. Fry quickly on both sides for about 5 minutes until brown. Season well.
4. Stir the parsley and mint into the fresh cream and pour over the chicken.
5. Cover the dish and cook in the oven at 200°C (400°F) mark 6 for about 1 hour, until tender. Turn the chicken pieces in the fresh cream once or twice during cooking. Serve hot.

Variations

Use fresh rosemary or tarragon to replace the mint.
Serves 4

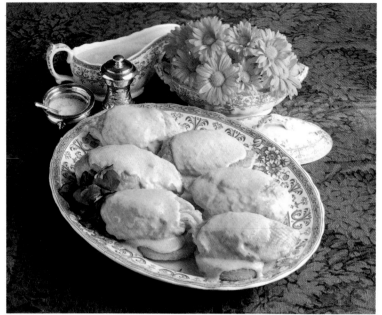

Above:
CHICKEN WITH APRICOTS AND BRANDY
Just one forkful of this elegant supper dish contains the crispness and richness of croûtons cooked in butter, firm delicately flavoured chicken meat and a fresh cream sauce.

CHICKEN SUNNYSIDE

4 chicken portions
50 g (2 oz) English butter
25 g (1 oz) flour
pinch of mustard powder
300 ml ($\frac{1}{2}$ pint) milk
300 ml ($\frac{1}{2}$ pint) dry cider
100 g (4 oz) English Cheddar cheese, grated
salt and freshly ground pepper
25 g (1 oz) potato crisps, crushed

1. Place the chicken portions in a flameproof dish with half the butter in the oven and bake at 160°C (325°F) mark 3 for 1$\frac{1}{4}$ hours.
2. Melt the remaining butter in a pan, stir in the flour and mustard and cook gently for 1 minute stirring. Remove pan from the heat and gradually stir in the milk and cider. Bring to the boil and continue to cook, stirring all the time, until the sauce thickens. Simmer for a further 1–2 minutes. Remove from the heat and stir in 75 g (3 oz) cheese; season.
3. Pour the cheese sauce over the chicken. Sprinkle with the remaining cheese and crushed crisps. Place under a hot grill or in a hot oven until brown and serve hot.
Serves 4

CHICKEN AU GRATIN

4 chicken breasts
1 egg, beaten
100 g·(4 oz) fresh breadcrumbs
100 g (4 oz) English butter
50 g (2 oz) flour
568 ml (1 pint) milk
salt and freshly ground pepper
100 g (4 oz) English Cheddar cheese, sliced

1. Dip each chicken breast in egg and breadcrumbs, shaking off any excess crumbs.
2. Heat 75 g (3 oz) butter in a large frying pan and when bubbling, add the chicken. Turn over when golden brown and cook on the other side. Drain on absorbent kitchen paper.
3. Melt the remaining butter in a pan, stir in the flour and cook gently for 1 minute, stirring. Remove pan from the heat and gradually stir in the milk. Bring to the boil slowly and continue to cook, stirring, until the sauce thickens. Season with salt and pepper. Put the chicken pieces in an ovenproof dish and cover with the sauce.
4. Place the sliced cheese on top and bake in the oven at 220°C (425°F) mark 7 for 10–15 minutes, until golden brown.
Serves 4

CHICKEN WITH APRICOTS AND BRANDY

125 g (4 oz) dried apricots
4–6 chicken breasts, boned
45 ml (3 level tbsp) flour
125 g (4 oz) English butter
60 ml (4 tbsp) dry white wine or cider
15–30 ml (1–2 tbsp) brandy (optional)
125 g (4 oz) streaky bacon, chopped
125 g (4 oz) mushrooms, wiped and sliced
125 g (4 oz) onion, skinned and chopped
300 ml ($\frac{1}{2}$ pint) chicken stock
salt and freshly ground pepper
3 juniper berries (optional)
1 bay leaf
150 ml (5 fl oz) fresh single cream
4–6 thick round slices of bread
fresh parsley or watercress to garnish

1. Soak the apricots overnight in cold water.
2. Dust the chicken with a little flour. Melt 40 g (1$\frac{1}{2}$ oz) butter in a heavy frying pan and gently brown the chicken on all sides, then remove to a large casserole.
3. Add the wine and brandy to the pan, bring to the boil, then pour over the chicken.
4. Melt 40 g (1$\frac{1}{2}$ oz) butter, fry the bacon, mushrooms and onion slowly together until the onion is soft and starting to brown. Blend in 45 ml (3 level tbsp) flour and gradually stir in the stock. Season well, add the juniper berries, drained apricots and bay leaf.

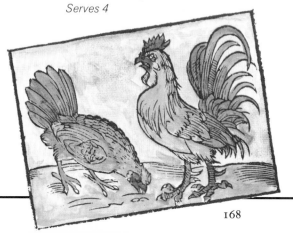

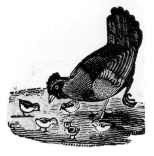

5. Pour the sauce over the chicken, cover and cook in the oven at 160°C (325°F) mark 3 for about 1½ hours, until tender.
6. Meanwhile, fry the bread in remaining butter until crisp and golden. Drain and keep hot.
7. When the chicken is cooked, remove from casserole and keep hot. Remove the bay leaf then rub through a sieve or purée the sauce in a blender. Add the fresh cream, adjust seasoning and reheat gently without boiling.
8. On a serving dish, arrange a chicken breast on each bread croûton and spoon over some sauce. Garnish with parsley or watercress. Serve remaining sauce separately.

Serves 4–6

CHICKEN AND STILTON ROULADES

125 g (4 oz) Blue Stilton cheese, crumbled

75 g (3 oz) English butter, softened

4 chicken breasts, skinned and boned

8 rashers smoked back bacon

15 ml (1 tbsp) vegetable oil

25 g (1 oz) English butter

1 glass red wine made up to 300 ml (½ pint) with chicken stock

salt and freshly ground pepper

5 ml (1 level tsp) arrowroot

watercress to garnish

1. Whisk the cheese and butter to a smooth paste.
2. Beat out the chicken breasts between two sheets of damp greaseproof paper. Spread the butter mixture evenly on one side of each breast.
3. Roll up the chicken breasts and wrap in rinded bacon rashers. Secure with wooden cocktail sticks.
4. In a heavy-based pan, heat the oil and butter and brown chicken rolls well.
5. Pour in the red wine and stock, season, bring to the boil, cover and simmer gently for 35–40 minutes, turning occasionally. Remove the cocktail sticks and place the chicken in a serving dish and keep warm.
6. Blend the arrowroot with a little water until smooth, pour into the pan juices and heat, stirring, until thickened. Season and spoon sauce over the chicken. Garnish with watercress sprigs.

Serves 4

MINTED CHICKEN BAKE

1 onion, skinned and chopped

75 g (3 oz) English butter

100 g (4 oz) fresh white breadcrumbs

finely grated rind and juice of 1 lemon

30 ml (2 tbsp) chopped fresh parsley

5 ml (1 tsp) concentrated mint sauce, or chopped fresh mint

salt and freshly ground pepper

4 chicken joints

1. Fry the onion in 50 g (2 oz) butter for about 5 minutes, until soft. Remove from the heat and mix in the breadcrumbs, rind and juice of lemon, parsley, mint and seasoning.
2. Gently lift as much skin as possible from the chicken joints and fill pockets with stuffing; secure with wooden cocktail sticks.
3. Put in a baking tin and brush with remaining butter, melted. Cook in the oven at 200°C (400°F) mark 6 for 45–50 minutes, until the chicken is golden brown. Remove the cocktail sticks. Serve with gravy made from the pan juices.

Serves 4

Below:
CHICKEN AND STILTON ROULADES
Chicken breasts spread with Blue Stilton and butter, wrapped in bacon and cooked in a red wine sauce make a sensational centre to a dinner party. Serve them with triangles of fried bread and garnish with watercress.

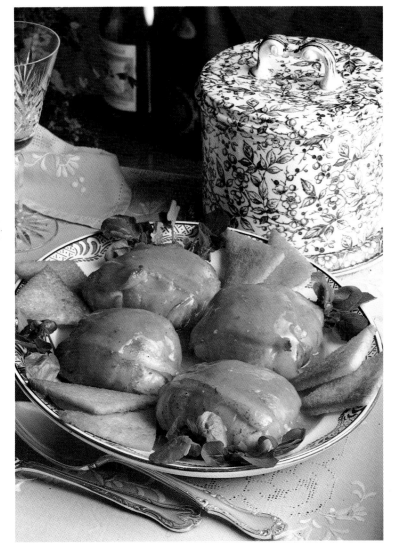

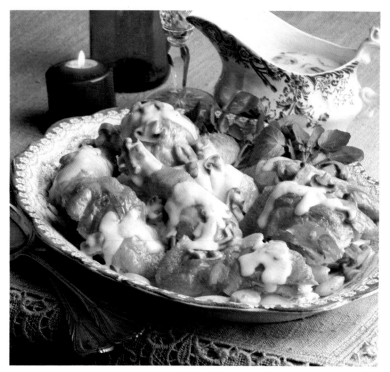

Above:
CHICKEN WITH LEMON
AND ALMONDS
Lemons and almonds are
traditional ingredients of the old
Lancashire dish, Hindle Wakes,
but there the similarity ends.
This recipe is simpler and
includes mushrooms and a fresh
cream sauce. It is a welcome
change from plain roast chicken.

Opposite:
CORONATION
CHICKEN
This delicious recipe was created
in 1953 by the Cordon Bleu
school in London in honour of
the Queen's Coronation – hence
its name.

CHICKEN WITH LEMON AND ALMONDS

1.4 kg (3 lb) chicken

50 g (2 oz) blanched almonds

1 lemon, thinly sliced

1 garlic clove, skinned

25 g (1 oz) English butter, softened

salt and freshly ground pepper

400 ml (¾ pint) stock made from the giblets

125 g (4 oz) button mushrooms, wiped and sliced

15 ml (1 level tbsp) cornflour

60 ml (4 tbsp) fresh single cream

watercress to garnish

1. Wipe chicken and loosen skin all over breast with fingertips. Slip almonds under skin.
2. Stuff the lemon into chicken cavity with garlic. Truss or tie bird securely.
3. Place chicken in roasting tin and spread butter all over its surface. Season well. Pour stock around, roast in the oven at 200°C (400°F) mark 6 for 1 hour, basting frequently.
4. Add mushrooms to roasting tin. Lay a piece of foil over bird, continue cooking for a further 20 minutes, until bird is tender.
5. Drain bird, discard lemon and garlic. Joint, so that each person has a breast and leg or thigh portion.
6. Blend the cornflour with a little water until smooth, pour into the pan juices and heat, stirring, until thickened. Add the fresh cream without re-boiling sauce. Adjust seasoning and spoon over bird for serving. Garnish with watercress.

Serves 4

LEMON AND TURMERIC CHICKEN

4 chicken breasts, skinned

rind and juice of 1½ lemons

1 onion, skinned and chopped

2.5 ml (½ level tsp) dried thyme

1 chicken stock cube, dissolved in 150 ml (¼ pint) boiling water

300 ml (½ pint) milk

40 g (1½ oz) flour

5 ml (1 level tsp) turmeric, or to taste

lemon slices and fresh parsley to garnish

1. Place the chicken breasts in a roasting tin. Sprinkle with a few curls of lemon peel, onion and thyme. Add lemon juice to stock and pour round chicken. Cover with foil and bake in the oven at 190°C (375°F) mark 5, for about 45 minutes until tender.
2. Keep chicken warm. Strain stock into measuring jug and add milk. Blend the flour and turmeric with a little of the milk and stock mixture; gradually add all the liquid.
3. Whisk continuously over a low heat until sauce thickens. Season to taste.
4. Place the chicken on a warmed serving dish, pour over sauce. Garnish with lemon slices and parsley. Serve with rice.

Serves 4

CORONATION CHICKEN

2.3 kg (5 lb) chicken, cooked

25 g (1 oz) English butter

1 small onion, skinned and finely chopped

15 ml (1 level tbsp) curry paste

15 ml (1 level tbsp) tomato purée

100 ml (4 fl oz) red wine

1 bay leaf

juice of ½ lemon

4 canned apricots, finely chopped

300 ml (½ pint) mayonnaise

150 ml (5 fl oz) fresh whipping cream

salt and freshly ground pepper

cucumber, sliced, to garnish

1. Remove all the flesh from the chicken and dice.
2. In a small pan, heat the butter, add the onion and cook for 3 minutes, until softened. Add the curry paste, tomato purée, wine, bay leaf and lemon juice.
3. Simmer, uncovered, for about 10 minutes, until well reduced. Strain and cool.
4. Sieve the chopped apricot to produce a purée. Beat the cooked sauce into the mayonnaise with the apricot purée.
5. Whip the fresh cream until softly stiff and fold into the mixture. Season, adding a little lemon juice if necessary.
6. Toss the chicken pieces into the sauce and garnish with sliced cucumber.

Serves 8

CHICKEN IN MUSHROOM SAUCE

6 chicken joints

225 g (8 oz) button mushrooms, wiped

bouquet garni

300 ml (½ pint) chicken stock

40 g (1½ oz) English butter

40 g (1½ oz) flour

100 g (4 oz) liver pâté

150 ml (¼ pint) milk

30 ml (2 tbsp) fresh single cream

salt and freshly ground pepper

lemon juice

25 g (1 oz) flaked almonds, toasted

1. Skin and halve the chicken joints. Place in a large ovenproof casserole with the mushrooms and bouquet garni.
2. Pour over the stock, cover dish and cook in the oven at 200°C (400°F) mark 6 for 1 hour.
3. Drain the stock from the chicken pieces and reserve. Discard bouquet garni.
4. Melt the butter in a pan, stir in the flour and cook gently for 2 minutes. Beat in the liver pâté and gradually stir in the milk and the reserved chicken stock. Bring to the boil, stirring continuously.
5. Remove from the heat and stir in the fresh cream. Season to taste and sharpen with a little lemon juice.
6. Pour the sauce over the chicken and sprinkle with the almonds. Serve with boiled rice and broccoli spears.

Serves 6

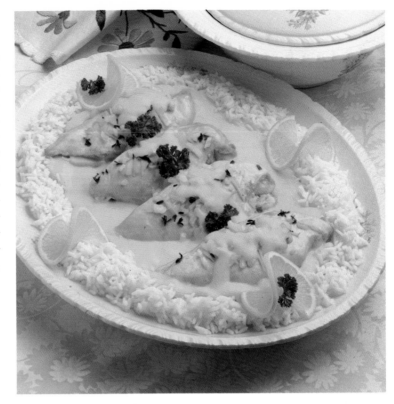

3. Meanwhile, prepare the sauce. Melt the butter in a pan and stir in the flour. Remove from the heat and gradually stir in 600 ml (1 pint) of the retained stock with the horseradish and seasoning.
4. Return to heat, bring to the boil, stirring, until the sauce thickens. Simmer gently for 5 minutes. Add the parsley and fresh cream, adjust seasoning and spoon over chicken for serving.

Serves 6

Above:
LEMON AND TUMERIC CHICKEN
Tumeric comes from the root of a plant belonging to the ginger family. It is used a great deal in Middle Eastern and Indian cookery and gives a mild but spicy flavour to this delightful chicken dish.

POACHED CHICKEN WITH HORSERADISH CREAM SAUCE

2 kg (4½ lb) boiling chicken

1 onion, skinned

1 carrot, peeled

1 bay leaf

6 peppercorns

50 g (2 oz) English butter

50 g (2 oz) flour

60 ml (4 level tbsp) grated horseradish

salt and freshly ground pepper

30 ml (2 tbsp) chopped fresh parsley

150 ml (5 fl oz) fresh double cream

1. Place the chicken in a large pan with onion, carrot, bay leaf and peppercorns. Add sufficient salted water to just cover, bring to the boil, reduce heat, cover and simmer for 2–2½ hours until tender.
2. Remove the chicken from pan, strain off stock and retain. Skin and joint chicken and keep warm in a covered dish.

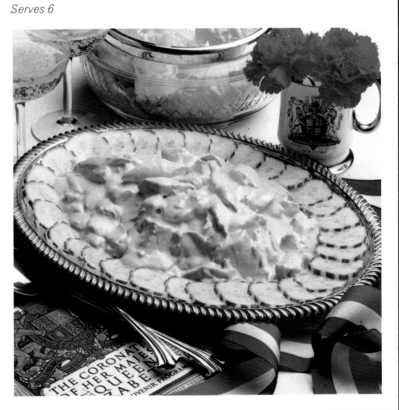

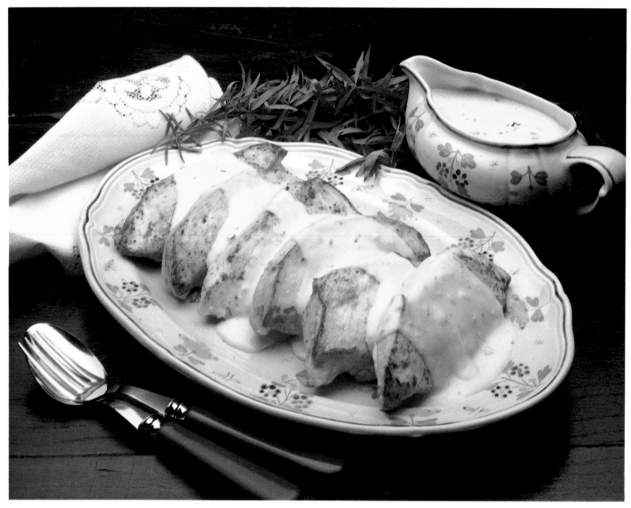

Above:
CHICKEN WITH TARRAGON SAUCE
Tarragon, a herb which the French are very fond of, has an unusual, original flavour. It is strong, so should be used sparingly, as in this recipe where the herb marries perfectly with chicken.

CHICKEN WITH TARRAGON SAUCE

6 chicken breasts
75 g (3 oz) English butter
25 g (1 oz) flour
400 ml (¾ pint) chicken stock
30 ml (2 tbsp) tarragon vinegar
10 ml (2 level tsp) French mustard
5 ml (1 level tsp) fresh tarragon, chopped, or 2.5 ml (½ level tsp) dried tarragon
50 g (2 oz) English Cheddar cheese, grated
salt and freshly ground pepper
150 ml (5 fl oz) fresh single cream

1. In a covered pan, slowly cook the chicken breasts in 50 g (2 oz) butter, for about 20 minutes, until tender, turning once.
2. Meanwhile, melt the remaining butter in a pan, stir in the flour and gradually stir in the stock and vinegar.
3. Stir in the mustard, tarragon and cheese; bring to the boil, stirring. Season, simmer for 3 minutes. Remove from heat and add the fresh cream.
4. Heat gently without boiling. Place drained chicken on a serving dish and spoon over sauce.

Serves 6

CHICKEN FRICASSÉE WITH ALMONDS

25 g (1 oz) English butter
1 medium onion, skinned and chopped
10 ml (2 level tsp) flour
300 ml (½ pint) chicken stock
450 g (1 lb) cooked chicken, cut into strips
300 ml (10 fl oz) soured cream
50 g (2 oz) flaked almonds, toasted
salt and freshly ground pepper

1. Melt the butter in a frying pan and cook the onion for about 5 minutes, until soft.
2. Stir in the flour and cook for 1–2 minutes. Gradually stir in the stock.
3. Add the chicken strips and soured cream, bring to the boil, stirring, then simmer for 5–10 minutes.
4. Stir in the almonds and season to taste. Serve with buttered noodles or boiled rice.

Serves 4

CHEESY CHICKEN FRICASSÉE

225 g (8 oz) long grain rice

100 g (4 oz) English butter

1 onion, skinned and chopped

225 g (8 oz) button mushrooms, wiped and sliced

40 g (1½ oz) flour

568 ml (1 pint) milk

salt and freshly ground pepper

275 g (10 oz) cooked chicken, cut into 2.5–5-cm (1–2-inch) pieces

200-g (7-oz) can sweetcorn, drained

15 ml (1 tbsp) chopped fresh parsley

175–225 g (6–8 oz) English Cheddar cheese, grated

fresh parsley to garnish

1. Cook the rice in a saucepan of boiling salted water for 12–15 minutes.
2. Melt half the butter in a frying pan, and fry onion gently until tender but not browned. Add mushrooms to onions in pan and fry for 2–3 minutes, until just cooked. Drain.
3. Melt remaining butter in a pan, stir in the flour and cook for 1 minute, stirring. Remove from the heat and gradually stir in the milk. Return to the heat and bring to the boil, stirring.
4. Season sauce and stir in the chicken, corn, parsley, mushrooms and onions. Cook for 3–4 minutes, then remove from heat, add the cheese and stir until cheese has melted.
5. Drain rice and arrange around edge of serving dish. Turn chicken mixture into centre. Garnish with parsley.

Serves 4–5

TURKEY ESCALOPES WITH HAZELNUT CREAM SAUCE

450 g (1 lb) turkey fillet

50 g (2 oz) English butter

60 ml (4 tbsp) sweet sherry

60 ml (4 tbsp) fresh double cream

25 g (1 oz) hazelnuts, finely chopped

salt and freshly ground pepper

paprika to garnish

1. Thinly slice the turkey fillet. Beat out the slices between two sheets of damp greaseproof paper or non-stick paper into small escalopes.
2. Melt the butter in a frying pan and cook the escalopes quickly for 4–5 minutes, turning once. Remove from the pan and keep warm.
3. Reduce heat and stir in the sherry, fresh cream and hazelnuts. Season. Cook, stirring, for 1 minute. Pour over escalopes and serve immediately with a light dusting of paprika.

Serves 4

TURKEY STROGANOFF

450 g (1 lb) turkey fillet

15 ml (1 tbsp) corn oil

50 g (2 oz) English butter

30 ml (2 tbsp) brandy

1 garlic clove, skinned and crushed

salt and freshly ground pepper

1 green pepper, seeded and thinly sliced

225 g (8 oz) button mushrooms, wiped and thinly sliced

60 ml (4 tbsp) soured cream

1. Thinly slice the turkey.
2. Heat the oil and butter in a large sauté pan and brown the turkey strips. Flame with the brandy, add crushed garlic and seasoning.
3. Cover the pan and simmer for 4–5 minutes until the turkey is just tender.
4. Increase the heat, add the mushrooms and pepper and cook for 3–4 minutes, turning occasionally.
5. Reduce the heat, stir in the soured cream (if on the thick side, stir before adding to the pan) and adjust seasoning. Serve hot with rice.

Serves 4

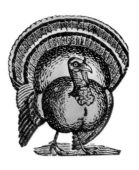

Below:
TURKEY ESCALOPES WITH HAZELNUT CREAM SAUCE
Hazelnuts and sherry give this quickly prepared supper dish a very classy touch! Buttered noodles and a green salad with lemon dressing are very good with it.

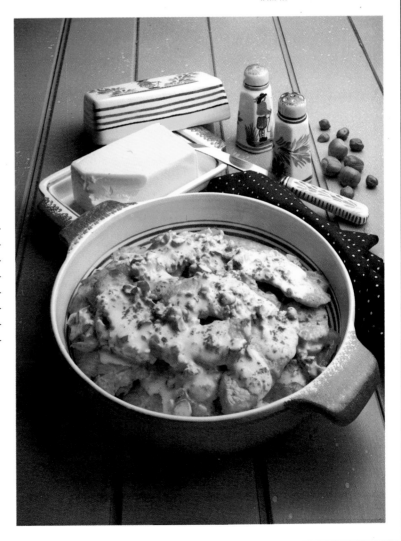

TURKEY IN SPICED YOGURT

about 1.1 kg (2½ lb) turkey leg meat on the bone

7.5 ml (1½ level tsp) ground cumin

7.5 ml (1½ level tsp) ground coriander

2.5 ml (½ level tsp) ground turmeric

2.5 ml (½ level tsp) ground ginger

salt and freshly ground pepper

300 g (10 fl oz) natural yogurt

30 ml (2 tbsp) lemon juice

225 g (8 oz) onion, skinned and sliced

45 ml (3 tbsp) vegetable oil

45 ml (3 level tbsp) desiccated coconut

30 ml (2 level tbsp) flour

150 ml (¼ pint) chicken stock or water

chopped fresh parsley to garnish

1. Cut the turkey meat off the bone into large fork-sized pieces, discarding the skin; there should be about 900 g (2 lb) meat.
2. In a large bowl, mix the spices with the seasoning, yogurt and lemon juice. Stir well until evenly blended.
3. Fold through the turkey meat until coated with the yogurt mixture. Cover tightly with cling film and refrigerate for several hours.
4. Lightly brown the onion in the hot oil in a medium flameproof casserole. Add the coconut and flour and fry gently, stirring, for about 1 minute.
5. Remove from the heat and stir in the turkey with its marinade and the stock. Return to the heat and bring slowly to the boil, stirring all the time. Cover tightly and cook in the oven at 170°C (325°F) mark 3 for 1–1¼ hours until the turkey is tender.
6. Adjust the seasoning and serve garnished with parsley.

Serves 6

CASSEROLED PIGEONS

100 g (4 oz) bacon, diced

50 g (2 oz) English butter

4 pigeons or 2 wood pigeons

4 medium onions, skinned and chopped

4 medium carrots, peeled and chopped

1 bay leaf

10 ml (2 tsp) chopped fresh parsley

1.25 ml (¼ tsp) dried thyme

salt and freshly ground pepper

25 g (1 oz) flour

300 ml (½ pint) meat stock

2 sherry glasses of red wine

1. Fry the diced bacon for 2 minutes, add the butter and the pigeons and brown quickly on all sides.
2. Remove and add the chopped vegetables, herbs, salt, freshly ground pepper and flour. Mix well.

3. Replace the birds, pour on the stock and the wine, bring to the boil and simmer very gently for 1½ hours, until the birds are tender. Serve with red currant jelly.

Serves 6

FISH

HALIBUT AND PRAWN BAKE

4 halibut steaks

juice of ½ lemon

2 bay leaves

150 ml (¼ pint) white wine or stock

6 peppercorns

salt and freshly ground pepper

oil

50 g (2 oz) English butter

50 g (2 oz) flour

milk

170 g (6 oz) prawns or shrimps

5 ml (1 tsp) fresh parsley, finely chopped

30 ml (2 tbsp) fresh single cream

fresh parsley to garnish

1. Butter an ovenproof dish. Place the halibut in dish, add the lemon juice, bay leaves, wine or stock, peppercorns and seasonings and cover with foil. Bake in the oven at 180°C (350°F) mark 4 for 15–20 minutes.
2. Strain liquid from the fish and reserve. Place the fish on a serving dish, cover and keep warm.
3. Place the butter, flour and liquid, made up to 450 ml (¾ pint) with milk, in a medium saucepan. Season. Heat, whisking all the time, until the sauce thickens and is cooked. Simmer for 2–3 minutes.
4. Add the prawns, parsley and cream to the sauce, heat through gently without boiling. Check seasoning and pour over fish. Garnish with parsley.

Serves 4

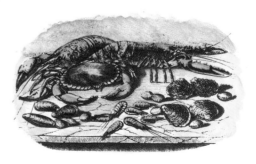

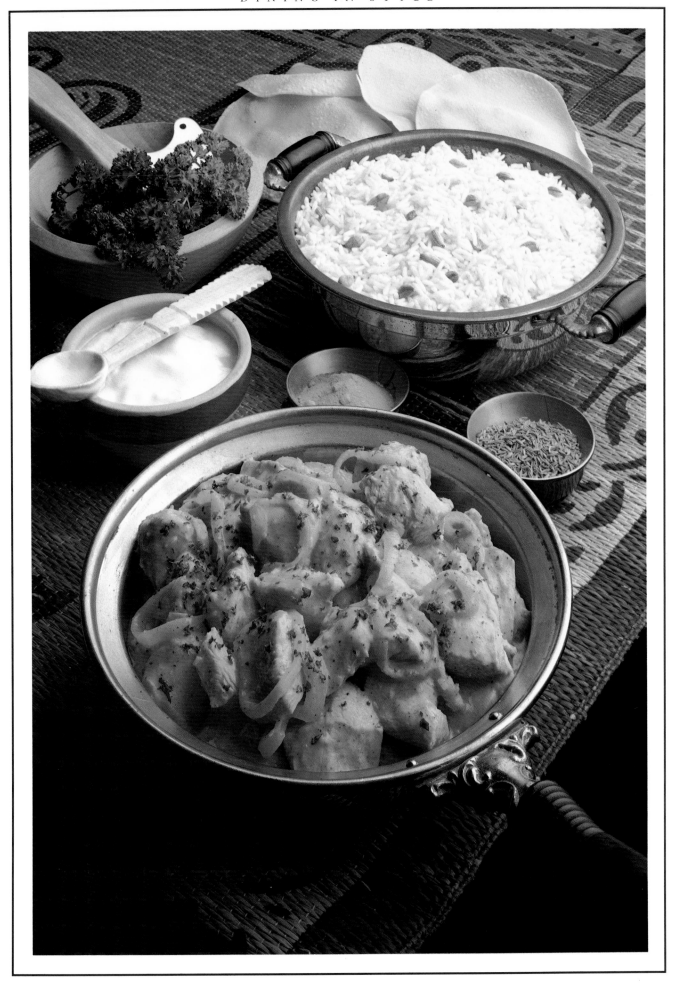

MUSHROOM-STUFFED PLAICE

50 g (2 oz) English butter

1 small onion, skinned and finely chopped

225 g (8 oz) flat mushrooms, wiped and finely chopped

grated nutmeg

salt and freshly ground pepper

30 ml (2 tbsp) fresh parsley, finely chopped

4 large plaice fillets, skinned

25 g (1 oz) flour

150 ml (¼ pint) milk

lemon juice

15 ml (1 tbsp) fresh double cream

chopped fresh parsley to garnish

1. Melt half the butter in a pan and fry the onion gently until soft and golden. Add the mushrooms and cook for about 20 minutes until all the juices have evaporated and the remaining mixture is a dryish, spreadable paste.
2. Remove from the heat, season with nutmeg, salt and freshly ground pepper, then transfer all but 30 ml (2 tbsp) of the mixture to a basin and mix with 15 ml (1 tbsp) of the parsley.
3. Cut the fish fillets in half lengthways and spread an equal quantity of the mushroom mixture on the skinned side of each piece of fish. Roll up the fillets from the head to the tail end and place them closely together in a baking dish.

4. Pour in 150 ml (¼ pint) water and place a piece of buttered foil on top of the fish. Bake in the oven at 180°C (350°F) mark 4 for 20–25 minutes until tender.
5. Melt the remaining butter in a saucepan, stir in the flour and cook for 2 minutes, stirring continuously. Remove from the heat and gradually stir in the cooking liquid. Stir in the milk. Bring to the boil, stirring all the time. Add the remaining mushroom mixture, season with salt, freshly ground pepper and a few drops of lemon juice and stir in the fresh cream.
6. When the fish is cooked, transfer it to a warmed serving dish. Pour the sauce over the fish and serve with new potatoes, if liked.

Serves 4

FISH WELLINGTON

100 g (4 oz) mushrooms, wiped and chopped

50 g (2 oz) onion, skinned and finely chopped

25 g (1 oz) English butter

175 g (6 oz) smooth liver pâté, or liver sausage

60 ml (4 tbsp) fresh double cream

salt and freshly ground pepper

2 large fillets of cod or haddock, about 900 g (2 lb)

368-g (13-oz) packet puff pastry

beaten egg to glaze

1. Fry the chopped mushrooms and onion in the butter until soft. Remove pan from heat.
2. Mash the liver pâté or sausage in a bowl. Stir in the fresh cream, onion and mushrooms. Season to taste.
3. Remove skin from fish. Roll out the pastry to a rectangle 35 × 30 cm (14 × 12 inches). Place one fillet in the centre of the pastry, spread filling mixture over fillet, then top with the other fillet. Trim pastry round, allowing a good 10-cm (4-inch) border. Reserve the trimmed pastry.
4. Brush round the edges of the pastry with beaten egg, then carefully fold it over the fish and neatly wrap it up like a parcel.
5. Place the parcelled fish on a baking sheet with the sealed edges down. Brush with beaten egg. Roll pastry trimmings into decorative fish shapes and seal on top of the pastry parcel.
6. Bake in the oven at 220°C (425°F) mark 7 for about 25 minutes, until the pastry is golden brown and the fish is cooked through.

Serves 6–8

Below:
MUSHROOM-STUFFED PLAICE
Plaice is found in abundance in the waters of the continental shelf – those taken from sandy bottoms are regarded as the best. This delicious flatfish is excellent rolled and stuffed with mushrooms.

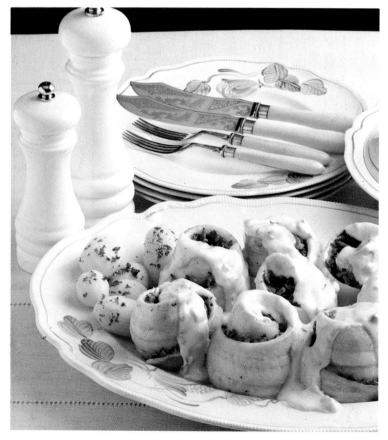

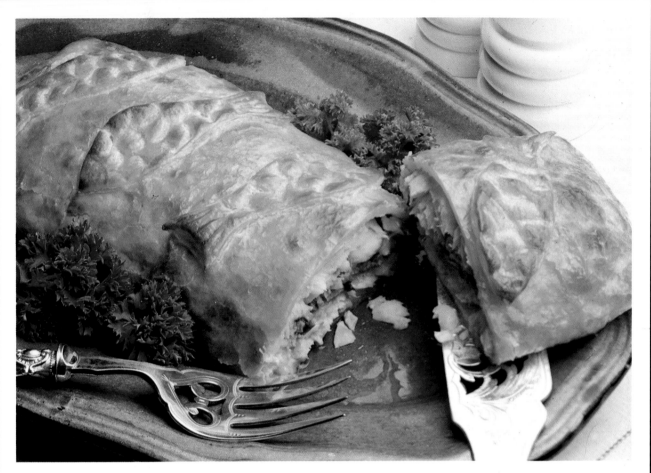

HADDOCK AND CUCUMBER SOUFFLÉ

450 g (1 lb) smoked haddock fillet

568 ml (1 pint) milk

salt and freshly ground pepper

50 g (2 oz) English butter

50 g (2 oz) flour

½ small cucumber, diced

3 eggs, separated

30 ml (2 tbsp) chopped fresh chives

1. Put the fish in a saucepan with 450 ml (¾ pint) milk. Season. Cook very gently for 10 minutes, until fish is cooked. Drain, reserving liquid. Flake fish, discarding all the skin and any bones.
2. Melt the butter in a pan, add flour and cook, stirring, for 1 minute. Gradually stir in the reserved liquid and remaining milk. Bring to the boil and cook, stirring, for 2 minutes. Season.
3. Pour half the mixture into a buttered 1.25-litre (2½-pint) soufflé dish and stir in the flaked fish and cucumber.
4. Add the egg yolks and 15 ml (1 tbsp) chives to remaining sauce. Whisk the egg whites until stiff and fold into the sauce.
5. Pour over fish in dish, sprinkle with remaining chopped chives and bake in the oven at 200°C (400°F) mark 6 for 40–45 minutes, until well risen and golden.
Serves 6

COD WITH ORANGE AND WALNUTS

50 g (2 oz) English butter

75 g (3 oz) fresh breadcrumbs

1 garlic clove, skinned and finely chopped (optional)

25 g (1 oz) walnuts, finely chopped

finely grated rind and juice of 1 orange

4 cod cutlets, each about 100–175 g (4–6 oz)

salt and freshly ground pepper

watercress to garnish

1. Melt the butter in a pan. Stir in the breadcrumbs, garlic if used, walnuts and orange rind. Leave over a low heat, stirring frequently, until the breadcrumbs have absorbed the butter.
2. Season the fish. Stand in a buttered shallow ovenproof dish. Moisten with orange juice and cover with the breadcrumb mixture.
3. Bake in the oven uncovered, at 190°C (375°F) mark 5 for 20–30 minutes, until the fish is tender. Garnish with watercress.
Serves 4

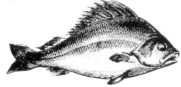

Above:
FISH WELLINGTON
Like its beef counterpart, Fish Wellington is one of those regal dishes to serve on an important occasion.

Right:
*COD WITH CORIANDER
IN CREAM*
Cod has firm, delicate flesh and is one of the world's most delicious fish when eaten fresh. In Britain we tend to take cod for granted. Often we automatically associate cod with chips and underestimate how tasty it also is when served in other ways than just deep fried.

In this mouthwatering recipe, tasty cod fillets are dipped in flour and spicy ground coriander before being gently cooked in bubbling golden butter. The finishing touch is tangy lemon juice, capers and a velvety cream sauce spooned over just before serving.

Opposite, top:
*COD IN CREAM AND
CELERY SAUCE*
Topped with a garnish of bright tomato slices, these cod steaks are coated with a well-seasoned cheese and celery sauce before being browned under the grill.

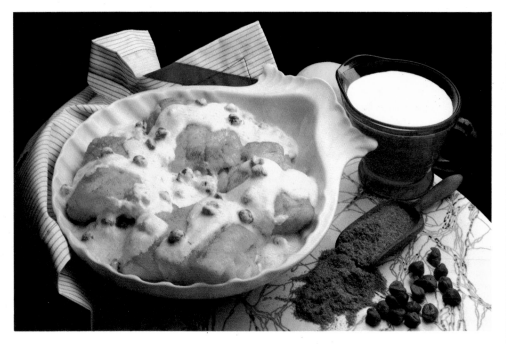

COD WITH CORIANDER
IN CREAM

450 g (1 lb) thick cut cod fillet

30 ml (2 level tbsp) flour

10 ml (2 level tsp) ground coriander

salt and freshly ground pepper

50 g (2 oz) English butter

15–30 ml (1–2 tbsp) lemon juice

15 ml (1 level tbsp) capers

1 egg yolk

90 ml (6 tbsp) fresh single cream

1. Skin the fish and divide into four portions. Mix the flour, ground coriander and seasoning together. Coat the fish pieces with this mixture.
2. Heat the butter in a medium sauté pan and sauté the fish gently until golden on both sides, turning only once.
3. Add 15 ml (1 tbsp) lemon juice to the pan with the capers, cover tightly and continue cooking for a further 4–5 minutes, until the fish is tender. Place the fish on a warm serving dish.
4. Mix the egg yolk and fresh cream together, stir into the pan juices and heat gently until the sauce thickens – do not boil. Adjust seasoning, adding extra lemon juice if wished and spoon the sauce over the fish.
Serves 4

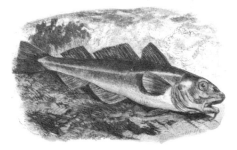

COD IN CREAM AND
CELERY SAUCE

4 cod steaks or cutlets

15 ml (1 tbsp) lemon juice

salt and freshly ground pepper

25 g (1 oz) English butter

*3 sticks of celery, cleaned, trimmed and
  chopped*

25 g (1 oz) flour

225 ml (8 fl oz) milk

75 ml (2½ fl oz) fresh double cream

2.5 ml (½ level tsp) dried thyme

50 g (2 oz) Lancashire cheese, crumbled

2 tomatoes, sliced

fresh parsley to garnish

1. Sprinkle the fish with lemon juice and season. Place under the grill or bake in the oven at 200°C (400°F) mark 6 for 20 minutes. Place in a serving dish and keep warm.
2. Melt the butter in a pan and fry the celery until tender. Stir in the flour and cook gently for 1 minute, stirring. Remove the pan from the heat and gradually stir in the milk and fresh cream. Heat and continue to stir, until the sauce thickens.
3. Add seasoning, thyme and 25 g (1 oz) cheese. Pour sauce over fish and sprinkle with remaining cheese.
4. Arrange tomatoes on the dish and place under the grill to brown. Serve hot garnished with parsley.

Variations
If celery is not available, use 1 large leek; any white fish is suitable for this recipe.
Serves 4

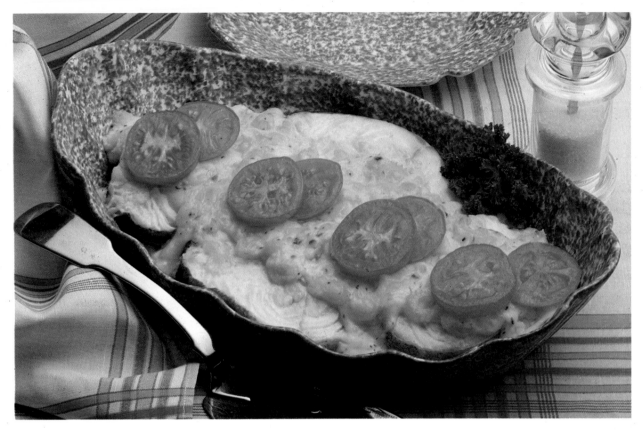

SOLE BONNE FEMME

2 fillets of sole

2 shallots, or 2–3 slices of onion, skinned and finely chopped

100 g (4 oz) button mushrooms, wiped

45 ml (3 tbsp) dry white wine

salt and freshly ground pepper

1 bay leaf

40 g (1½ oz) English butter

30 ml (2 level tbsp) flour

about 150 ml (¼ pint) milk

45 ml (3 tbsp) fresh single cream

1. Trim off the fins, wash and wipe the fillets and fold each into three. Put the shallots or onion in the bottom of an ovenproof dish with the stalks from the mushrooms, finely chopped. Cover with the fish, pour round the wine and 15 ml (1 tbsp) water, season and add the bay leaf.
2. Cover with foil or a lid and bake in the oven at 180°C (350°F) mark 4 for about 15 minutes, until tender. Strain off the cooking liquid and keep the fish warm.
3. Fry the mushroom caps lightly in half the butter. Melt the remaining butter in a pan, stir in the flour and cook gently for 1 minute, stirring. Remove the pan from the heat and gradually stir in the cooking liquid from the fish, made up to 300 ml (½ pint) with milk.

4. Bring to the boil and continue to cook, stirring, until the sauce thickens, then remove from the heat and stir in the fresh cream. Pour the sauce over the fish and serve garnished with the mushroom caps

Serves 4

Below:
SOLE BONNE FEMME
This delicate and delicious dish is a classic French way of finishing tender poached sole in a creamy sauce garnished with mushrooms.

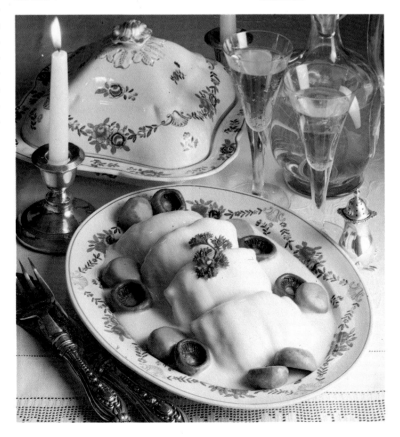

TROUT IN CREAM

4 trout

juice of 1 lemon

15 ml (1 tbsp) chopped fresh chives

15 ml (1 tbsp) chopped fresh parsley

150 ml (5 fl oz) fresh single cream

30 ml (2 level tbsp) fresh breadcrumbs

a little English butter, melted

Below:

TROUT IN CREAM

Fresh trout has a delicate and unique flavour which is greatly prized by those who know and love good food.

In this recipe very fresh trout are gently baked in their own juices with a sprinkling of zesty lemon and herbs. They are then finished under the grill with a coating of single cream, melted butter and a crispy brown breadcrumb topping.

1. Clean the fish, leaving the heads on if wished. Wash and wipe the fish, lay them in a buttered shallow flameproof dish.
2. Sprinkle over the lemon juice, herbs and about 15 ml (1 tbsp) water. Cover with foil
3. Cook in the oven at 180°C (350°F) mark 4 for 10–15 minutes, until tender.
4. Heat the fresh cream gently and pour over the fish. Sprinkle with breadcrumbs and melted butter and brown under a hot grill. Serve immediately.

Serves 4

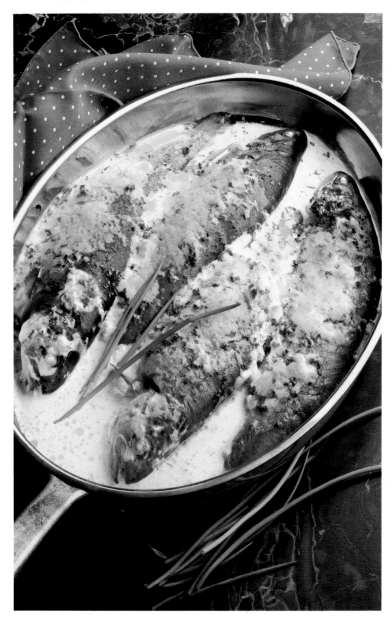

MOUSSELINE OF SOLE WITH PRAWNS

450 g (1 lb) fillets of sole, skinned and chopped

50 g (2 oz) shelled prawns

1 egg white

1.25 ml ($\frac{1}{4}$ level tsp) salt

1.25 ml ($\frac{1}{4}$ level tsp) white pepper

450 ml (15 fl oz) fresh double cream

3 egg yolks

75 g (3 oz) English butter, softened

10 ml (2 tsp) lemon juice

5 ml (1 level tsp) tomato purée

whole prawns to garnish

1. Combine the chopped fish with the prawns, egg white and seasoning. Purée half the mixture in a blender with 150-ml ($\frac{1}{4}$-pint) fresh cream. Remove from the goblet and purée the rest of the fish with another 150 ml ($\frac{1}{4}$ pint) fresh cream.
2. Butter six 150 ml ($\frac{1}{4}$ pint) ovenproof ramekins and press the mixture well down into the dishes. Chill, covered, for 3 hours.
3. Cook in the oven in a water bath at 150°C (300°F) mark 3 for 30–40 minutes. Turn out on to a wire rack to drain. Keep warm.
4. In a double boiler or a bowl over a pan of hot water, combine the yolks, a knob of butter and the lemon juice. Stir until of a coating consistency.
5. Remove from the heat and slowly beat in the rest of the butter and the tomato purée. Whip the remaining fresh cream until softly stiff. Fold into the sauce, return to the heat to thicken without boiling.
6. Place the moulds in a warm dish and cover with the sauce. Garnish with the whole prawns. Serve hot.

Serves 6

FILLETS OF SOLE DUGLÉRÉ

2 sole, filleted, or 4 fillets of plaice

1–2 shallots, skinned and chopped

$\frac{1}{2}$ bay leaf

few sprigs of fresh parsley

150 ml ($\frac{1}{4}$ pint) dry white wine

salt and freshly ground pepper

25 g (1 oz) English butter

45 ml (3 level tbsp) flour

150 ml (5 fl oz) fresh single cream

2 tomatoes, skinned and diced with seeds removed

30 ml (2 tbsp) chopped fresh parsley

1. Rinse and dry the fish, remove the dark skin and put in an ovenproof dish with the shallots, herbs, wine, 45 ml (3 tbsp) water and seasoning; cover.

2. Cook in the oven at 180°C (350°F) mark 4 for 15 minutes. Strain off the cooking liquid and keep the fish warm.

3. Melt the butter in a pan, stir in the flour and cook gently for 1 minute, stirring. Remove from the heat and gradually stir in the fish stock.

4. Bring to the boil and continue to cook, stirring, until the sauce thickens. Remove from the heat and stir in the fresh cream, tomatoes and parsley. Reheat gently but do not boil. Check the seasoning and pour over the fish to serve.

Serves 4

SOURED CREAM SALMON PIE

450 g (1 lb) salmon
60 ml (4 tbsp) dry white wine
salt and freshly ground pepper
165 g (6½ oz) English butter
40 g (1½ oz) plain flour
225 g (8 oz) English Cheddar cheese, grated
3 eggs, hard-boiled and roughly chopped
142 ml (5 fl oz) soured cream
30 ml (2 tbsp) chopped fresh parsley
50 g (2 oz) lard
450 g (1 lb) self-raising flour
milk to bind
beaten egg to glaze

1. Cover the salmon sparingly with cold water, add the wine, season and simmer for about 20 minutes. Reserve fish stock, flake fish, discarding bones and skin.

2. Melt 40 g (1½ oz) butter in a pan and stir in the plain flour. Remove pan from the heat and gradually stir in 300 ml (½ pint) reserved fish stock. Bring to the boil and continue to cook, stirring, for 2 minutes. Remove from the heat and stir in 200 g (7 oz) grated cheese, chopped eggs, soured cream, parsley and seasonings; cool.

3. Make shortcrust pastry by rubbing the remaining butter and lard into the self-raising flour and remaining cheese until the mixture resembles fine breadcrumbs. Add a little cold milk to bind the mixture together.

4. Roll out one-third of pastry to a 35.5 × 10 cm (12 × 4 inches) oblong, place on a baking sheet. Top with the sauce mixture, salmon and more sauce.

5. Cover with remaining pastry, sealing edges well. Garnish with pastry trimmings.

6. Glaze with beaten egg and bake in the oven at 190°C (375°F) mark 5 for about 40 minutes. Serve warm.

Serves 8

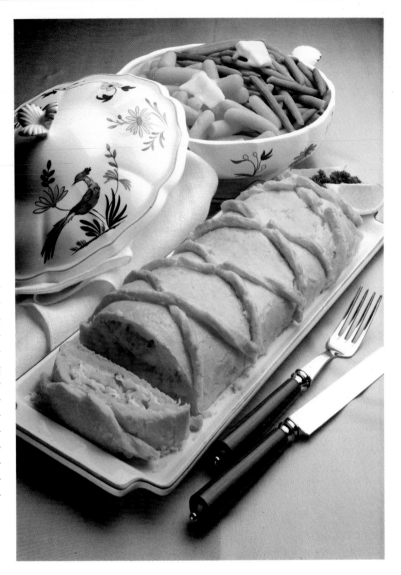

VEGETABLES WITH A LUXURY TOUCH

COURGETTES SAUTÉED IN BUTTER

75 g (3 oz) English butter
450 g (1 lb) courgettes, trimmed and cut into diagonal slices
salt and freshly ground pepper
lemon juice
chopped fresh parsley to garnish

1. Heat the butter in a large pan and when hot add the courgettes. Cook over a high heat until well browned, moving them round in the pan. Reduce heat and cook for a further 2 minutes. It is best if they retain a little crispness.

2. Transfer to a warmed serving dish, season well, sprinkle with lemon juice and parsley. Serve immediately.

Serves 4

Above:
SOURED CREAM
SALMON PIE
This delicious fish pie combines freshly poached salmon, grated Cheddar cheese, chopped hard-boiled eggs and tangy soured cream in a crisp pastry case.

This dish makes an attractive and tasty centre to a late summer dinner party and is based on Kulebiaka or Salmon Pie, one of the classic fish dishes from old Russia.

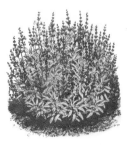

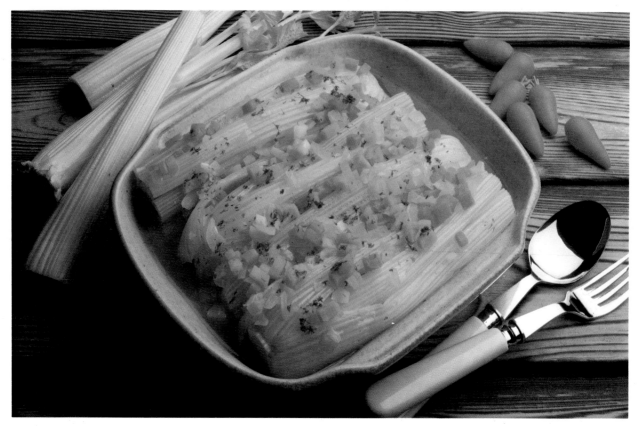

Above:
BRAISED CELERY
Celery is an extremely versatile vegetable, full of flavour and just as good raw or cooked. For a tasty way of serving celery hot, try this rich and savoury dish in which celery hearts are browned in English butter and then braised slowly in chicken stock.

JUGGED PEAS

2 kg (4½ lb) peas, shelled
25 g (1 oz) English butter
2.5 ml (½ level tsp) salt
5 ml (1 level tsp) caster sugar
12 mint leaves
freshly ground pepper

1. Put all the ingredients in a screw-top jar. Screw the lid on tightly and stand in a saucepan of boiling water coming half way up the jar.
2. Boil for 30 minutes. Take out the mint leaves before serving. If the peas are old, they may take a little longer, but cooked this way peas are delicious and tender.
Serves 8

BRAISED CELERY

1 small onion, skinned and very finely chopped
50 g (2 oz) carrot, peeled and very finely chopped
50 g (2 oz) English butter
1 garlic clove, skinned and crushed
4 small celery hearts
150 ml (¼ pint) chicken stock
chopped fresh parsley

1. Sauté the onion and carrot in half the butter for 5 minutes, add the garlic and transfer to an ovenproof casserole.

2. Evenly brown the celery hearts in the remaining butter and put on top of the vegetables. Spoon over the stock and season well.
3. Cover tightly and bake in the oven at 180°C (350°F) mark 4 for about 1½ hours. Turn the celery hearts in the juices to glaze. Serve hot, scattered with lots of chopped fresh parsley.
Serves 4

BAKED COURGETTES WITH MUSHROOMS

50 g (2 oz) English butter
1.1kg (2½ lb) courgettes, trimmed and cut into 0.5-cm (¼-inch) slices
salt and freshly ground pepper
225 g (8 oz) button mushrooms, wiped
142 g (5 fl oz) soured cream

1. Melt the butter in a medium roasting tin, add the courgettes and turn over in the butter; season well. Roast in the oven at 200°C (400°F) mark 6 for 20 minutes.
2. Meanwhile, stir the sliced mushrooms into the courgettes and return to the oven for a further 10–15 minutes,
3. Stir the soured cream and then mix through the vegetables. Heat on top of the stove until bubbling and adjust seasoning. Spoon the vegetables into a serving dish and serve hot.
Serves 6

SCALLOPED KOHLRABI

175 g (6 oz) onion, skinned and thinly sliced

40 g (1½ oz) English butter

900 g (2 lb) kohlrabi

200 ml (7 fl oz) milk

salt and freshly ground pepper

chopped fresh parsley to garnish

1. Soften the onion in 25 g (1 oz) butter in a covered pan.
2. Thickly peel the kohlrabi to remove all the woody outer layer. Slice thinly and layer with the onions and seasoning in a 1.7-litre (3-pint) lightly buttered shallow ovenproof dish, topping with a neat layer of kohlrabi.
3. Pour over the milk and dot with remaining butter. Place on a baking tray and cook in the oven at 200°C (400°F) mark 6 for about 1½ hours, until tender. Garnish with chopped parsley for serving.

Serves 6

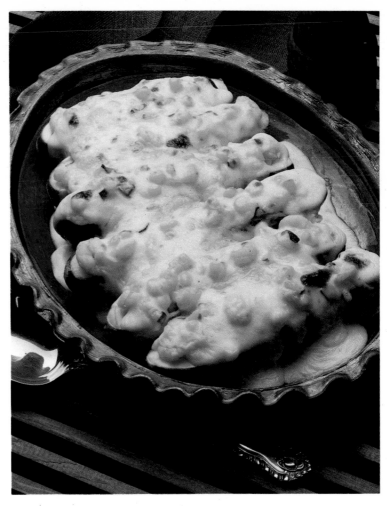

COURGETTES AU GRATIN

6 medium courgettes – about 700 g (1½ lb)

1 small onion, skinned and chopped

50 g (2 oz) English butter

198-g (7-oz) can sweetcorn, drained

100 g (4 oz) peeled prawns

salt and freshly ground pepper

30 ml (2 level tbsp) flour

300 ml (½ pint) milk

150 g (5 oz) English Cheddar cheese, grated

1. Wipe the courgettes, then blanch in boiling salted water for 8 minutes; drain well. Cut a slice off the top of each and scoop out the flesh, leaving a 0.5-cm (¼-inch) rim around the edge. Roughly chop the flesh, including the top slices. Turn shells upside down, drain.
2. Fry the onion in half the butter until lightly browned. Stir in the chopped courgette flesh and cook over a high heat for a few minutes. Mix in the sweetcorn, the prawns and plenty of seasoning.
3. Place the courgette shells in a shallow ovenproof dish and fill with the prawn mixture. Melt the remaining butter in a pan, stir in the flour and cook gently for 1 minute stirring. Remove from the heat and gradually stir in the milk.
4. Season, then bring to the boil and continue to cook stirring, until the sauce thickens. Remove from the heat and stir in 125 g (4 oz) cheese, adjust seasoning.
5. Spoon the cheese sauce over the courgettes and sprinkle with the remaining cheese. Cook in the oven at 200°C (400°F) mark 6 for 15–20 minutes, until golden.

Serves 6

CREAMED MUSHROOMS

75 g (3 oz) English butter

700 g (1½ lb) button mushrooms, wiped and trimmed

45 ml (3 level tbsp) chopped onion

30 ml (2 level tbsp) flour

450 ml (15 fl oz) fresh single cream

2 egg yolks

45 ml (3 tbsp) sherry

few grains of cayenne pepper

good pinch of grated nutmeg

salt

1. Heat 50 g (2 oz) butter until it bubbles, add the mushrooms and onion and sauté until almost tender. Drain well.
2. Melt the remaining butter in a pan, stir in the flour and cook gently for 1 minute, stirring. Remove from the heat. Warm the fresh cream and stir it gradually into the pan. Stir over a gentle heat until the mixture thickens. Mix the egg yolks with the sherry and stir into the sauce
3. Stir the mushrooms and onions into the sauce with the cayenne, nutmeg and a good pinch of salt and heat through gently. Spoon on to slices of hot toast and serve immediately.

Serves 6

Above:
COURGETTES AU GRATIN
Courgettes are small deliciously flavoured members of the marrow family, which have become much better known in Britain in recent years. In this sophisticated recipe, courgettes are blanched before being scooped out and stuffed with a mouthwatering filling of sweetcorn and prawns. They are then topped with a tempting cheese sauce and baked in the oven until golden brown.

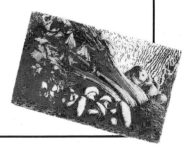

Right:
CARROTS IN LEMON
CREAM SAUCE
Bright orange-gold carrots are one of the most popular vegetables we have. Whatever the time of year they add colour, flavour or crunch to a wide variety of dishes, from warming winter stews to tangy summer party dips.

Try this unusual recipe for a delicious new way of presenting carrots at a dinner party. Cooked gently in butter and finished with tangy lemon juice and soured cream, they turn taken-for-granted carrots into a very special treat.

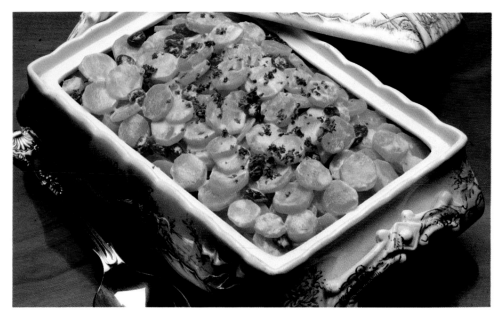

CARROTS IN LEMON CREAM SAUCE

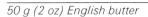

50 g (2 oz) English butter

700 g (1½ lb) carrots, peeled and thinly sliced

juice of ½ lemon

pinch of grated nutmeg

50 g (2 oz) sultanas

142 ml (5 fl oz) soured cream

chopped fresh parsley to garnish

1. Melt the butter in a pan and add the carrots. Cover and sauté gently for about 20 minutes, until just tender, shaking the pan occasionally to prevent sticking.
2. Stir in the lemon juice, nutmeg, sultanas and soured cream, season to taste and heat through gently. Serve immediately, garnished with chopped parsley.
Serves 4

KOHLRABI IN CREAM DILL SAUCE

350 g (12 oz) kohlrabi

225 g (8 oz) carrots

25 g (1 oz) English butter

1 chicken stock cube

15 ml (1 level tbsp) cornflour

2.5 ml (½ tsp) dried dill

150 ml (5 fl oz) fresh single cream

salt and freshly ground pepper

1. Thickly peel the kohlrabi to remove all the woody outer layer. Slice thinly and cook with the carrots, butter, 300 ml (½ pint) water and stock cube for about 10 minutes, until tender.
2. Blend the cornflour with very little cold water and strain in the vegetable liquid, stirring.
3. Return to the boil, stir in the dill and the fresh cream, then adjust seasoning. Bring almost to the boil and pour over the vegetables.
Serves 4

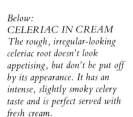

Below:
CELERIAC IN CREAM
The rough, irregular-looking celeriac root doesn't look appetising, but don't be put off by its appearance. It has an intense, slightly smoky celery taste and is perfect served with fresh cream.

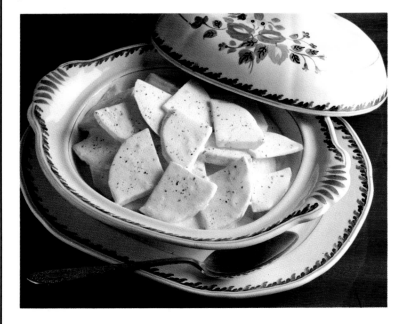

CELERIAC IN CREAM

450 g (1 lb) celeriac

salt

slice of lemon and lemon juice

40 g (1½ oz) English butter

150 ml (5 fl oz) fresh single cream

pinch of grated nutmeg

1. Wash and trim the celeriac; cover with cold, salted water in a pan with the lemon slice. Simmer, covered for about 50 minutes until almost tender; drain, peel and slice.
2. Melt the butter in a clean pan, add the celeriac with a little lemon juice; cover and

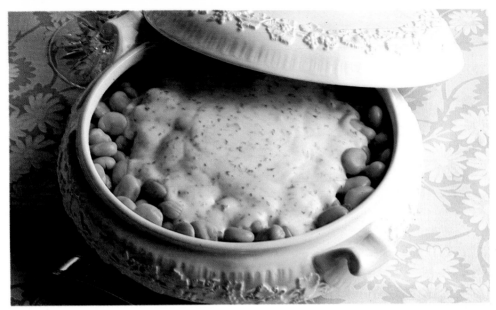

Left:
BROAD BEANS IN
PARSLEY SAUCE
Broad beans have been grown in the Western world since ancient times and they are best eaten when young and tender, when they have a delicate taste and flavour. All vegetables benefit from the extra care that comes from being served with a well-made sauce. In this simple but delicious recipe, the beans are presented with a savoury parsley sauce, enriched with fresh cream and egg yolks and a zesty taste of lemon juice.

cook for 8–10 minutes, shaking the pan occasionally.

3. Take from the heat and add the fresh cream. Simmer gently for 5 minutes and serve sprinkled with grated nutmeg.

Serves 4

BROAD BEANS IN PARSLEY SAUCE

1.8 kg (4 lb) broad beans, shelled
50 g (2 oz) English butter
75 ml (5 level tbsp) flour
400 ml (¾ pint) chicken stock
salt and freshly ground pepper
2 egg yolks
90 ml (6 tbsp) fresh single cream
45 ml (3 tbsp) chopped fresh parsley
30 ml (2 tbsp) lemon juice

1. Wash the beans well and drain. Cook in a large pan of boiling salted water for about 15 minutes until tender. Drain and place in a vegetable dish. Keep warm, covered.

2. Meanwhile, prepare the sauce. Melt the butter in a pan, stir in the flour and cook gently for 1 minute, stirring. Remove from the heat and gradually stir in the stock.

3. Bring to the boil, and continue to cook, stirring, until the sauce thickens. Season and simmer for about 5 minutes.

4. Beat the egg yolks with the fresh cream in a small basin, add about 90 ml (6 tbsp) hot sauce and stir until blended.

5. Remove the pan from the heat, add the egg mixture and stir well. Cook over a low heat without boiling until the sauce thickens a little more. Remove from the heat and stir in the parsley and lemon juice. Adjust seasoning and pour over the broad beans.

Serves 6

SAVOURY SPRING CABBAGE

50 g (2 oz) English butter
700 g (1½ lb) young cabbage, finely shredded
1 medium onion, skinned and grated
2 rashers streaky bacon, chopped
pinch of grated nutmeg

1. Heat the butter in a large saucepan. Add all remaining ingredients, cover pan and cook very gently for 20–30 minutes, until the cabbage is just tender, shaking the pan frequently.

Serves 4

Below:
SAVOURY SPRING
CABBAGE
Cabbage is a delicious vegetable when cooked with care and not just carelessly boiled to a pulp so that it loses both flavour and food value.
When cooked gently in good English butter with chopped bacon, onion and a pinch of nutmeg, fresh young cabbage is a tempting vegetable dish worthy of a special dinner party.

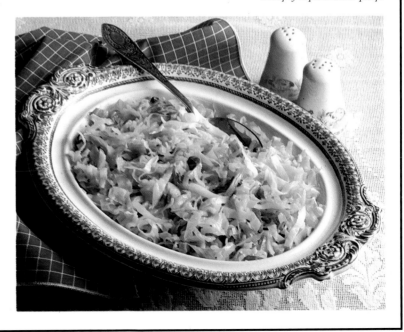

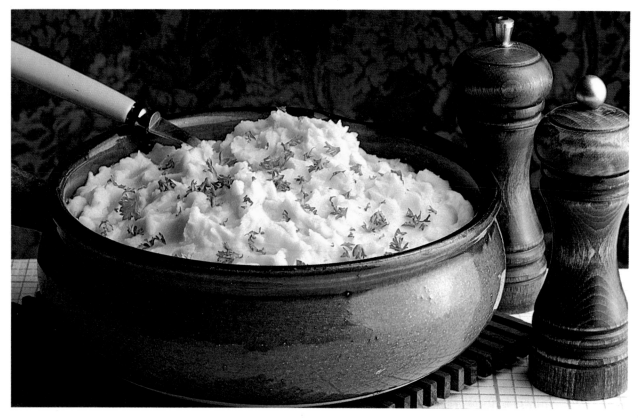

Above:
CREAMED BUTTER
BEANS
A delicious savoury purée is one
of the classic French ways of
making simple vegetables into
something special. Use
flavoursome English butter and
plenty of chopped fresh parsley
to give these delicious creamed
butter beans their extra appeal.

CREAMED BUTTER BEANS

350 g (12 oz) fresh butter beans, or three
425-g (15-oz) cans butter beans

50 g (2 oz) English butter

salt and freshly ground pepper

chopped fresh parsley to garnish

1. If using fresh butter beans, cover with plenty of cold water and soak overnight.
2. Drain off the water and cover with fresh cold unsalted water, bring to the boil, cover and simmer for $1\frac{1}{2}$–$1\frac{3}{4}$ hours, until the beans are quite tender. If using canned butter beans, cook as directed on the can.
3. Drain, then return to the pan and mash until smooth with a potato masher.
4. Push purée to one side of pan, melt butter in other side, then stir into the purée with seasoning. Stir over a low heat until thoroughly hot.
5. Spoon into a serving dish and scatter generously with parsley for serving.
Serves 6

CREAMED SWEDE

900 g (2 lb) swede, peeled and cut into
small pieces

salt and freshly ground pepper

50 g (2 oz) English butter

chopped fresh parsley to garnish

1. Put the swede into a large pan, cover with

cold salted water and bring to the boil. Cover the pan and boil gently for about 40 minutes, until quite tender. Drain well in a colander.
2. Return to the pan. Mash the swede, add the butter and seasoning and cook over a high heat, stirring frequently to drive off all excess moisture.
3. When a dry, stiffish purée is formed, adjust seasoning and spoon into a serving dish. Garnish with parsley.
Serves 6

CREAMED CARROT AND PARSNIP

900 g (2 lb) carrots, peeled and cubed

450 g (1 lb) parsnips, peeled and cut into
small pieces

50 g (2 oz) English butter

salt and freshly ground pepper

pinch of ground nutmeg

chopped fresh parsley to garnish

1. Boil the carrots and parsnips together in salted water for about 25 minutes until tender; drain well and mash using a potato masher.
2. Return to the pan with the butter and seasoning and cook over a high heat, stirring frequently, to drive off any moisture.
3. Beat well to mix the vegetables and pile into a serving dish. Garnish with parsley to serve.
Serves 6

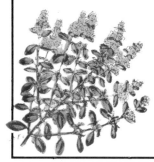

SPINACH WITH NUTMEG

1.8 kg (4 lb) fresh spinach

salt and freshly ground pepper

50 g (2 oz) English butter

large pinch of grated nutmeg

1. Trim the spinach, removing any coarse stalks and brown or damaged leaves. Wash well in several changes of cold water, making sure all the grit is removed. Drain in a colander.
2. Place the minimum of water – 1 cm ($\frac{1}{2}$ inch) is ample – in the bases of one or two large saucepans. Add the spinach and season generously.
3. Cover tightly and cook over a moderate heat for about 10 minutes, until tender. Push down and turn the spinach over once or twice during cooking.
4. Drain in a colander and press firmly with a potato masher to extract all moisture; chop roughly.
5. Melt the butter in a medium saucepan, add the spinach with plenty of seasoning and cook over a moderate heat, stirring occasionally, until piping hot.
6. Add a generous grating of nutmeg and spoon into a serving dish.
Serves 6

CREAMED BRUSSELS

1 kg (2.2 lb) brussels sprouts

salt and freshly ground pepper

300 ml ($\frac{1}{2}$ pint) milk

slice of carrot and onion

1 bay leaf

6 peppercorns

50 g (2 oz) English butter

30 ml (2 level tbsp) flour

large pinch of grated nutmeg

2 eggs

25 g (1 oz) fresh breadcrumbs

1. Trim the sprouts and wash well. Cook in boiling salted water for about 12 minutes, until tender; drain and chop finely.
2. Meanwhile, bring the milk to the boil with the carrot, onion, bay leaf and peppercorns; remove from heat and infuse for 10 minutes.
3. Melt 25 g (1 oz) butter in a medium saucepan, stir in the flour and cook gently for 1 minute, stirring. Remove from the heat and gradually stir in the strained milk and seasoning.
4. Bring to the boil and continue to cook, stirring, until the sauce thickens; simmer for 2 minutes. Remove from the heat, stir in the chopped sprouts with a generous grating of nutmeg. Adjust the seasoning and beat in the eggs.
5. Spoon into the lightly buttered 1.7-litre (3-pint) shallow soufflé dish and sprinkle with breadcrumbs. Dot with remaining

butter and bake in the oven at 180°C (350°F) mark 4 for about 50 minutes, until set and golden.
Serves 6

CREAMED BROAD BEANS

450 g (1 lb) broad beans, shelled

50 g (2 oz) mushrooms, wiped and sliced

25 g (1 oz) English butter

150 ml (5 fl oz) fresh double cream

1. Cook the beans in boiling salted water for 15–20 minutes, until tender.
2. Meanwhile, fry the mushrooms in the butter and keep warm.
3. Drain the beans in a colander. Return to the pan. Add the mushrooms and pan juices with the fresh cream. Mix well and reheat gently.
Serves 4

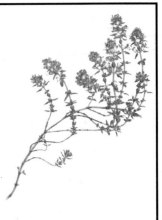

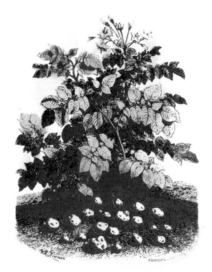

GOLDEN OVEN-FRIED POTATOES

1.1 kg (2$\frac{1}{2}$ lb) medium potatoes

60 ml (4 tbsp) vegetable oil

25 g (1 oz) English butter

salt and freshly ground pepper

1. Peel the potatoes, cover with cold salted water and bring to the boil. Simmer for 8–10 minutes. Drain, cut into 0.5–1-cm ($\frac{1}{4}$–$\frac{1}{2}$-inch) slices and score the surfaces of each piece by running a sharp-pronged fork in both directions across the surface.
2. Heat the oil and butter in a large roasting tin, about 30.5 × 23 cm (12 × 9 inches) and add the potato slices. Turn over in the hot oil and butter and season.
3. Bake in the oven at 200°C (400°F) mark 6 for about 1$\frac{1}{4}$ hours, turning once. Drain and place in a shallow serving dish to serve.
Serves 6–8

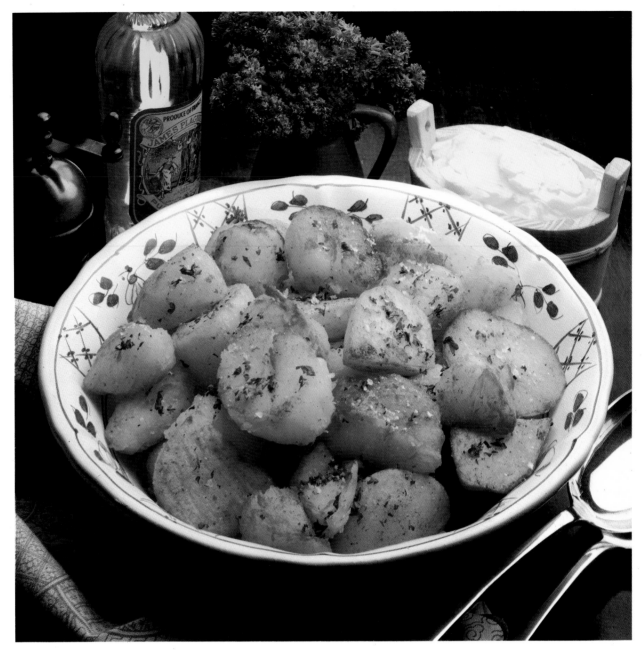

Above:
SAUTÉ POTATOES
When sprinkled with chopped parsley and perhaps a little freshly ground sea salt, these crisp, golden potatoes are a popular and mouthwatering accompaniment to a wide variety of savoury dishes from plain grills and family stews to elegant fish dishes for special occasions.

When frying these potatoes it is important to use good English butter as well as vegetable oil. The butter adds a special rich flavour and the oil stops the butter from burning.

SAUTÉ POTATOES

1.4 kg (3 lb) medium potatoes
salt and freshly ground pepper
60 ml (4 tbsp) vegetable oil
50 g (2 oz) English butter
60 ml (4 tbsp) chopped fresh parsley

1. Scrub the potatoes, but do not peel. Place in a large pan of cold salted water, bring to the boil and cook steadily for 20 minutes, until almost tender.
2. Drain and keep warm. Peel and cut into large wedge-shaped pieces. Heat the oil in a large frying pan, add the butter and, when bubbling spoon in the potatoes.
3. Fry over a moderate heat, turning occasionally, until golden brown and flaky. Season well, add the parsley and serve.

Serves 8

FONDANT POTATOES

700 g (1½ lb) small new potatoes
40 g (1½ oz) English butter
salt

1. Scrape the new potatoes – choose ones of even size. Wash and dry well.
2. Melt the butter in a deep frying pan with lid or sauté pan. Add the potatoes, cover and cook over a low heat. Shake the pan from time to time but do not lift the lid for the first 10 minutes as the steam inside helps the cooking and prevents sticking.
3. Test for tenderness, cook further if necessary. Serve sprinkled with salt.

Serves 4

CHÂTEAU POTATOES

900 g (2 lb) small new potatoes

50 g (2 oz) English butter

salt and freshly ground pepper

1. Scrape the potatoes, wash and drain well.
2. Melt the butter in a shallow flameproof casserole. When bubbling, add the potatoes and fry gently until golden brown on all sides.
3. Season well, cover the pan and cook in the oven at 180°C (350°F) mark 4 for 20–25 minutes until quite tender.

Serves 4–6

SLICED POTATOES WITH PARSLEY AND CELERY SEEDS

1.4 kg (3 lb) medium potatoes

salt and freshly ground pepper

50 g (2 oz) English butter

10 ml (2 level tsp) celery seeds

45 ml (3 tbsp) chopped fresh parsley

1. Scrub the potatoes. Cover with cold salted water and bring to the boil. Boil for about 30 minutes until tender.
2. Drain well then cut the potatoes into 0.5-cm ($\frac{1}{4}$-inch) slices and place in a shallow serving dish.
3. Melt the butter in a pan, add the celery seeds, parsley and plenty of seasoning and spoon over the potatoes. Serve hot.

Serves 8

SCALLOPED POTATOES WITH NUTMEG

900 g (2 lb) potatoes

40 g (1$\frac{1}{2}$ oz) English butter

1.25–2.5 ml ($\frac{1}{4}$–$\frac{1}{2}$ level tsp) ground nutmeg

salt and freshly ground pepper

scant 568 ml (1 pint) milk

50 g (2 oz) English Cheddar cheese, grated

1. Peel, rinse, pat dry and thinly slice the potatoes. (Don't leave them in water.)
2. Rub a little butter over a 1.1-litre (2-pint) shallow ovenproof dish. Layer three-quarters of the potatoes with the nutmeg and seasoning. Pour over the milk.
3. Arrange the remaining potatoes in neat overlapping layers on the top of the dish and dot the remaining butter over the surface.
4. Stand the dish on an edged baking sheet and cook in the oven at 180°C (350°F) mark 4 for about 1$\frac{1}{2}$ hours, until tender with a golden brown top and all the milk is absorbed. Sprinkle with the grated cheese 15 minutes before the end of cooking.

Serves 4–6

POTATOES WITH FENNEL AND SOURED CREAM

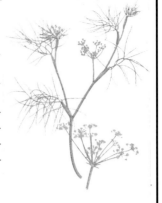

700 g (1$\frac{1}{2}$ lb) potatoes, peeled and thinly sliced

225 g (8 oz) fennel, cleaned, trimmed and thinly sliced

142 ml (5 fl oz) soured cream

75 g (3 oz) English butter

salt and freshly ground pepper

1. Place a layer of potato in a shallow ovenproof dish, cover with half the fennel, then spread with the soured cream.
2. Dot with one-third of the butter and season liberally, then cover with another layer of potato and the rest of the fennel.
3. Finish with a final layer of sliced potato and dot with another third of the butter. Season again.
4. Cover and bake in the oven at 190°C (375°F) mark 5 for about 45 minutes. Uncover and bake for a further 35 minutes, until golden brown. Serve with bacon chops for a main meal.

Serves 4

CREAMED POTATO

1.1 kg (2$\frac{1}{2}$ lb) potatoes, peeled

salt and freshly ground pepper

50–75 g (2–3 oz) English butter

300 ml ($\frac{1}{2}$ pint) milk

1. Cut any large potatoes into even-sized pieces. Cook in salted water for about 15 minutes, until tender – test with point of a knife. Drain off all the water, return pan to a gentle heat for the potatoes to dry.
2. Add the butter in pieces and use a potato masher or a fork to mash well. Season to taste.
3. Pour over the hot milk and beat the potatoes well with an electric mixer or balloon whisk until fluffy. Adjust seasoning.

Serves 6–8

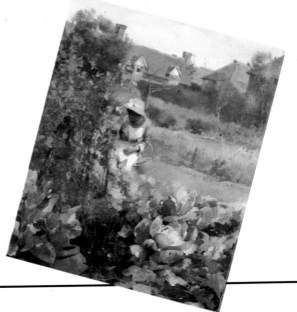

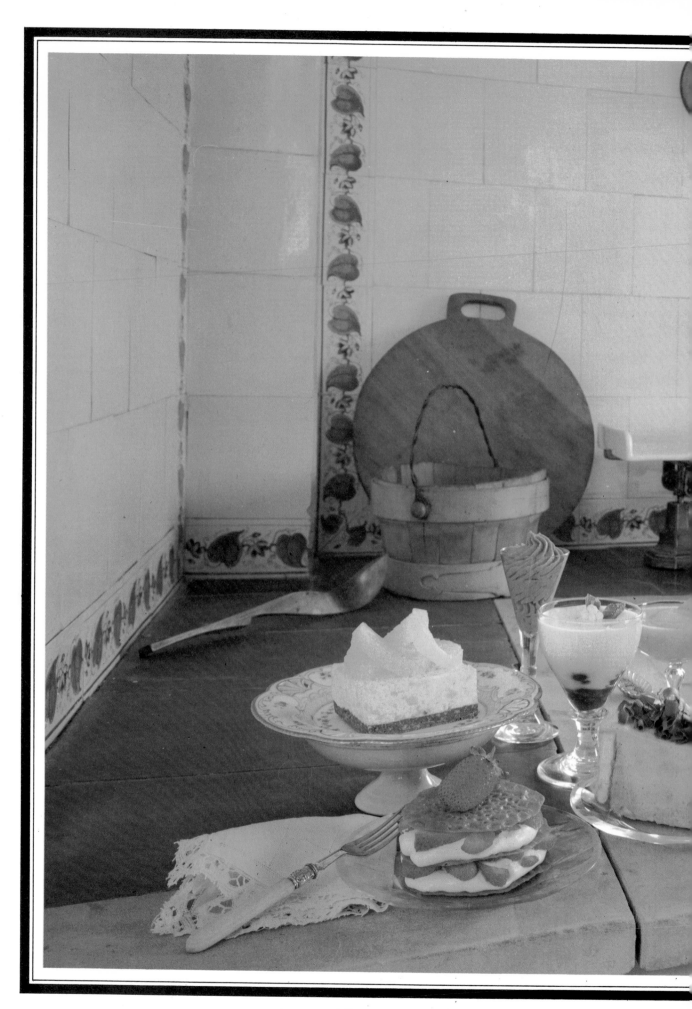

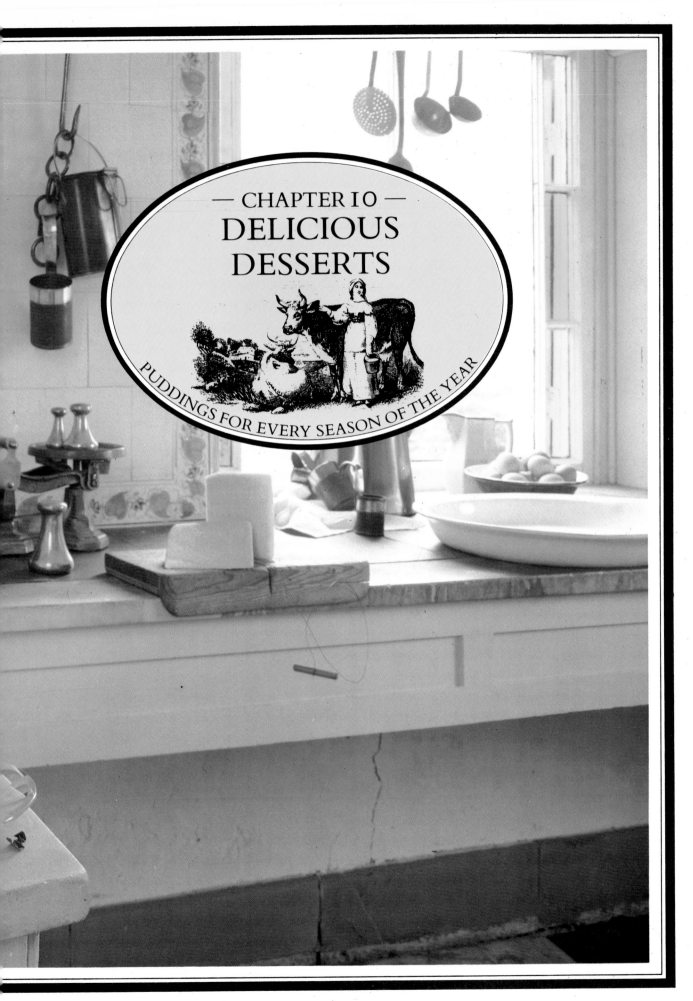

— CHAPTER 10 —
DELICIOUS
DESSERTS

PUDDINGS FOR EVERY SEASON OF THE YEAR

Opposite, top:
POOR KNIGHTS OF
WINDSOR
This unusual pudding, based on bread, fresh milk and eggs, with an added dash of sherry, is a light and delicate ending to a meal. The dish is named after the Poor Knights, an order of military pensioners founded in 1349.

Throughout the world, England is famous for its delicious desserts. In the seventeenth century, and even earlier, cold sweets and hot puddings were mentioned by travellers as one of the glories of the English kitchen.

Then – and now – hot winter puddings such as Lemon Layer Pudding and Apricot and Ginger Upside-Down Pudding were unique to England and almost unknown everywhere else. Fruit pies, made from whatever is in season, have long been a part of our cooking repertoire, are less fussy than their French counterparts and equally good. What could be better than ending a meal with a pie of fresh gooseberries or apples and blackberries in a double-crust pastry made of pure farm fresh butter?

There is also no doubt about the variety and pleasure we can get from our equally incomparable, cold desserts. Delicious fruit fools – deceptively simple and so very very elegant – come to us in an unbroken line from the sixteenth century, as do creams and snows. Charlottes, moulds, tansies and betties – their very names evoke the forgotten glories of the English table – are less common these days. Another very important sweet is the syllabub. In its earliest form it was liquid and drunk from a tall glass or a silver cup. It was considered essential that a mixture of wine and sugar should be made in the bottom of a large bowl and then that a cow should be milked directly into it! The liquid foamed up as it was stirred and was ladled into tall glasses or cups.

PUDDINGS ROUND THE REGIONS

POOR KNIGHTS OF WINDSOR

| 8 slices of white bread, about 2.5-cm ($\frac{1}{2}$-inch) thick |
| 300 ml ($\frac{1}{2}$ pint) milk |
| 75 g (3 oz) caster sugar |
| 30 ml (2 tbsp) sweet sherry |
| 2 egg yolks |
| 125 g (4 oz) English butter |
| 2.5 ml ($\frac{1}{2}$ level tsp) ground cinnamon |

1. Remove the crusts from the bread and cut each slice into two triangles.
2. Pour half the milk into a shallow dish and add 25 g (1 oz) caster sugar and the sherry. Stir well together.
3. Dip the bread into the sherry mixture until each slice has been soaked completely then drain on a wire rack.
4. Beat the egg yolks and remaining milk together and dip the bread in this mixture.
5. Heat the butter in a large pan and fry the bread slices until golden. Place on a warmed serving dish. Mix the remaining caster sugar with the cinnamon and sprinkle over the dish. Delicious served with chilled whipped fresh cream.
Serves 4

SUSSEX POND PUDDING

| 350 g (12 oz) self-raising flour |
| 2.5 ml ($\frac{1}{2}$ level tsp) salt |
| 175 g (6 oz) shredded suet |
| 100 g (4 oz) English butter |
| 100 g (4 oz) demerara sugar |
| 1 large lemon |

1. Mix together the flour, salt and suet. Add enough cold water – about 175 ml (6 fl oz) – to make a light, elastic dough. Knead lightly until smooth. Set aside a quarter of the pastry for the lid.
2. On a floured surface roll out large piece of pastry to a circle, 2.5 cm (1 inch) larger all round than the top of a 1.5-litre (2$\frac{1}{2}$-pint) pudding basin.
3. Use the large piece to line the pudding basin. Put half the butter, cut up into pieces, into the centre, with half the sugar.
4. Prick the lemon all over with a skewer. Put the whole lemon on top of the butter and sugar. Add the remaining butter and sugar.
5. Roll out the reserved quarter of the pastry to a circle to fit the top of the pie. Dampen

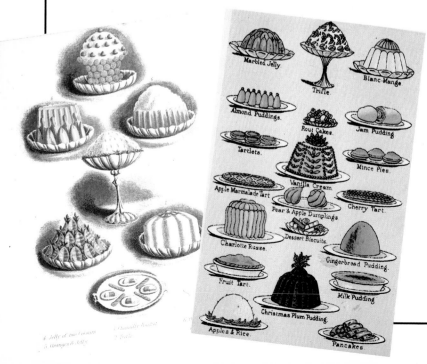

the edges and seal the lid. Cover with greaseproof paper and foil.

6. Steam for about 4 hours. Remove wrapping and turn out on to a warm serving dish.

Serves 4–6.

CRÈME BRÛLÉE

600 ml (1 pint) fresh whipping cream

4 eggs yolks

75 g (3 oz) caster sugar

5 ml (1 tsp) vanilla flavouring

1. Put the fresh cream in the top of a double saucepan or in a bowl over a pan of hot water and heat gently – but do not boil.

2. Meanwhile, put the egg yolks, 50 g (2 oz) of the caster sugar and the vanilla flavouring in a mixing bowl and beat thoroughly. Add fresh cream and mix well together.

3. Pour the mixture into six individual ramekin dishes and place in a roasting tin containing sufficient water to come half way up the sides of the dishes. Bake in the oven at 150°C (300°F) mark 2 for about 1 hour or until set; remove from the roasting tin and leave until cold.

4. Chill in the refrigerator for several hours, preferably overnight. Sprinkle the top of each Crème Brulée with the remaining sugar and put under a preheated hot grill until the sugar turns to caramel. Chill for 2–3 hours before serving.

Serves 6

NOTTINGHAM APPLE BATTER PUDDING

100 g (4 oz) flour

pinch of salt

2 eggs, separated

300 ml (½ pint) milk

4 small Bramley apples, peeled and cored

50 g (2 oz) English butter

50 g (2 oz) demerara sugar

2.5 ml (½ level tsp) ground cinnamon

icing sugar

1. Sift the flour and salt into a bowl. Beat the egg yolks and milk into the flour.

2. Arrange the apples in a buttered 1.1-litre (2-pint) ovenproof pie dish. Whisk together the butter and sugar and add cinnamon, then stuff the mixture into the apples.

3. Whisk the egg whites to soft peaks and fold into the batter. Pour the mixture over the apples and bake in the oven at 180°C (350°F) mark 4 for about 1¼ hours until the apples are tender and the batter well risen and golden. Serve immediately, dusted with icing sugar.

Serves 4

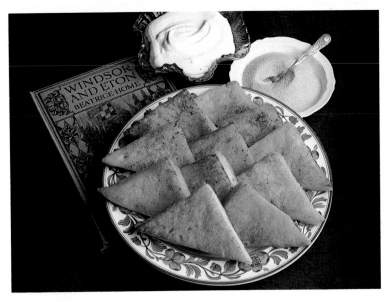

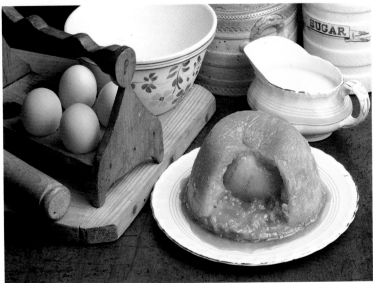

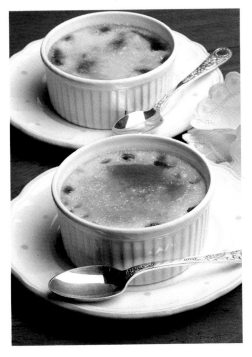

Above:
SUSSEX POND PUDDING
Named after a moat of buttery lemon sauce, this deceptively clever pudding has a whole lemon inside! The bitter citrus flavour is wonderful with the richness of the melted butter and sugar.

Left:
CRÈME BRÛLÉE
The name of this exquisite pudding literally means 'burnt cream' and it refers to the crisp layer of caramelised sugar which tops a very rich chilled custard made from fresh cream and egg yolks. The origins of this dish are lost in the mists of time, but it is usually credited to the kitchens of Trinity College, Cambridge, where it has been a favourite for well over a century.

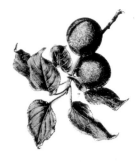

COUNTRY PLUM MOULD

450 g (1 lb) plums

30 ml (2 level tbsp) stem ginger, finely chopped

30 ml (2 level tbsp) sugar

15 ml (3 level tsp) gelatine

300 ml (10 fl oz) fresh whipping cream

2 egg whites

1. Stew the plums in very little water until soft. Discard stones and purée the flesh. Stir in the ginger and sugar.

2. In a small bowl sprinkle the gelatine over 150 ml (¼ pint) water. Place the bowl over a pan of hot water and stir until dissolved. Stir into the warm plum purée – allow to cool but not set.

3. Whip the fresh cream until softly stiff. Whisk the egg whites until stiff but not dry. Fold the fresh cream and then the egg whites into the plum mixture.

4. Turn into a 1.4-litre (2½-pint) fancy jelly mould. Refrigerate. When set, unmould and serve with sponge fingers.

Serves 6–8

GOOSEBERRY CHARLOTTE

Below:
GOOSEBERRY
CHARLOTTE
Gooseberries – one of the first fruits of spring – sharpen our taste buds for all the other good things to come. But what could be more welcome than this pretty pale charlotte served on your most delicate china?

450 g (1 lb) gooseberries, topped and tailed

75 g (3 oz) caster sugar

10 ml (2 level tsp) gelatine

2 egg yolks

300 ml (½ pint) milk

300 ml (10 fl oz) fresh double cream

20 langue de chats biscuits

1. Place the gooseberries in a small saucepan with 60 ml (4 tbsp) water. Cover the pan and simmer until the fruit softens to a pulpy consistency. Purée in a blender, then sieve to remove the pips. Stir in 50 g (2 oz) of the sugar.

2. Spoon 30 ml (2 tbsp) water into a small basin and sprinkle the gelatine over the surface. Allow the gelatine to soak until it has become spongy.

3. Beat the egg yolks with the remaining sugar until light in colour, pour on the warmed milk stirring until evenly blended. Return to the pan and cook over a low heat, stirring all the time, until the custard thickens sufficiently to lightly coat the back of the spoon – do not boil. Remove from the heat and immediately add the soaked gelatine. Stir until dissolved.

4. Pour the custard out into a large bowl and mix in the gooseberry purée, leave to cool. Whip the fresh cream until softly stiff. When the gooseberry mixture is cold, but not set, stir in half the fresh cream.

5. Butter and base-line a 15-cm (6-inch) soufflé type non-metal straight sided dish and pour in the gooseberry mixture. Refrigerate to set. When firm turn out on to a flat serving plate.

6. Spread a thin covering of the remaining fresh cream around the edge of the charlotte and spoon the rest into a piping bag fitted with a 1-cm (½-inch) star vegetable nozzle and pipe the cream around the top edge. Just before serving, arrange the langue de chats carefully around the outside.

Serves 6

OLDE ENGLISH EGG-NOG PIE

125 g (4 oz) English butter

175 g (6 oz) flour

45 ml (3 level tbsp) ground almonds

90 ml (6 level tbsp) caster sugar

300 ml (½ pint) milk, plus 30 ml (2 tbsp)

1.25 ml (¼ level tsp) ground nutmeg

2 eggs, separated

15 ml (3 level tsp) gelatine

45 ml (3 tbsp) rum

90 ml (6 tbsp) fresh double cream

grated chocolate to decorate

1. Rub the butter into the flour, stir in the ground almonds with 45 ml (3 level tbsp) sugar. Add about 30 ml (2 tbsp) milk to bind the mixture to a soft dough.

2. Roll out the pastry and use to line a deep 20.5-cm (8-inch) loose bottomed flan tin. Bake 'blind' in the oven at 200°C (400°F) mark 6 for 10–15 minutes. Leave to cool.

3. Gently heat the milk and nutmeg in a saucepan. Beat the egg yolks, one egg white and remaining sugar together. Pour on the heated milk, return to the pan and cook

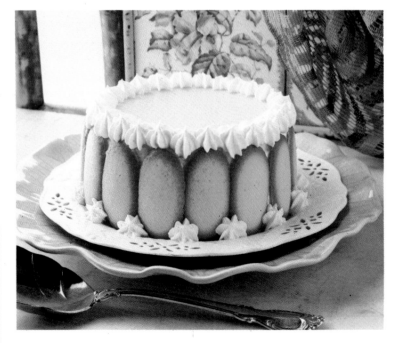

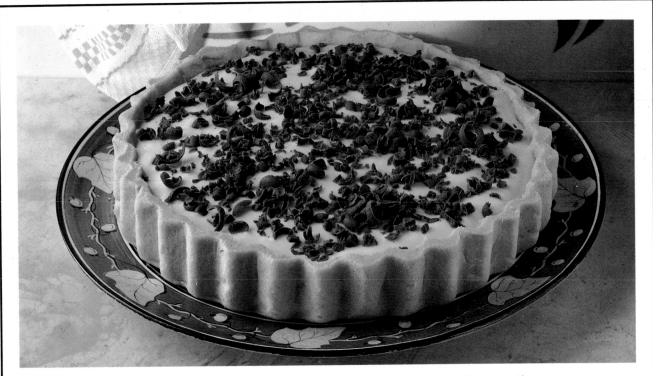

gently until it thickens. Do not allow the mixture to boil.

4. Soak the gelatine in the rum. Stir into the hot custard to dissolve.

5. Whip the fresh cream until softly stiff, then whisk the remaining egg white until stiff. Fold the fresh cream then egg white into the cool, half-set custard. Turn into a flan case and refrigerate to set.

6. Remove the flan ring, leave for 30 minutes at room temperature. Decorate with grated chocolate.

Serves 6

MANCHESTER PUDDING

450 ml (¾ pint) milk
25 g (1 oz) English butter
finely grated rind of 1 lemon
3 eggs, separated
75 g (3 oz) caster sugar
75 g (3 oz) fresh breadcrumbs
soured cream to serve

1. Warm the milk, butter and lemon rind in a saucepan. Lightly beat the yolks and 25 g (1 oz) caster sugar. When the butter has melted pour the milk mixture on to the yolks.

2. Stir in the breadcrumbs and turn into a buttered 1.1-litre (2-pint) pie or soufflé dish. Leave to stand for 15 minutes.

3. Whisk the egg whites until stiff but not dry looking. Whisk in the rest of the sugar. Pipe or spread the meringue over the pudding to cover completely.

4. Bake in the oven at 170°C (325°F) mark 3 for 40 minutes, reduce heat to 150°C (300°F) mark 2 for about a further 20 minutes. Serve warm with soured cream.

Serves 4

THE DEAN'S CREAM

8 small sponge cakes or trifle sponges
50 g (2 oz) strawberry jam
50 g (2 oz) orange jelly marmalade
50 g (2 oz) ratafia biscuits or small macaroons
150 ml (5 fl oz) sherry
grated rind and juice of a lemon
50 g (2 oz) caster sugar
45 ml (3 tbsp) white wine
45 ml (3 tbsp) brandy
300 ml (10 fl oz) fresh double cream
glacé cherries, angelica and toasted almonds to decorate

1. Spread the sponge cakes half with jam and half with marmalade. Arrange in a deep dish in alternate layers. Scatter over the ratafia biscuits or macaroons and soak with sherry.

2. Put the lemon rind into a pan, add the lemon juice and sugar. Warm gently to dissolve the sugar, add the wine and brandy.

3. Whip the fresh cream until stiff and fold in the cool wine mixture. Spoon this syllabub over the sponge cakes and chill for several hours or overnight.

4. Decorate before serving with cherries, angelica and toasted almonds.

Serves 6–8

Above:
OLDE ENGLISH EGG-NOG PIE
More sophisticated than any egg-nog you'd dream of having for breakfast, this pie, with its almond and rum flavour, is in fact fit for the fanciest feast.

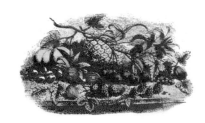

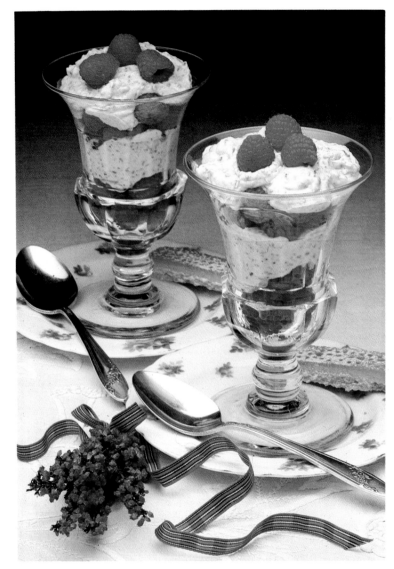

CREAM CROWDIE

50 g (2 oz) medium oatmeal
300 ml (10 fl oz) fresh double cream
60 ml (4 tbsp) clear honey
45 ml (3 tbsp) whisky
350 g (12 oz) fresh raspberries

1. Place the oatmeal in a grill pan (without the rack) and toast until golden brown, turning occasionally with a spoon.
2. Whip the fresh cream until softly stiff, then stir in the honey, whisky and cool oatmeal.
3. Pick over the raspberries; reserve a few for decoration.
4. Layer up the raspberries and fresh cream mixture in four tall glasses, cover with cling film and refrigerate.
5. Allow to come to room temperature for 30 minutes before serving. Decorate with reserved raspberries.
Serves 4

BLANCMANGE

60 ml (4 level tbsp) cornflour
568 ml (1 pint) milk
strip of lemon rind
45 ml (3 level tbsp) sugar

1. Blend the cornflour to a smooth paste with 30 ml (2 tbsp) of the milk.
2. Boil the remaining milk with the lemon rind and strain it on to the blended mixture, stirring well.
3. Return the mixture to the pan and bring to the boil, stirring all the time, until the mixture thickens and cook for a further 3 minutes. Add sugar to taste.
4. Pour into a 600-ml (1-pint) dampened jelly mould and leave for several hours until set. Turn out to serve with fresh fruit.

Variations
Chocolate Omit the lemon rind and add 50 g (2 oz) melted chocolate to the cooked mixture.
Coffee Omit the lemon rind and add 15–30 ml (1–2 tbsp) coffee essence.
Orange Substitute the lemon rind with 5 ml (1 level tsp) grated orange rind.
Honey Use 15 ml (1 tbsp) honey instead of the caster sugar.
Serves 4

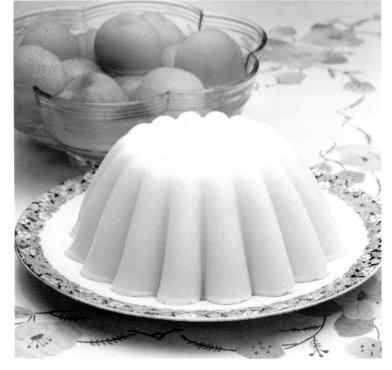

Left:
BLANCMANGE
The name Blancmange originally meant 'white food' and in medieval times it was a savoury dish combining finely diced chicken with almond milk and rice! The Elizabethans had a sweet tooth and they refined it, omitting the chicken and serving it as the delicious sweet we know today.

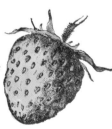

SUMMER PUDDING WITH CHANTILLY CREAM

6 large slices of stale bread

100 g (4 oz) sugar

750 g (1½ lb) soft summer fruit (either raspberries, strawberries, stoned cherries, blackcurrants or red currants, or a mixture)

150 ml (5 fl oz) fresh double cream

½ an egg white

15 g (½ oz) icing sugar, sifted

vanilla flavouring

1. Remove the crusts from the bread. Cut slices into neat fingers.
2. Put the sugar and 75 ml (5 tbsp) water into a pan and heat slowly, stirring, until the sugar dissolves. Add the fruit and simmer gently for about 7–10 minutes. (Gooseberries and blackcurrants may take a few minutes longer.)
3. Line the base and sides of a 1-litre (2-pint) pudding basin with bread fingers. Add half the hot fruit mixture. Cover with more bread fingers. Pour in the rest of the fruit mixture and top with the remaining bread fingers.
4. Cover with a saucer or plate. Put a heavy weight on top. Refrigerate or leave in a cold pantry overnight.
5. To make the Chantilly Cream, whip the fresh cream until softly stiff. In another bowl, whisk the egg white until stiff and fold into the fresh cream with the icing sugar and a few drops of vanilla flavouring. Chill well until required.
6. Turn the pudding out on to a plate and serve with the Chantilly Cream. Decorate with fresh fruit.

Serves 4–6

CHERRY BATTER PUDDING

45 ml (3 level tbsp) flour

pinch of salt

3 eggs, beaten

75 ml (5 level tbsp) caster sugar

450 ml (¾ pint) milk

15 ml (1 tbsp) rum (optional)

50 g (2 oz) English butter

675 g (1½ lb) black cherries, stoned and washed

1. Sift the flour and salt into a bowl then blend in the eggs. Add 45 ml (3 tbsp) of sugar.
2. Heat the milk until lukewarm and gradually stir it into the egg mixture, with the rum, if used.
3. Butter a shallow dish, put in the cherries, pour in the batter and dot with the remaining butter. Bake in the oven at 220°C (425°F) mark 7 for 25–30 minutes. Sprinkle the pudding with the remaining sugar and serve lukewarm.

Serves 6

Opposite, top:
CROWDIE
This delectable Scottish pudding consists of toasted oatmeal, fresh cream, delicate heather honey and a liberal splash of whisky combined with the sharp full taste of raspberries.

Below, left:
SUMMER PUDDING
One of the great English classics. Use good quality bread for a Summer Pudding and serve it very cold with lots of thick fresh cream.

Below:
CHERRY BATTER PUDDING
Cherries baked in a rich egg batter, makes a mouthwatering pudding served with lashings of fresh cream.

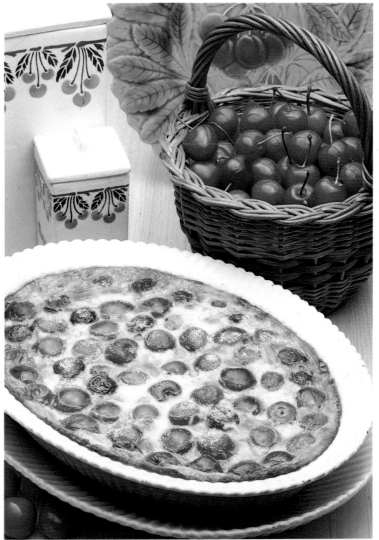

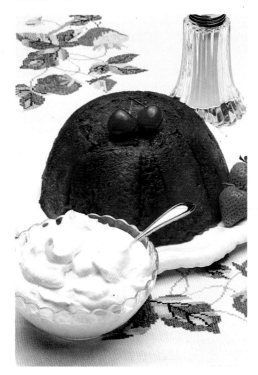

TRIFLE: THE GREAT BRITISH PUDDING

OLDE ENGLISH TRIFLE

568 ml (1 pint) milk

½ vanilla pod

2 eggs, plus 2 egg yolks

30 ml (2 level tbsp) caster sugar

1 Victoria sandwich cake (see page 247)

175 g (6 oz) raspberry or strawberry jam

100 g (4 oz) macaroons, lightly crushed

100 ml (4 fl oz) medium sherry

300 ml (10 fl oz) fresh double cream

40 g (1½ oz) flaked almonds, toasted and
    50 g (2 oz) glacé cherries to decorate

1. Scald the milk with the vanilla pod. Cover the pan and leave to infuse for 20 minutes.
2. Beat together the eggs, egg yolks and sugar and strain on the milk. Cook over a gentle heat, without boiling, stirring all the time until the custard thickens slightly. Pour into a bowl; lightly sprinkle the surface with sugar and cool.

3. Spread the sponge cake with jam, cut up and place in a 2-litre (3½-pint) shallow serving dish with the macaroons. Spoon over the sherry and leave for 2 hours. Pour over the cold custard.
4. Whip the cream until softly stiff. Top the custard with half the fresh cream. Pipe the remaining cream on top and decorate with the almonds and cherries.
Serves 6

GAELIC COFFEE TRIFLE

1 packet of trifle sponges (about 8)

30 ml (2 tbsp) coffee essence

60 ml (4 tbsp) whisky

25 g (1 oz) caster sugar

15 ml (1 level tbsp) cornflour

568 ml (1 pint) milk

2 egg yolks

25 g (1 oz) English butter

300 ml (10 fl oz) fresh double cream

walnut halves to decorate

1. Put the trifle sponges into a glass bowl. Mix half the coffee essence with 45 ml (3 tbsp) whisky and pour over the sponges.
2. Place the sugar, cornflour and milk in a saucepan. Heat, stirring continuously until the sauce thickens and boils. Cook gently for 3 minutes.
3. Remove from the heat and stir in the egg yolks and remaining coffee. Cook for a further minute then remove from the heat and mix in the butter and remaining whisky. Cool.
4. Whip the fresh cream until softly stiff. Fold half the fresh cream into the coffee mixture. Spoon over the trifle sponges. Decorate with the remaining fresh cream and walnuts.
Serves 6

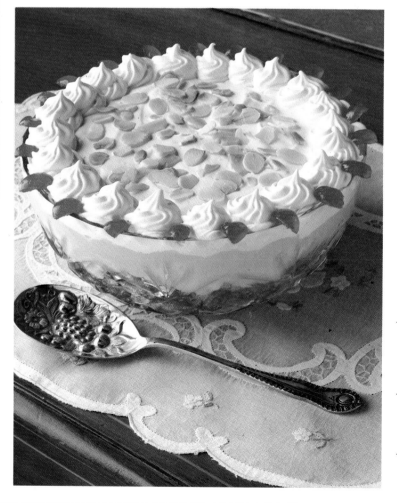

Left:
OLDE ENGLISH TRIFLE
When it is properly made with
fresh ingredients, a trifle
deserves its reputation as one of
the finest and most popular of
all English puddings. Trifle
dates from the sixteenth century.
It was served in palaces and
farmhouses alike on special
occasions and could be as
elaborately or as simply
decorated as circumstances
demanded. Topped with toasted
flaked almonds and fresh double
cream, this lovely recipe uses a
real egg custard in the traditional
way.

SAINT CLEMENT'S TRIFLE

300 ml (10 fl oz) fresh double cream

25 g (1 oz) icing sugar

grated rind and juice of 1 lemon

grated rind and juice of 2 oranges

6 trifle sponges

thin slices of orange and lemon to decorate

1. Whip the fresh cream until softly stiff and fold in the icing sugar. Add the lemon and orange rind and juice and stir together.
2. Crumble the trifle sponges in the cream mixture and blend evenly through the cream.
3. Turn the trifle into a serving dish, cover and chill for at least 2 hours. The trifle may seem rather floppy. During the chilling period it thickens up considerably to a light, foamy and very refreshing dessert. Decorate, with very thin alternating slices of orange and lemon.

Serves 6–8

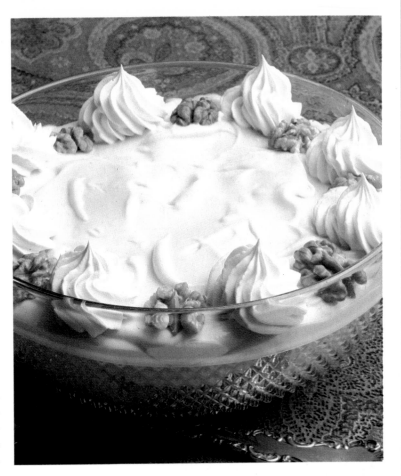

GINGER AND ORANGE TRIFLE

350 g (12 oz) Jamaica ginger cake

4 oranges

120 ml (8 tbsp) orange-flavoured liqueur

4 egg yolks

50 g (2 oz) caster sugar

45 ml (3 level tbsp) cornflour

vanilla flavouring

568 ml (1 pint) milk

45 ml (3 tbsp) stem ginger syrup

300 (10 fl oz) fresh double cream

chopped almonds, browned, and few pieces of stem ginger to decorate

1. Thinly slice the cake and line the base of a 26-cm (10-inch) fluted flan dish or a shallow serving dish.
2. Peel and segment the oranges, placing the segments on top of the cake.
3. Spoon the liqueur evenly over the cake and orange.
4. In a saucepan, combine the egg yolks, sugar, cornflour and vanilla flavouring. Gradually stir in the milk and ginger syrup; bring the mixture almost to the boil and simmer for 4–5 minutes until thickened.
5. Pour the custard evenly into the dish. Leave to cool.
6. Whip the fresh cream until softly stiff. Use to decorate the top of the trifle, finishing with the browned chopped almonds and stem ginger.

Serves 8

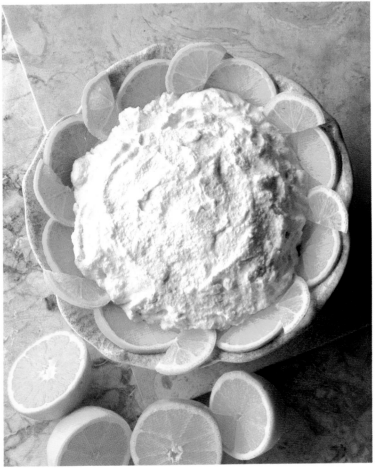

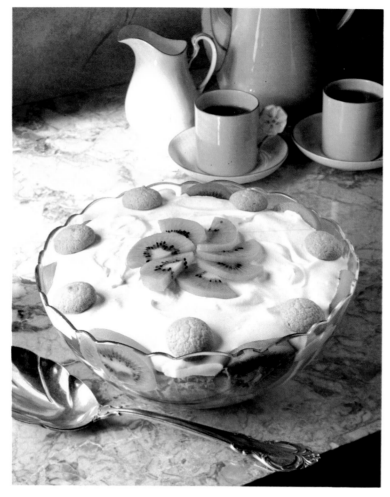

Above:
KIWI TRIFLE
An excellent trifle made from broken macaroons and a brandy-flavoured syllabub, topped with the exotic beautiful green fruit named after New Zealand's national bird.

the kiwi fruit over the swiss roll with broken macaroons.
2. Whisk the egg whites until stiff, then gradually beat in the sugar until firm and glossy. Pour in the vermouth, brandy and lemon juice and gently fold through the meringue. Whip the fresh cream until softly stiff and fold through the meringue mixture.
3. Pour over the swiss roll and fruit, cover and refrigerate for about 2 hours. Just before serving, decorate with fresh whipped cream, ratafias and slices of kiwi fruit.
Serves 8

SYLLABUBS AND POSSETS

SYLLABUB

150 ml (¼ pint) dry white wine
30 ml (2 tbsp) lemon juice
10 ml (2 level tsp) finely grated lemon rind
75 g (3 oz) caster sugar
300 ml (10 fl oz) fresh double cream

1. Put the wine, lemon juice, rind and sugar into a bowl. Leave to infuse for a minimum of 3 hours.
2. Add the fresh cream and whip until the mixture is softly stiff and holds its shape. Do not overwhip as the mixture may curdle.
3. Transfer to six glass dishes. Leave in a cool place for several hours before serving.
Serves 6

KIWI TRIFLE

1 large jam swiss roll
medium sweet sherry
6 kiwi fruit, peeled and sliced
100 g (4 oz) macaroons, broken
3 egg whites
125 g (4 oz) caster sugar
150 ml (¼ pint) dry white vermouth
30 ml (2 tbsp) brandy
15 ml (1 tbsp) lemon juice
300 ml (10 fl oz) fresh double cream
fresh whipped cream, ratafias and slices of kiwi fruit to decorate

1. Slice the swiss roll and arrange in a large trifle bowl. Moisten with some sherry. Place

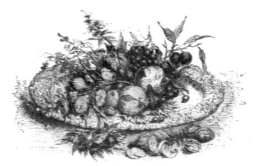

WHITE WINE POSSET

finely grated rind of 1 lemon
300 ml (10 fl oz) fresh double cream
45 ml (3 tbsp) lemon juice
75 ml (5 tbsp) Riesling or White Bordeaux
2 egg whites
25 g (1 oz) icing sugar
sponge fingers to serve

1. Put the grated lemon rind into a large, deep bowl. Pour in the fresh cream, stir and leave to chill in the refrigerator for 1 hour.
2. Combine the lemon juice with the wine.
3. Whip the fresh cream until softly stiff. Gradually whisk in the wine until the mixture holds its shape. Do not overwhip as the mixture may curdle.
4. In a clean bowl, whisk the egg white until softly stiff, add the sifted sugar and whisk again. Fold evenly into the fresh cream.
5. Divide the mixture between six stemmed glasses. Chill for up to 1 hour. Serve with sponge fingers.

Variation:
For a pretty pink posset, use rosé wine.
Serves 6

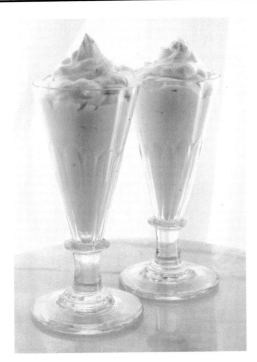

CIDER SYLLABUB

1 medium orange
150 ml (¼ pint) medium-dry cider
45 ml (3 level tbsp) caster sugar
300 ml (10 fl oz) fresh double cream

1. Pare off a few strips of orange peel using a potato peeler. Cut into really fine shreds and blanch in boiling water for 2 minutes, strain and cool.

2. Finely grate the remaining rind, then place in a small bowl with 60 ml (4 tbsp) orange juice, the cider and sugar. Stir well, cover and leave to stand for 2–3 hours.

3. Whip the fresh cream until softly stiff. Gradually whisk in the cider until the mixture holds its shape. Do not overwhip as the mixture may curdle.

4. Spoon into six glass dishes, cover and chill well before serving. Decorate with a few shreds of orange rind.

Serves 6

CALEDONIAN CREAM

90 ml (6 level tbsp) thin shred marmalade
25 g (1 oz) caster sugar
60 ml (4 tbsp) whisky liqueur
juice of 1 lemon
300 ml (10 fl oz) fresh double or whipping cream

1. Mix together the marmalade, sugar, liqueur and lemon juice. Whip the fresh cream until softly stiff.

2. Gently whisk in the marmalade mixture until the fresh cream stands in soft peaks – take care not to overwhip. Serve in small glasses.

Serves 6

FOOLS AND FLUFFS

YOGURT GOOSEBERRY FOOL

450 g (1 lb) gooseberries, topped and tailed
30 ml (2 tbsp) clear honey
30–60 ml (2–4 level tbsp) caster sugar
20 ml (4 level tsp) gelatine
142 g (5 oz) natural yogurt
green food colouring
soft sponge fingers to serve

1. Place the gooseberries in a saucepan with 250 ml (½ pint) water. Cover the pan and cook gently until the fruit is soft.

2. Purée in a blender and press through a sieve to remove seeds. Return to the pan with the honey and sugar. Bring to the boil.

3. Meanwhile, in a small basin, sprinkle the gelatine over 60 ml (4 tbsp) water. When the gelatine has swollen, stir into the hot puréed gooseberries until dissolved. Leave to cool.

4. When the gooseberry mixture is beginning to set, fold in the yogurt. Add a few drops of edible green colouring if necessary.

5. Divide between six stemmed glasses. Refrigerate to set. Serve with sponge fingers.

Serves 6

Left:
SYLLABUB
One of the best and simplest of sweets, this syllabub is what was known in the seventeenth century as an everlasting syllabub – the other type was a liquid mixture of milk and cider or wine.

Below:
CALEDONIAN CREAM
Another treat which gets its inspiration from north of the border! Richly flavoured with whisky liqueur and thin shred marmalade, this delectable cream has the advantage of being made in a minute.

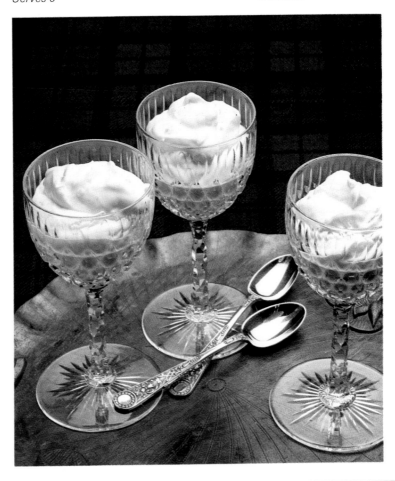

MANDARIN CREAM FLAN

50 g (2 oz) sponge fingers

75 g (3 oz) English butter, softened

100 g (4 oz) icing sugar

1 egg, beaten

311-g (11-oz) can mandarin segments, drained

150 ml (5 fl oz) fresh double cream

finely grated rind of $\frac{1}{2}$ a lemon

fresh whipped cream to decorate

1. Crush the sponge fingers into fine crumbs by placing them in a polythene bag and firmly rolling with a rolling pin. Scatter half of the crumbs into a 20-cm (8-inch) flan dish.
2. Whisk the butter and sugar together until pale and fluffy, then gradually beat in the egg, beating well after each addition. Spoon the mixture evenly over the crumbs in the flan dish.
3. Roughly chop the mandarins, reserving three segments. Whip the fresh cream until stiff, then stir in the mandarin segments and the lemon rind. Spread this evenly over the butter mixture.
4. Sprinkle the remaining crumbs around the top edge of the flan. Cover the dish with cling film, then refrigerate for 36 hours before decorating with additional fresh whipped cream and mandarin segments.
Serves 6

NUTTY FRUIT CREAM

75 g (3 oz) dessert apples, cored, peeled and chopped

75 g (3 oz) pears, cored, peeled and chopped

2 bananas, sliced

juice of 1 lemon

150 ml (5 fl oz) fresh double cream

75 g (3 oz) hazelnut yogurt

100 g (4 oz) hazelnuts, chopped

1. Place the apples, pears and bananas in a bowl. Toss in lemon juice, cover and leave aside.
2. Whip the fresh cream until stiff and fold in the yogurt. Stir in all but 15–20 ml (3–4 tsp) of the chopped hazelnuts.
3. Place the fruit mixture in the bottom of four glass dishes. Cover with the cream mixture and sprinkle the remaining nuts on top. Serve chilled.
Serves 4

RHUBARB ORANGE FOOL

1 orange

900 g (2 lb) rhubarb, trimmed and cut into 2.5-cm (1-inch) lengths

75 ml (5 level tbsp) red currant jelly

30 ml (2 level tbsp) thick honey

150 ml (5 fl oz) fresh double cream

sponge fingers to serve

1. Pare a few strips of rind off the orange using a potato peeler. Slice each one into *very* thin strips. Blanch in boiling water for 2 minutes, drain and dry with absorbent kitchen paper; keep covered until required.
2. Put the rhubarb into a saucepan with 90 ml (6 tbsp) strained orange juice, the red currant jelly and honey.
3. Cover tightly and simmer gently until the fruit is soft and pulpy. Stir occasionally to prevent the rhubarb sticking to the pan. Cool slightly, then rub through a sieve or purée in a blender. Pour into a large bowl and leave to cool.
4. Whip the fresh cream until softly stiff and fold through the cold fruit purée. Spoon into individual glass dishes, cover and chill well. Decorate with shredded rind. Serve with sponge fingers.
Serves 6

APPLE-BERRY FOOL

2 dessert apples

lemon juice

450 g (1 lb) raspberries, hulled

45 ml (3 level tbsp) sugar

15 ml (1 level tbsp) custard powder

150 ml ($\frac{1}{4}$ pint) milk

300 ml (10 fl oz) fresh double cream

1. Cut four thin slices of apple for decoration, sprinkle with lemon juice to prevent browning. Reserve four whole raspberries for decoration.
2. Peel, core and roughly chop the remaining apples and place in a saucepan with the raspberries and sugar. Cook gently to a pulp, then sieve to remove the pips.
3. Blend the custard powder with a little milk, and heat the remaining milk. Pour the hot milk on to the blended custard powder, stirring, then return to the pan and stir over a gently heat until thick.
4. Beat the custard into the fruit pulp; allow to cool.
5. Whip the fresh cream until softly stiff, fold into the fruit mixture reserving half to decorate. Spoon into glasses. Chill.
6. Decorate each glass with a spoonful of reserved fresh cream, an apple slice and a whole raspberry.
Serves 4

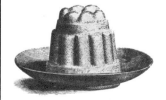

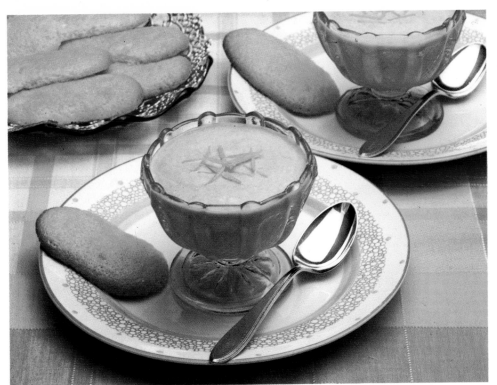

BLACKCURRANT FLUFF

450 g (1 lb) blackcurrants

100 g (4 oz) caster sugar

15 ml (3 level tsp) gelatine

45 ml (3 tbsp) blackcurrant liqueur

150 ml (5 fl oz) fresh double cream

3 egg whites

fresh whipped cream and chopped nuts or
    grated chocolate to decorate

1. Cook the fruit gently with the sugar until
pulpy. Sieve to remove the pips.
2. Dissolve the gelatine in 45 ml (3 tbsp)
water, in a bowl over a pan of hot water. Stir
into the fruit purée with the blackcurrant
liqueur. Cool until beginning to set.
3. Whip the fresh cream until softly stiff.
Fold into the half-set mixture.
4. Whisk the egg whites until stiff and fold
into the fruit mixture
5. Spoon into individual glasses and
decorate with fresh whipped cream and nuts
or chocolate. Chill lightly before serving.

Serves 6

HONEY POT FOOL

350 g (12 oz) dried fruit – apricots, peaches,
    pears, prunes, apples

2 ripe bananas, peeled

lemon juice

15 ml (1 tbsp) clear honey

150 ml (5 fl oz) fresh double cream

chopped walnuts to decorate

1. Soak the dried fruit in cold water
overnight. Drain.
2. Reserve twelve thin slices of banana for
decoration and dip in lemon juice.
3. Place the remaining banana in a blender
with the dried fruit and honey. Blend until
smooth. (It may be necessary to blend the
mixture in two batches.)
4. Whip the fresh cream until softly stiff then
fold into the fruit mixture.
5. Spoon into six individual dishes and chill.
Serve decorated with banana slices and
chopped nuts.

Serves 6

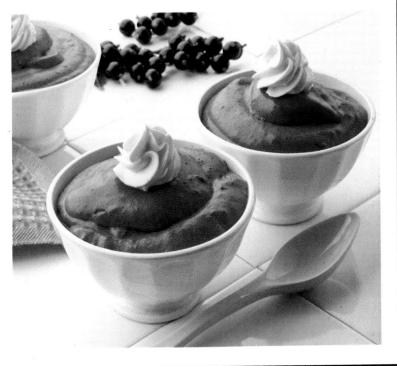

SPICED PLUM FOOL WITH COCONUT WAFERS

538 g (1 lb 3 oz) can red plums, with syrup

whole nutmeg

30 ml (2 level tbsp) thick honey

15 ml (1 tbsp) lemon juice

20 ml (4 level tsp) arrowroot

142 ml (5 fl oz) soured cream

red food colouring

25 g (1 oz) English butter

25 g (1 oz) caster sugar

7.5ml (1½ level tsp) golden syrup

25 g (1 oz) flour

15 g (½ oz) desiccated coconut

1. Cook the plums with the syrup from the can, a generous grating of nutmeg, the honey and lemon juice until pulpy and reduced. Drain and return the purée to the pan.
2. Blend the arrowroot to a smooth paste with a little water, add to the purée and bring to the boil. Boil for 1 minute, stirring, turn into a bowl; cool.
3. Stir the soured cream and enough colouring to give an attractive pink into the purée. Spoon into individual glasses. Chill well.

Below: clockwise from top CINNAMON AND RAISIN FLAN (on page 231), SPICED PLUM FOOL WITH COCONUT WAFERS (above), AND APPLE FLAPJACK (on page 229)
Three delicious puddings blending fruit and spice. Spiced Plum Fool is an exotic South Sea dessert made from meltingly delicious plums, spiced with a touch of nutmeg and served with buttery coconut biscuits. The flan is cheerfully flavoured with cinnamon while ginger adds a special touch to the Apple Flapjack.

4. Meanwhile, make the Coconut Wafers. Whisk the butter and sugar until pale and fluffy. Beat in the golden syrup. Then fold in the flour, desiccated coconut and remaining lemon juice.
5. Place the mixture in about eight teaspoonfuls, well apart on buttered baking sheets. Bake in the oven at 180°C (350°F) mark 4 until brown tinged. Remove while warm. Cool on wire racks.
6. Serve the plum fool with the wafers.
Serves 4

LEMON YOGURT WHIPS

two 127-g (4½-oz) packets lemon jelly tablets

90 ml (6 tbsp) lemon juice

300 g (10 oz) natural yogurt

3 individual trifle sponge cakes

1. Break up the jelly tablets and place in a large heatproof measuring jug. Make up to 600 ml (1 pint) with boiling water and stir until dissolved.
2. Add the strained lemon juice and make up to 900 ml (1½ pints) with ice cubes. Stir until the cubes dissolve.
3. Pour half the jelly into a large mixing bowl and refrigerate until it is on the point of setting. Leave the other half out of the refrigerator.
4. Whisk the setting jelly vigorously. Stir the yogurt until smooth and then whisk into the jelly.
5. Pour into six stemmed glasses and refrigerate until set.
6. Cut the trifle sponges into small cubes and scatter over the set lemon mixture. Spoon over the remaining liquid jelly, cover with cling film and refrigerate to set.
Serves 6 *(illustration on page 210)*

PEACH CREAM DESSERT

6 peaches, peeled and sliced, or 850-g (30-oz) can sliced peaches, drained

300 ml (10 fl oz) fresh double cream

3–4 pieces of stem ginger, chopped

50 g (2 oz) chopped almonds

225 g (8 oz) caster sugar

1. Arrange the peaches in the bottom of the soufflé dish.
2. Whip the fresh cream until softly stiff. Cover the peaches with half the cream. Sprinkle with the ginger and nuts, then the remaining fresh cream. Refrigerate for 1–2 hours.
3. Sprinkle the sugar evenly over the mixture. Put under a very low grill to caramelise the sugar. Cool, then chill in the refrigerator until ready to serve.
Serves 6

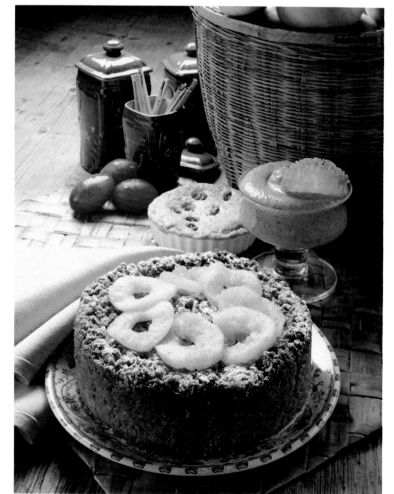

BARBADOS FRUIT

15 g (½ oz) English butter

2 bananas, sliced

125 g (4 oz) seedless grapes, halved

175 g (6 oz) dessert apple, peeled, cored and diced

25 g (1 oz) glacé cherries

25 g (1 oz) mixed peel, chopped

25 g (1 oz) blanched almonds, coarsely chopped

100 g (4 oz) pineapple, chopped

grated rind and juice of ½ lemon

300 ml (10 fl oz) fresh double cream

30 ml (2 level tbsp) rum

175 g (6 oz) demerara sugar

1. Melt the butter in a pan and fry the sliced bananas until lightly brown. Remove from the heat and stir in the prepared grapes, apple, cherries, peel, almonds, pineapple, lemon rind and juice. Place the mixture in six small ovenproof dishes.
2. Whip the fresh cream with the rum until stiff and spread over the fruit in each dish.
3. Completely cover each dish with a layer of brown sugar. Just before serving, quickly brown the sugar under a hot grill. Serve immediately.
Serves 6

CHESTNUT AND ORANGE WHIRL

440-g (15½-oz) can sweetened chestnut purée

finely grated rind and juice of 1 orange

50 g (2 oz) icing sugar, sifted

30 ml (2 tbsp) orange-flavoured liqueur

150 ml (5 fl oz) fresh double cream

1. Place the chestnut purée in a large bowl and beat in the orange rind. Beat until really smooth.
2. Stir in the icing sugar with the liqueur and 30 ml (2 tbsp) strained orange juice.
3. Whisk the fresh cream until stiff and stir through the chestnut mixture. Whisk the two together until thick enough to pipe.
4. Spoon into a piping bag fitted with a large star vegetable nozzle. Pipe into six tall glasses and chill well.
Serves 6

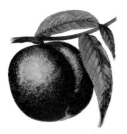

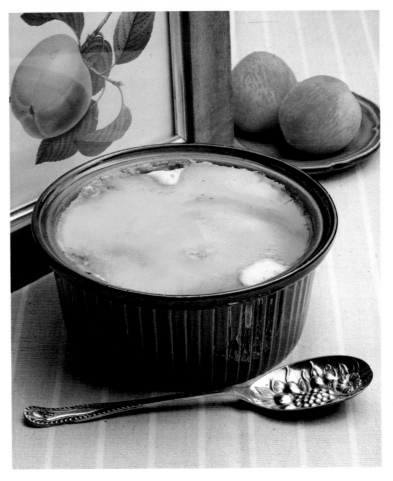

LEMON CHERRY CHIFFONS

350 g (12 oz) black or dark red cherries, stoned

30 ml (2 tbsp) cherry-flavoured liqueur

3 eggs, separated

175 g (6 oz) caster sugar

finely grated rind and juice of 2 lemons

15 ml (3 level tsp) gelatine

150 ml (5 fl oz) fresh whipping cream

mimosa balls and angelica to decorate

1. Divide the cherries between six individual glass dishes. Spoon a little liqueur over each.
2. Place the egg yolks in a deep bowl, add the caster sugar and lemon rind and whisk until thick.
3. Add 75 ml (5 tbsp) strained lemon juice and continue whisking until thick.
4. Soak the gelatine in 45 ml (3 tbsp) water in a small bowl. Dissolve by standing the bowl over a pan of hot water. Stir into the lemon mixture.
5. Whip the cream until softly stiff. Whisk the egg whites until stiff. Fold the fresh cream and egg whites into the lemon mixture.
6. Spoon the mixture into the glasses and refrigerate to set. Decorate with mimosa balls and angelica.
Serves 6

Above:
PEACH CREAM DESSERT
Choose fresh, firm peaches with velvety skin and a fragrant perfume for this delicate cream which is layered with ginger and almonds.

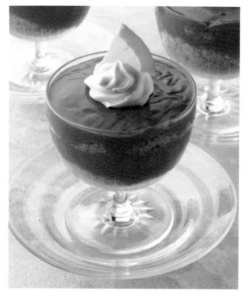

Right:
ORANGE CHOCOLATE
CREAM DESSERTS
Everyone loves chocolate
desserts! This one is a delicious
Jaffa flavour, rich with fresh
cream and is mixed with crunchy
biscuit crumbs.

3. Make up the orange juice to 75 ml (2½ fl oz). Stir the rind and juice into the chocolate with 50 g (2 oz) of the sugar.
4. Beat the egg, then fold into the chocolate mixture. Remove from the heat.
5. Place the cornflour, fresh single cream, milk and remaining sugar in a saucepan. Whisk over a gentle heat until the sauce boils and thickens. Simmer gently for 2 minutes.
6. Add the sauce to the chocolate mixture and then whisk with a rotary or electric whisk, until the mixture is completely smooth and blended. Add the orange liqueur to taste, if used.
7. Layer the biscuit mixture and chocolate mixture in six glasses, finishing with a chocolate layer. Whip the fresh double cream until stiff. Decorate the desserts with piped fresh cream and the orange slices.
Serves 6

ORANGE CHOCOLATE CREAM DESSERTS

100 g (4 oz) English butter
225 g (8 oz) digestive biscuits, crushed
150 g (5 oz) sugar
100 g (4 oz) plain chocolate
grated rind and juice of 1 orange
1 egg
25 g (1 oz) cornflour
150 ml (5 fl oz) fresh single cream
150 ml (¼ pint) milk
orange-flavoured liqueur (optional)
150 ml (5 fl oz) fresh double cream
1 orange, sliced to decorate

1. Melt the butter in a pan then add the crushed biscuits and 50 g (2 oz) sugar.
2. Place the chocolate in a basin, standing over a pan of hot water. Heat gently until melted, stirring occasionally.

STRAWBERRY FOAM

225 g (8 oz) strawberries, hulled
1 egg white
75 g (3 oz) icing sugar, sifted
150 ml (5 fl oz) fresh double cream

1. Do not wash the strawberries, wipe only if really necessary as the berries should be very dry.
2. Turn into a deep bowl and squash with a stainless potato masher.
3. Add the egg white and the icing sugar and with an electric beater whisk for about 10 minutes until thick and frothy – with a hand rotary whisk this will take about twice as long. Whip the fresh cream until stiff. Gently fold into the strawberry mixture.
4. Turn into glasses, piling the mixture well up. Chill for up to 6 hours before serving. Serve with fresh cream.
Serves 4–6

MOUSSES AND BAVAROIS

VANILLA AND APRICOT BAVAROIS

100 g (4 oz) dried apricots
pinch of allspice
450 ml (¾ pint) milk
vanilla pod
3 egg yolks
75 ml (5 level tbsp) vanilla sugar (see below)
20 ml (4 level tsp) gelatine
300 ml (10 fl oz) fresh double cream
canned apricot halves to decorate

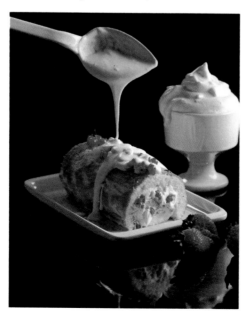

Right:
REDCURRANT
GRIESTORTE AND
STRAWBERRY FOAM
A fluffy foamy favourite, made
from the queen of fruits,
Strawberry Foam has a fragrant
smell and taste. Serve it in your
palest, prettiest china.
  Redcurrant Griestorte (page
236) can also be served with
fresh double cream.

1. Soak the apricots in cold water overnight. Simmer in fresh water with allspice, covered, for about 1 hour until tender. Drain, reserving 60 ml (4 tbsp) liquid and purée fruit in a blender with the reserved juice. Cool.

2. Heat the milk with the vanilla pod until almost boiling. Remove the pod. Whisk together the yolks and sugar until thick; add the milk, stirring. Return to the pan and cook over a low heat without boiling until the custard thickens. Cool.

3. Soak the gelatine in 60 ml (4 tbsp) water in a small bowl. Dissolve by standing the bowl in a pan of gently simmering water. Stir into the cooled custard with the apricot purée.

4. Chill until on point of setting. Whip the fresh cream until softly stiff then quickly fold half into the apricot custard. Turn into a dampened 900-ml (1½-pint) mould or soufflé dish and chill to set.

5. Turn out and decorate with the remaining fresh cream and apricots.

Note: To make vanilla sugar, leave a vanilla pod in the caster sugar jar (kept specially).

Serves 4

LEMON PRUNE MOUSSE

225 g (8 oz) dried plump prunes

pared rind of 1 lemon

10 ml (2 level tsp) gelatine

45 ml (3 tbsp) lemon juice

30 ml (2 level tbsp) thick honey

150 ml (5 fl oz) fresh double cream

1 egg white

flaked almonds, toasted, to decorate

1. Soak the prunes in cold water overnight.
2. In a lidded saucepan, simmer the prunes gently with the pared lemon rind and enough soaking liquid to cover well, for about 20 minutes until tender.
3. Soak the gelatine in a small basin with the strained lemon juice. Drain the prunes, reserving 150 ml (¼ pint) cooking liquid. While still hot, stone the prunes, place the flesh in a blender with the reserved juice, gelatine and honey. Blend until really smooth; turn into a bowl to cool.
4. Whip the fresh cream until softly stiff. Whisk the egg white until stiff. As prune mixture begins to set, fold in fresh cream then the egg white. Turn mousse into a glass serving bowl, refrigerate until set. Decorate with browned flaked almonds.

Serves 4–6

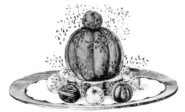

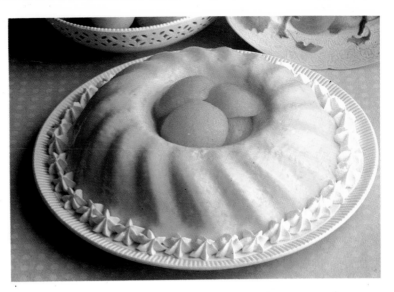

HONEY MOUSSE

3 eggs, separated

100 g (4 oz) caster sugar

finely grated rind of 2 lemons

90 ml (6 tbsp) lemon juice

10 ml (2 level tsp) gelatine

300 ml (10 fl oz) fresh whipping cream

30 ml (2 tbsp) clear honey

pistachio nuts or coarsely grated chocolate to decorate

1. Whisk together the egg yolks, sugar and lemon rind until thick, add 45 ml (3 tbsp) lemon juice and place over a pan of simmering water until thick and mousse-like. Remove from the heat and whisk occasionally until cold.
2. Soak the gelatine in the remaining lemon juice in a small bowl. Place the bowl over a pan of hot water and stir until dissolved.
3. Whip the fresh cream until softly stiff. Whisk the egg whites until stiff. Fold half the fresh cream into the mousse with the gelatine, honey and whisked egg whites. Turn into a 1.1-litre (2-pint) glass bowl.
4. Decorate with the remaining fresh whipped cream and chopped pistachio nuts.

Serves 6

Above:
VANILLA AND APRICOT BAVAROIS
This creamy apricot-coloured sweet is also known as Bavaroise Pompadour.

Below:
HONEY MOUSSE
Honey, fresh eggs and cream flavoured with lemon are the essence of this mousse which is lighter than air! It is very beautiful scattered with pale green pistachio nuts.

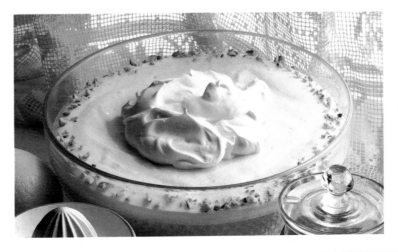

MOUSSE AU CHOCOLAT

225 g (8 oz) plain chocolate
15 ml (1 tbsp) rum
125 g (4 oz) English butter
125 g (4 oz) caster sugar
4 eggs, separated
150 ml (5 fl oz) fresh double cream
chocolate curls to decorate

1. Break the chocolate into pieces and place in a bowl over simmering water, with 30 ml (2 tbsp) water and rum. Stir until smooth. Cool slightly.
2. Whisk together the butter and sugar until pale and fluffy, then beat in the egg yolks one at a time.
3. Add the chocolate to the butter mixture and beat for 5 minutes until light.
4. Whisk the whites until stiff but not dry and fold into the chocolate. Pour into a serving dish or individual glasses and chill until set. Whip the fresh cream until stiff. Decorate the mousse with fresh piped cream and chocolate curls.
Serves 6

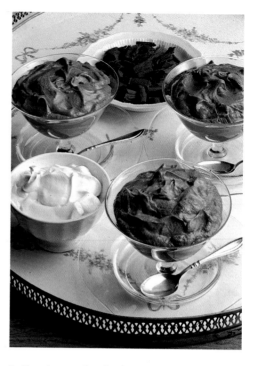

CRANBERRY MOSCOVITE

225 g (8 oz) cranberries
75 g (3 oz) sugar
3 egg yolks
30 ml (2 level tbsp) caster sugar
400 ml (¾ pint) milk
15 ml (3 level tsp) gelatine
30 ml (2 tbsp) lemon juice
60 ml (4 tbsp) fresh double cream
'frosted' cranberries and fresh cream to decorate (see below)

1. Put the cranberries in a small heavy-based pan with 90 ml (6 tbsp) water; boil then simmer gently until the fruit 'pops'. Remove from the heat and add the sugar, stir until dissolved; cool.
2. Beat the egg yolks and caster sugar together in a bowl. Heat the milk gently then pour on to the egg mixture. Return to the saucepan and cook until the custard thickens but do not boil. Leave to cool. Purée the custard and fruit in a blender and sieve out the skin or pips.
3. Soak the gelatine in the strained lemon juice and 30 ml (2 tbsp) of water in a small basin. Dissolve by standing it in a pan of gently simmering water.
4. Stir the gelatine into the cold purée. Whip the fresh cream until softly stiff and fold into the fruit custard. Pour into glass dishes, refrigerate, then decorate before serving.

Note: To 'frost' cranberries, dip in lightly beaten egg white, roll in sugar and leave to harden on non-stick paper.
Serves 4

GINGER BAVAROIS

3 egg yolks
50 g (2 oz) caster sugar
400 ml (¾ pint) milk
30 ml (2 level tbsp) gelatine
60 ml (4 tbsp) stem ginger syrup
300 ml (10 fl oz) fresh double cream
75 g (3 oz) stem ginger, finely chopped
chopped stem ginger to decorate

1. Beat the egg yolks with the sugar until pale and fluffy.
2. Heat the milk gently without boiling and whisk into the egg mixture.

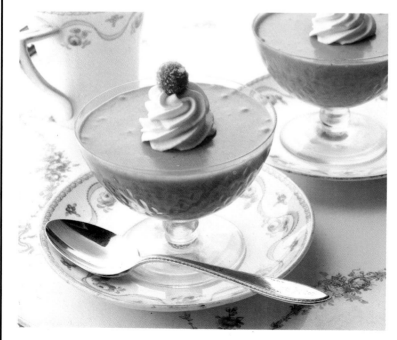

3. Return to the pan and stir over a gentle heat until it is thick enough to coat the back of the spoon.
4. Sprinkle the gelatine over the stem ginger syrup; when it swells, stir into the hot custard until dissolved. Cool until beginning to set.
5. Whip the fresh cream until softly stiff and fold into the custard with 75 g (3 oz) ginger. Turn into a dampened 1.4-litre (2½-pint) ring mould and chill until set.
6. Turn out on to a flat serving plate and decorate the top with chopped ginger.
Serves 6

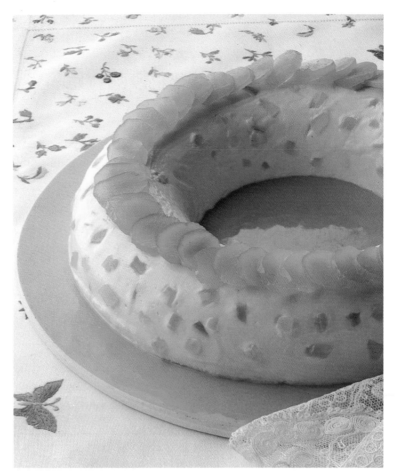

CRUSHED RASPBERRY CREAMS

450 g (1 lb) raspberries
60 ml (4 tbsp) icing sugar
45 ml (3 tbsp) orange-flavoured liqueur
3 eggs, separated
75 g (3 oz) caster sugar
300 ml (10 fl oz) fresh whipping cream
10 ml (2 level tsp) gelatine

1. Pick over the raspberries, reserving six berries for decoration. Place the remainder in a flat dish. Sprinkle with the icing sugar and spoon over the liqueur. Leave to stand for 1 hour. Purée in a blender then push through a sieve to remove the pips.
2. Whisk the egg yolks and caster sugar until really thick; gradually whisk in the raspberry purée.
3. Whip the fresh cream until softly stiff and fold a quarter into the raspberry mixture. Spoon the remainder into a piping bag fitted with a small star nozzle and refrigerate.
4. Soak the gelatine in 30 ml (2 tbsp) of water in a small bowl. Dissolve by standing the bowl in a pan of gently simmering water. Stir quickly into the raspberry mixture.
5. When the raspberry mixture begins to set whisk the egg whites until stiff then fold into the mixture. Pour into stemmed glasses and refrigerate to set.
6. Decorate with the remaining fresh whipped cream and whole raspberries.
Serves 6

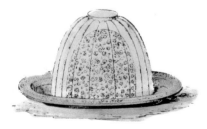

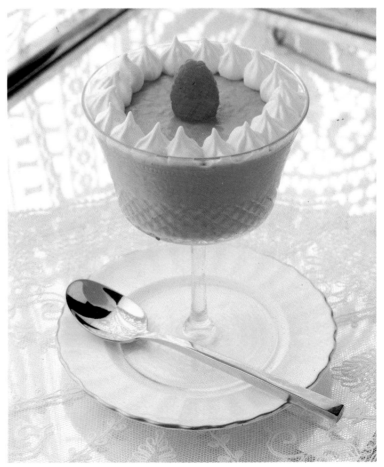

HONEY POT CREAMS

grated rind and juice of 1 lemon

45 ml (3 tbsp) clear honey

30 ml (2 tbsp) whisky

300 ml (10 fl oz) fresh double cream

1 egg white

flaked almonds, toasted, to decorate

1. Soak the grated rind in the lemon juice with the honey and whisky for 20 minutes.
2. Whip the fresh cream until softly stiff and gradually beat in the lemon mixture. Whisk the egg white until stiff then fold into the mixture.
3. Pile into individual glasses. Chill well and decorate with browned flaked almonds.

Serves 4

Below:
STRAWBERRY AND ORANGE MOUSSE, LEMON YOGURT WHIPS
Sweet delicious strawberries instantly spell summer magic. This mouthwatering mousse is decorated with fresh fruit and cream, the flavour of the strawberries delicately blended with the complementary taste of freshly squeezed orange juice.

The recipe for Lemon Yogurt Whips is given on page 204. A fresh light dessert served in individual glasses, it is a summer favourite with people who dislike rich heavy puddings.

STRAWBERRY AND ORANGE MOUSSE

700 g (1½ lb) strawberries, hulled

1 large orange

45 ml (3 level tbsp) icing sugar

2 eggs, separated, plus 1 egg yolk

125 g (4 oz) caster sugar

15 ml (3 level tsp) gelatine

450 ml (15 fl oz) fresh whipping cream

1. Thinly slice enough hulled strawberries to line the sides of a 2.3-litre (4-pint) shallow glass dish.

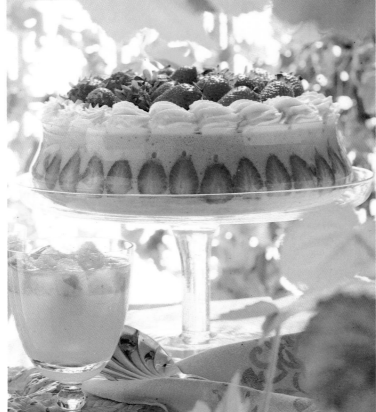

2. Purée half the remainder in a blender with the finely grated orange rind, 75 ml (5 tbsp) orange juice and the icing sugar. Then pass through a nylon sieve to give a very smooth texture. Reserve the rest of the strawberries for decoration.
3. Whisk the three egg yolks and caster sugar until thick and light. Gradually whisk in the strawberry purée.
4. Soak the gelatine in 45 ml (3 tbsp) water in a small bowl. Dissolve by standing the bowl over a pan of hot water. Stir into the mousse mixture.
5. Whip the fresh cream until softly stiff. Fold one-third through the mousse. Keep the rest covered in the fridge. Whisk the egg whites until stiff then fold into the mixture. Turn carefully into glass dish. Refrigerate.
6. When set decorate with the reserved fresh cream. Refrigerate.
7. Decorate with the reserved strawberries. Remove from the refrigerator 20 minutes before eating.

Serves 6

CHOCOLATE COFFEE REFRIGERATOR SLICE

30 ml (2 level tbsp) instant coffee granules

45 ml (3 tbsp) brandy

125 g (4 oz) plain chocolate

125 g (4 oz) English butter, softened

50 g (2 oz) icing sugar

2 egg yolks

300 ml (10 fl oz) fresh whipping cream

50 g (2 oz) chopped almonds, toasted

about 30 boudoirs (sponge fingers)

1. Make up the coffee granules with 200 ml (7 fl oz) boiling water and stir in the brandy; cool.
2. Break up the chocolate and melt in a small basin with 15 ml (1 tbsp) water; cool.
3. Whisk the butter and icing sugar together until pale and fluffy. Add the egg yolks, beating well.
4. Stir in the cool chocolate. Whip the fresh cream until softly stiff and stir half into the chocolate mixture, with the nuts. Refrigerate the remaining fresh cream.
5. Butter and base-line a 21.5 × 11.5 cm (8½ × 4½ inch) top measurement loaf tin with non-stick paper and line the bottom with sponge fingers, cutting to fit if necessary. Spoon over one-third of the coffee mixture.
6. Layer up the tin with the chocolate mixture and sponge fingers soaking each layer with coffee, ending up with soaked sponge fingers. Weight down lightly and refrigerate for several hours.
7. Turn out on to serving dish. Decorate with remaining fresh whipped cream.

Serves 6–8

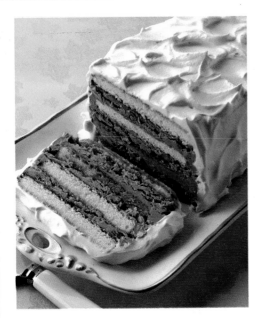

COFFEE PARFAIT

300 ml (½ pint) milk

25 g (1 oz) coffee beans

3 egg yolks

40 g (1½ oz) caster sugar

scant 15 g (½ oz) gelatine

300 ml (10 fl oz) fresh double cream

1. Heat the milk gently in a saucepan with the coffee beans, to release their flavour.
2. Whisk the egg yolks with the sugar and strain on to the milk. Return to the pan and stir over a gentle heat, without boiling, until thick. Strain into a bowl and cool.
3. Dissolve the gelatine in 75 ml (2½ fl oz) water in a small basin over a pan of hot water, then add to the custard. Leave to cool.
4. Whip the fresh cream until softly stiff and fold half into the coffee mixture when on the point of setting. Pour into a 900-ml (1½-pint) dampened mould.
5. Allow to set, then turn out and decorate with the remaining fresh cream.

Serves 4

BLENDER BERRY CHEESE MOUSSE

100 g (4 oz) caster sugar

125 g (4 oz) blackcurrants, topped and tailed

125 g (4 oz) red currants, topped and tailed

35 ml (7 level tsp) gelatine

125 g (4 oz) raspberries, hulled

grated rind and juice of 1 orange

grated rind and juice of 1 lemon

150 ml (5 fl oz) soured cream

350 g (12 oz) cottage cheese

2 eggs, separated

150 ml (5 fl oz) fresh double cream

1. In a saucepan dissolve 25 g (1 oz) sugar in 150 ml (¼ pint) water. Add the prepared currants and cook slowly until fruit is just tender, not mushy. Meanwhile, in a cup or small bowl, sprinkle 10 ml (2 level tsp) gelatine over 30 ml (2 tbsp) water, leave for a few minutes. Off the heat, stir into the fruit until dissolved. Cool and add the raspberries. When beginning to set pour into a 1.7-litre (3-pint) ring mould. Chill.
2. Using a large blender, combine the orange and lemon rind and juice, 50 g (2 oz) caster sugar, soured cream, cottage cheese and egg yolks; blend until smooth. Dissolve the remaining 25 ml (5 level tsp) gelatine in 45 ml (3 tbsp) water in a small bowl over a pan of hot water. Add to blender mixture, switch on for a few seconds. Turn into a bowl.
3. Whip the fresh cream until softly stiff. Fold into the cheese mixture. Whisk the egg whites until stiff, then whisk in the remaining 25 g (1 oz) sugar. Fold into the mixture and then pour into ring mould. Chill until set then unmould to serve.

Serves 8–10

Left:
CHOCOLATE COFFEE REFRIGERATOR SLICE
Layers of sponge fingers, brandied coffee and a rich chocolate mixture make Chocolate Coffee Refrigerator Slice an ideal ending to any summer meal.

Below:
BLENDER BERRY CHEESE MOUSE and ICED RASPBERRY SOUFFLÉS, Blender Berry Mousse is a delicious dessert which contrasts a smooth lemony cheese base with a piquant soft fruit topping. It is chilled in two stages for a striking two-tone effect.
The recipe for individual Iced Raspberry Soufflés is given on page 214.
Try them, decorated with fresh plump raspberries, for a perfect end to a summer dinner party.

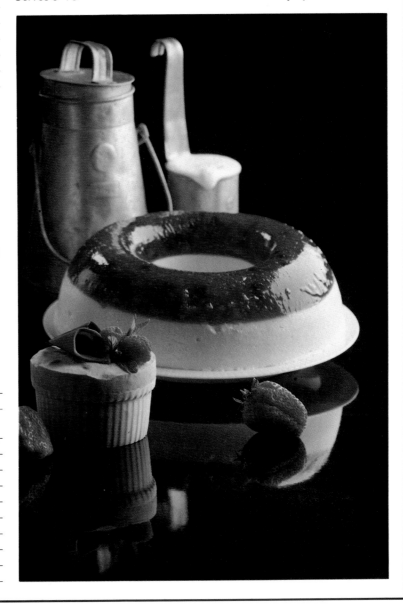

ICED COFFEE GÂTEAU

30 ml (2 level tbsp) apricot jam

10 boudoir biscuits, halved crosswise

2 eggs, separated

30 ml (2 tbsp) coffee essence

15 ml (1 tbsp) medium sherry

60 ml (4 level tbsp) icing sugar

150 ml (5 fl oz) fresh double cream

grated or curled chocolate to decorate

1. Warm the jam gently and brush around the edges of a 16-cm (6½-inch) round cake tin base-lined with non-stick paper. Stand the biscuits around the edge of the tin.
2. Beat the egg yolks, coffee essence and sherry well together.
3. Whisk the egg whites until stiff and gradually whisk in the sifted icing sugar. Stir the egg yolk mixture through the whites.
4. Whip the fresh cream until softly stiff. Fold into the mixture then pour into the lined cake tin.
5. Freeze for about 6 hours until firm. Turn out of the tin and serve straight away decorated with coarsely grated or curled chocolate.
Serves 6–8

ICED PINEAPPLE CRUSH

125 g (4 oz) English butter

125 g (4 oz) plain chocolate cake covering

30 ml (2 tbsp) golden syrup

225 g (8 oz) digestive biscuits, crushed

400 ml (15 fl oz) fresh double cream

three 250 g (8½ oz) cans crushed pineapple, drained

45 ml (3 tbsp) lemon juice

40 g (1½ oz) icing sugar, sifted

fresh or canned pineapple slices

Below:
CHILLED CHOC MINT
CHIP SOUFFLÉ
A scrumptious chocolate soufflé laced with the cool fresh taste of mint. Serve it with cups of freshly made coffee for a perfect ending to any meal.

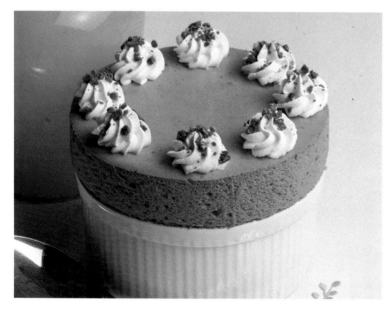

1. Melt the butter, chocolate and syrup together in a small pan. Stir in the crushed biscuits.
2. Base-line a 28×18×2.5 cm (11×7×1 inch) deep tin with non-stick paper and press the crumb mixture over this; refrigerate to set.
3. Whip the fresh cream until softly stiff and fold in the crushed pineapple, lemon juice and icing sugar.
4. Spread the pineapple mixture over the biscuit base and freeze for at least 3 hours, until firm.
5. Serve cut into wedges or squares topped with a twist of fresh pineapple. Cut off as many portions as required and return to the freezer. Allow portions to come to cool room temperature for 10–15 minutes.
Serves 10

SOUFFLÉS

CHILLED CHOC MINT CHIP SOUFFLÉ

400 ml (¾ pint) milk

50 g (2 oz) plain chocolate

113 g (¼ lb) packet mint Matchmakers, roughly chopped

3 eggs, separated, plus 1 egg white

75 g (3 oz) caster sugar

15 ml (3 level tsp) gelatine

300 ml (10 fl oz) fresh whipping cream

1. Prepare a 900-ml (1½-pint) soufflé dish with a paper collar.
2. Heat the milk, chocolate and 25 g (1 oz) Matchmakers. When melted, boil, whisking. Remove from the heat.
3. Beat the egg yolks with the sugar until light. Pour on the flavoured milk, return to the pan and cook over a gentle heat, without boiling, until the custard coats the back of a spoon, pour into a bowl, cool.
4. Soak the gelatine in 45 ml (3 tbsp) water in a small bowl. Dissolve by standing the bowl in a pan of gently simmering water. Stir into the custard and chill.
5. Whip the fresh cream until softly stiff. Stir half into the custard on the point of setting. Stir 50 g (2 oz) Matchmakers into the custard.
6. Whisk the four egg whites until stiff then fold into the mixture. Spoon into a soufflé dish, refrigerate to set.
7. Remove the paper, decorate with remaining cream and Matchmakers.
Serves 4

CHILLED APRICOT AND ALMOND SOUFFLÉ

125 g (4 oz) dried apricots
60 ml (4 tbsp) almond-flavoured liqueur
4 eggs, separated
125 g (4 oz) caster sugar
300 ml (10 fl oz) fresh whipping cream
20 ml (4 level tsp) gelatine
100 g (4 oz) ratafias

1. Soak the apricots overnight in cold water.
2. Prepare a 1.1-litre (2-pint) soufflé dish with a paper collar and stand a slim, well-oiled bottle in the centre.
3. Cook the apricots in their soaking liquid in a covered pan for about 45 minutes until tender.
4. Strain, reserving the liquid; purée the fruit in a blender with 60 ml (4 tbsp) of the juice and 30 ml (2 tbsp) of almond liqueur. Leave until cold.
5. Whisk the egg yolks and sugar until thick. Gradually whisk in the apricot purée, keeping the mixture thick. Whip the fresh cream until softly stiff and stir half into the apricot mixture..
6. Soak the gelatine in 60 ml (4 tbsp) of water in a small bowl. Dissolve by standing the bowl over a pan of gently simmering water. Fold into the soufflé mixture.
7. Whisk the egg whites until stiff, fold into the mixture and spoon into the prepared dish. Refrigerate to set. Soak 75 g (3 oz) ratafias in the remaining liqueur and crush the remainder. Remove the paper and bottle from the soufflé. Fill the centre with soaked ratafias. Decorate with the remaining fresh cream and crushed ratafias.

Serves 6

COFFEE CREAM SOUFFLÉS

15 ml (3 level tsp) gelatine
3 eggs, separated
75 g (3 oz) caster sugar
45 ml (3 tbsp) coffee essence
150 ml (5 fl oz) fresh single cream
300 ml (10 fl oz) fresh whipping cream
25g (1 oz) chopped almonds, toasted

1. Prepare six 100 ml (4 fl oz) soufflé dishes, by surrounding them with foil to come 2.5 cm (1 inch) above the top of the dish. Secure with adhesive tape.
2. Dissolve the gelatine in 45 ml (3 tbsp) water in a small basin over a pan of hot water.
3. In a deep bowl whisk the egg yolks and sugar together over a pan of hot water until thick. Cool to lukewarm.
4. Add the coffee essence and gelatine to the fresh single cream, whisk into the egg yolk mixture. Leave until beginning to set.

5. Whip the fresh whipping cream until softly stiff. Whisk the egg whites until stiff. Fold the fresh cream and egg whites into the coffee mixture. Turn into the prepared soufflé dishes.
6. Refrigerate until set, remove foil and decorate edges with almonds.

Serves 6

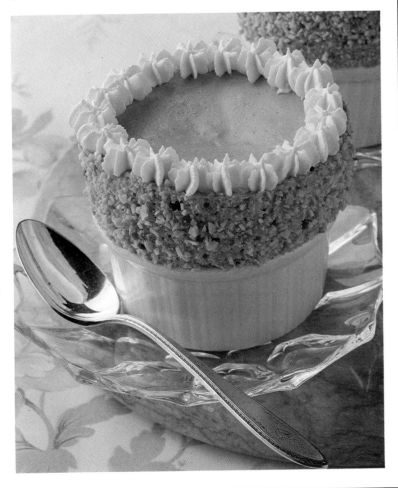

Left:
CHILLED APRICOT AND
ALMOND SOUFFLÉ
The combination of apricots and almonds is a very natural one, and in fact the kernels of apricots are sometimes used in the same ways that almonds are. This soufflé has an added treat – ratafia biscuits soaked in almond-flavoured liqueur.

Below:
COFFEE CREAM SOUFFLÉS
To some people coffee desserts are even more perfect than chocolate-flavoured ones. Served in individual dishes, at least you avoid the inevitable squabbling over seconds!

ORANGE SOUFFLÉ CRUNCH

50 g (2 oz) English butter

175 g (6 oz) digestive biscuits, crumbled

150 g (5 oz) demerara sugar

2 eggs

150 ml (5 fl oz) fresh double cream

grated rind and juice of 1 orange

15 ml (1 tbsp) orange-flavoured liqueur

1. Melt the butter and add the digestive biscuits and 50 g (2 oz) of the sugar. Stir and leave to cool.
2. Whisk together one whole egg and one yolk until thick. (For best results use an electric whisk.) Add 75 g (3 oz) of the sugar and continue to whisk until the mixture leaves a trail. Put to one side.
3. Whip the fresh cream until softly stiff. Add the orange rind and 30 ml (2 tbsp) of orange juice with the orange liqueur. Continue to whip the mixture until stiff. Leave to one side.
4. Whisk the egg white until stiff. Carefully fold the egg yolk mixture into the fresh cream followed by the egg white.
5. Starting with the biscuit crumb, layer the fresh cream mixture and crumbled biscuits into one large or individual serving dishes – but if glass dishes are being used, make sure they will withstand freezer temperature.
6. Place in the freezer until set and ready to serve.

Serves 4–6

FROSTED CREAM SOUFFLÉ

300 ml (10 fl oz) fresh double cream

30–45ml (2–3 tbsp) orange-flavoured liqueur

75 ml (5 tbsp) champagne, dry white wine or dry cider

30–45 ml (2–3 tbsp) lemon juice

finely grated rind of ½ lemon

4 eggs, separated

75 g (3 oz) caster sugar

lemon slices to decorate

1. Tie a collar of kitchen foil or greaseproof paper round the outside of six individual soufflé dishes to stand 5 cm (2 inches) above the rim. Secure with adhesive tape.
2. Whip the fresh cream until softly stiff, then gently whip the orange liqueur, champagne, lemon juice and grated lemon rind into the fresh cream. Leave in a cool place.
3. Whisk the egg yolks with caster sugar until thick and foamy. Gently fold into the fresh cream.
4. Whisk the egg whites until stiff then fold into the fresh cream mixture.

5. Turn the soufflé mixture into the prepared dishes. Smooth the top, then place in freezer until firm.
6. Remove the soufflés from the freezer and gently ease away the collar. Decorate with lemon slices.

Serves 8–10

GINGER WINE SOUFFLÉS

3 eggs, separated

40 g (1½ oz) demerara sugar

2.5 ml (½ tsp) ground ginger

300 ml (½ pint) milk

10 ml (2 level tsp) gelatine

60 ml (4 tbsp) ginger wine

300 ml (10 fl oz) fresh whipping cream

20 g (¾ oz) stem ginger, chopped

1. Tie a collar of kitchen foil or greaseproof paper around the outside of six individual soufflé dishes to stand 5 cm (2 inches) above the rim. Secure with adhesive tape.
2. Beat the egg yolks, sugar and ground ginger together in a bowl.
3. Heat the milk then pour on to egg mixture. Return to the saucepan and cook until the custard thickens but do *not* allow to boil.
4. Soak the gelatine in 30 ml (2 tbsp) water in a small bowl. Place the bowl over a pan of hot water and stir until dissolved. Stir into the cool custard and add the ginger wine.
5. Whip the fresh cream until softly stiff. Whisk the egg whites until stiff. Stir half the fresh cream and half the stem ginger into the nearly set ginger mixture. Fold in the whisked egg whites.
6. Spoon into the soufflé dishes. Chill in the refrigerator. To serve, remove the paper collars and decorate with the reserved fresh whipped cream and chopped ginger.

Serves 6

ICED RASPBERRY SOUFFLÉS

30 ml (2 level tbsp) cornflour

300 ml (½ pint) milk

75 g (3 oz) caster sugar

2 eggs, beaten

225 g (8 oz) raspberries, hulled

175 ml (6 fl oz) fresh double cream

chocolate cornets (see below) fresh raspberries and mint sprigs to decorate

1. Tie a collar of non-stick paper around the outside of four 7.5-cm (3-inch) individual soufflé dishes to stand 5 cm (2 inches) above the rim. Secure with adhesive tape. Put the dishes on a baking sheet.
2. Blend the cornflour with 30 ml (2 tbsp) cold milk. In a small pan, dissolve the sugar in the remaining milk over a low heat. Pour

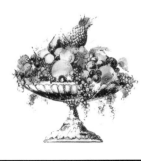

on to the blended cornflour, stirring, then pour slowly on to the beaten eggs, whisking. Return to the pan and cook for a few minutes without boiling. Allow mixture to cool.

3. Push the raspberries through a sieve to remove the seeds and stir into the cornflour sauce. Leave covered until cold.

4. Whip the fresh cream until softly stiff and the same consistency as the cornflour mixture. Then fold the cornflour mixture evenly through the fresh cream.

5. Spoon into the prepared soufflé dishes so that the mixture comes about 1 cm (½ inch) above the rim.

6. Freeze until firm but not solid, either in a freezer or the frozen food compartment of a refrigerator, set at lowest temperature. Just before serving, remove the paper collar and decorate with chocolate cornets, fresh raspberries and mint sprigs.

Serves 4   (illustration on page 211)

CHOCOLATE CORNETS

1. Cut non-stick paper into 10-cm (4-inch) squares then cut each into two triangles. With the base towards you, fold the right-hand corner up to the top point of the triangle and then turn round to take in the other point. Slightly overlap the points and secure with a staple or fold the tips over.

2. Melt 50–75 g (2–3 oz) chocolate in a small basin over a pan of hot, not boiling, water. Spoon a little of the chocolate, cool but still flowing, in the centre of each paper cornet, turn the cornet to evenly coat the sides. Chill, recoat if necessary. When set, carefully peel away the paper. Store in a cool place.

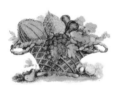

CHEESECAKES

PINEAPPLE CHEESECAKE

75 g (3 oz) English butter
175 g (6 oz) plain chocolate wholewheat biscuits, roughly crushed
225 g (8 oz) cottage cheese
100 g (4 oz) full fat soft cheese
pared rind and juice of 1 large lemon
150 ml (5 fl oz) soured cream
3 eggs, separated
50 g (2 oz) caster sugar
15 ml (3 level tsp) gelatine
two 432 g (14½ oz) cans sliced pineapple, with juice
60 ml (4 level tbsp) sieved apricot jam

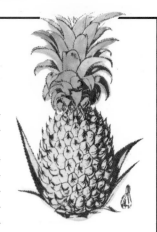

1. Melt the butter in a pan. Stir the biscuits into butter. Press the crumb mixture into a 23-cm (9-inch) spring-release cake tin and refrigerate to set.

2. Place the cottage and full fat soft cheeses, lemon rind, 45 ml (3 tbsp) lemon juice and the soured cream in a blender and switch on until smooth.

3. Whisk the egg yolks and sugar until thick. Soak the gelatine in 45 ml (3 tbsp) of water in a small bowl. Dissolve by standing the bowl in a pan of simmering water. Whisk into the egg yolks with the cheese mixture.

4. Drain and roughly chop three-quarters of the pineapple, reserve juices. Whisk the egg whites until stiff. Fold into the setting cheese mixture with the chopped pineapple. Pour into crust and refrigerate.

5. Carefully remove the sides of the cake tin then, using a fish slice, lift and slide the cheesecake off the base on to a serving plate.

6. Decorate with reserved pineapple. Boil down juices with the jam to a thick glaze, cool, spoon over pineapple.

Serves 10

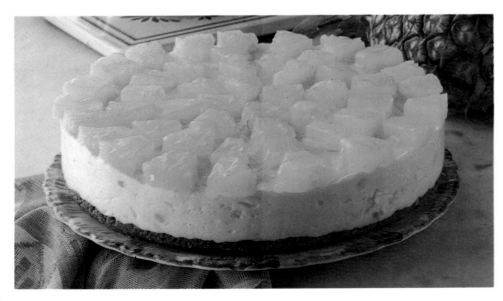

Left:
PINEAPPLE
CHEESECAKE
Pineapple looks and tastes fabulously exotic and has long been used to complement cheese. Enjoy its sundrenched sweetness in this mouthwatering cheesecake made of cottage cheese, soft cheese and tangy soured cream.

MAKING A CHEESECAKE

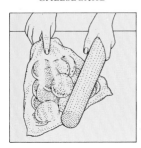

1 Crushing the biscuits with a rolling pin

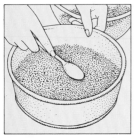

2 Pressing in the biscuit base

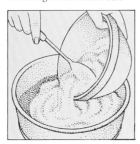

3 Spooning the cheesecake mixture into the tin

COFFEE CHEESECAKE

50 g (2 oz) English butter
175 g (6 oz) gingernut biscuits, finely crushed
15 ml (1 level tbsp) gelatine
20 ml (4 level tsp) instant coffee-flavoured powder
45 ml (3 tbsp) coffee-flavoured liqueur
150 g (5 oz) soft brown sugar
450 g (1 lb) full fat soft cheese
300 ml (10 fl oz) fresh whipping cream
coffee beans to decorate

1. Lightly butter a 20.5-cm (8-inch) loose bottomed deep cake tin or spring-release cake tin.
2. Melt the butter in a pan and stir in the biscuit crumbs. Press firmly into the base of the tin. Chill well.
3. Sprinkle the gelatine on to 45 ml (3 tbsp) of water. Leave to soak.
4. Stir the coffee and coffee liqueur into 300 ml (½ pint) of boiling water. Add the soaked gelatine, stirring until dissolved. Stir in the sugar.
5. In a blender whirl the coffee mixture and soft cheese until just smooth. Lightly whip the fresh cream until softly stiff and fold the cheese mixture into half of it.
6. Turn into the prepared tin. Chill to set. When set remove from the tin and decorate with remaining fresh ceam and coffee beans.
7. Allow the wedges to soften at cool room temperature for 1¼ hours before serving.

Serves 8

LEMON CHEESECAKE

75 g (3 oz) English butter
175 g (6 oz) digestive biscuits, finely crushed
15 ml (1 level tbsp) gelatine
finely grated rind and juice of 1 lemon
225 g (8 oz) cottage cheese, sieved
150 ml (5 fl oz) soured cream
75 g (3 oz) caster sugar
2 eggs, separated
fresh fruit such as strawberries, sliced, black and green grapes, halved and seeded, or kiwi fruit, skinned and sliced to decorate

1. Melt the butter in a pan and mix in the biscuit crumbs. Press down in an even layer in the base of a 20.5-cm (8-inch) spring-release tin. Chill in the refrigerator for 30 minutes until firm.
2. Sprinkle the gelatine in 60 ml (4 tbsp) water in a small bowl. Place the bowl in a pan of simmering water and stir until dissolved.
3. Put the lemon rind, juice and cottage cheese into a bowl and add the soured cream and sugar and mix well together. Add the egg yolks and cooled gelatine.
4. Whisk the egg whites until stiff and then fold lightly into the mixture. Carefully pour into the tin and chill for several hours, preferably overnight.
5. Remove the cheesecake from the tin and place on a flat serving plate. Decorate with fresh fruits.

Serves 6

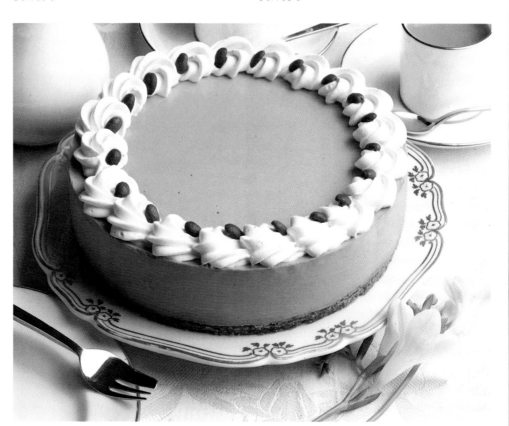

Right:
COFFEE CHEESECAKE
A crisp gingery crust with a rich coffee-flavoured cheesy filling makes this a cheesecake out of the ordinary. It is delicious!

Opposite:
LEMON CHEESECAKE
Everyone loves this classic cheesecake, decorated here with slices of kiwi fruit.

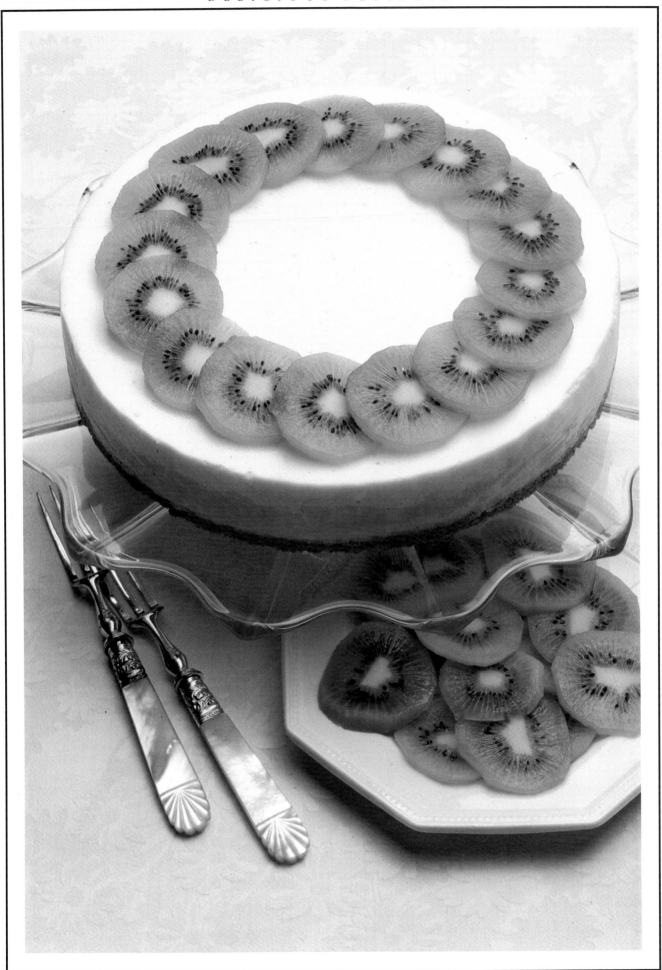

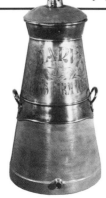

MILK PUDDINGS

BAKED RICE PUDDING

50 g (2 oz) pudding rice, or flaked rice,
    barley, tapioca, broken macaroni

568 ml (1 pint) milk

25 g (1 oz) caster sugar

1 strip of lemon rind

grated nutmeg

15 g (½ oz) English butter

1. Wash the rice and drain well. Put into a ¾-litre (1½-pint) buttered ovenproof dish and stir in the milk.
2. Leave the rice to soak and soften for 30 minutes. Add the sugar and lemon rind and stir well. Sprinkle with grated nutmeg and dot with butter.
3. Bake in the oven at 150°C (300 °F) mark 2 for 2–2½ hours. Stir it after about 30 minutes.

Serves 4

BAKED CUSTARD

568 ml (1 pint) milk

3 eggs

30 ml (2 level tbsp) caster sugar

grated nutmeg

1. Warm the milk in a saucepan but do not boil.
2. Whisk the eggs and sugar lightly in a bowl; pour on the hot milk, stirring all the time. Strain the mixture into a buttered ovenproof dish.
3. Sprinkle the nutmeg on top and bake in the oven at 170°C (325°F) mark 3 for about 45 minutes, until set and firm to the touch. Serve cold.

Serves 4

JUNKET

568 ml (1 pint) pasteurised milk

15 ml (1 level tbsp) caster sugar

5 ml (1 tsp) liquid rennet

grated nutmeg

1. Gently heat the milk until just warm to the finger. Remove from the heat and stir in the sugar until dissolved. Add the rennet, stirring gently.
2. Pour into a shallow dish and leave for 1–1½ hours in a warm place, undisturbed, until set.
3. Chill in the refrigerator and sprinkle the top with a little grated nutmeg to serve.

Note: It is important to use only ordinary pasteurised milk for junket making. In order not to kill the rennet enzyme, care must be taken not to overheat the milk, nor to cool the junket too rapidly. Junket should not be

Below: clockwise from top
BAKED RICE PUDDING,
JUNKET AND BAKED
CUSTARD
Three puddings – one hot and two cold – which illustrate just how deliciously versatile milk can be.

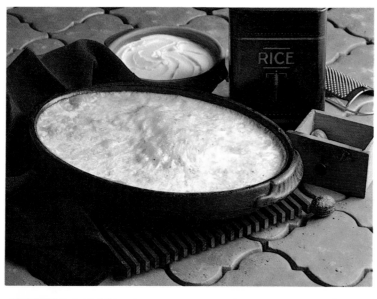

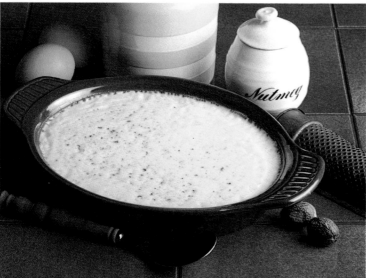

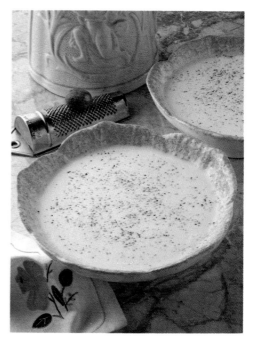

disturbed until it is served as once it is cut the whey runs out and separates from the curds.

Rennet is sold as a liquid or in a tablet without added colouring. There are also commercial preparations of rennet in tablet and liquid form, which are coloured and flavoured. Use according to the directions on the packet. Ensure that the rennet is not old as it loses its setting properties with age.

Variation
Cold Velvet Cream
Add 5–10 ml (1–2 tsp) rum to the milk.
Serves 4

HONEYED GOOSEBERRY DESSERT

350 g (12 oz) gooseberries, topped and tailed
150 g (5 oz) light brown sugar
10 ml (2 level tsp) arrowroot
grated rind and juice of 1 lemon
75 ml (5 level tbsp) honey
568 ml (1 pint) milk
50 g (2 oz) semolina

1. Simmer the gooseberries gently in a covered pan with 75 g (3 oz) sugar and 90 ml (6 tbsp) water. When soft but still whole, strain off the liquid and reserve. Set the berries aside.
2. In the saucepan, blend the arrowroot to a smooth paste with 15 ml (1 tbsp) lemon juice and the honey. Add the strained gooseberry juice and bring to the boil, stirring. Cook until clear. Cool in a bowl.
3. Wash the pan, bring milk nearly to the boil, sprinkle on the semolina, lemon rind and remaining sugar. Cook for about 10 minutes until thickened. Stir in 60 ml (4 tbsp) cooled gooseberry juice.

4. Layer the gooseberries and cool semolina in four glasses, finishing with gooseberries. Spoon over the rest of the gooseberry juice. Chill before serving.
Serves 4

CITRUS CONDÉ

3 satsumas
568 ml (1 pint) milk
60 ml (4 tbsp) clear honey
50 g (2 oz) pudding rice
15 ml (1 level tbsp) gelatine
150 ml (5 fl oz) fresh double cream
1 egg white
25 g (1 oz) blanched almonds, split and toasted

1. Remove the peel from the satsumas with a serrated knife and reserve; divide the flesh into segments, discarding all the pith.
2. Scald the milk in a heavy-based pan with the satsuma peel, cover and leave to infuse for 10 minutes. Strain.
3. Return the milk to the pan, add the honey and rice and bring to the boil. Simmer, uncovered, stirring occasionally for about 30 minutes until the rice is tender and the milk absorbed. Turn out into a bowl and cool.
4. Arrange a few fruit segments in the bottom of a dampened 1.1-litre (2-pint) ring mould.
5. Sprinkle the gelatine over 45 ml (3 tbsp) water in a small basin or cup. Dissolve by standing the basin in a pan of gently simmering water. Stir into the rice with the unwhipped fresh cream.
6. Whisk the egg white until stiff. Fold the remaining fruit into the rice with the whisked egg white. Spoon carefully into the mould. Refrigerate to set.
7. Turn out to serve; decorate with almonds.
Serves 4

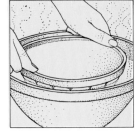

1 Dip the mould into hot water for a few seconds. Heat travels through a metal mould very quickly, but a china or glass mould may take a little longer.

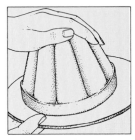

2 Put a plate on top of the mould and quickly turn them over together

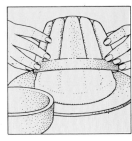

3 Lift the mould off carefully and put the unmoulded jelly into refrigerator immediately

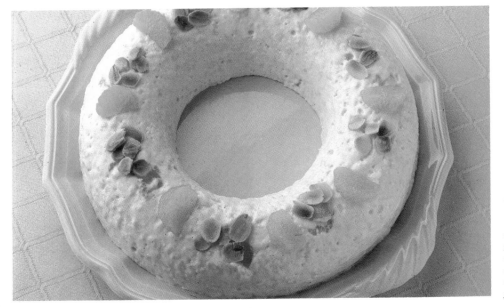

Left:
CITRUS CONDÉ
This delicious dish is a sophisticated variation on rice pudding. Fragrant with honey, crunchy with golden almonds and rich with fresh cream, it is an unusual sweet which could grace any party.

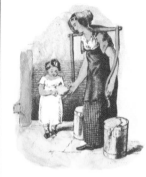

CABINET PUDDING

6 trifle sponge cakes
50 g (2 oz) glacé cherries coarsely chopped
25 g (1 oz) caster sugar
2 eggs
568 ml (1 pint) milk
5 ml (1 tsp) vanilla flavouring
fresh double cream to serve

1. Cut each cake into six cubes. Put cherries in a basin with the sugar and toss lightly together to mix.
2. Beat the eggs, milk and vanilla flavouring well together. Gently stir into the cake mixture.
3. Leave to stand for 30 minutes. Turn into a $\frac{3}{4}$-litre ($1\frac{1}{2}$-pint) well-buttered pudding basin. Cover securely with buttered greaseproof paper or buttered foil.
4. Steam very gently for 1 hour. Turn out carefully on to a warm plate. Serve with fresh double cream.
Serves 4

QUEEN OF PUDDINGS

4 eggs
568 ml (1 pint) milk
100 g (4 oz) fine breadcrumbs
45–60 ml (3–4 level tbsp) raspberry jam
75 g (3 oz) caster sugar

1. Separate three eggs and beat together the three egg yolks and one whole egg. Add to the milk and mix well. Add the breadcrumbs.
2. Put the jam on the bottom of a pie dish, making a layer of about 1 cm ($\frac{1}{2}$ inch). Pour over the milk, egg and crumb custard and leave for 30 minutes.
3. Bake in the oven at 150°C (300°F) mark 2 for 1 hour, until set.
4. Whisk the egg whites until stiff then fold in the sugar. Pile on top of the custard, sprinkle with a little sugar and return to the cool oven for a further 15–20 minutes until the meringue is set and delicately browned.
Serves 4

Below:
QUEEN OF PUDDINGS
How this most subtle and lovely of puddings got its name is a mystery, but everyone agrees that it is well deserved.

CREAMY APRICOT MERINGUE

50 g (2 oz) pudding rice
450 ml (¾ pint) milk
1.25 ml (¼ tsp) vanilla flavouring
100 g (4 oz) caster sugar, plus 30 ml (2 level tbsp)
150 ml (5 fl oz) fresh double cream
425 g (15 oz) can apricot pie filling
1 egg white
30 ml (2 level tbsp) ground almonds
30 ml (2 level tbsp) flaked almonds

1. Put the rice and milk in a saucepan and simmer for 25 minutes, until cooked. Add the vanilla flavouring, 100 g (4 oz) sugar and leave to cool.
2. Whip the fresh cream until softly stiff and fold into the cooled rice.
3. Place the apricot pie filling in a dish, spoon over the rice.
4. Whisk the egg white until stiff, add the ground almonds and remaining sugar and whisk again. Spoon on to the rice, sprinkle with flaked almonds. Place under a hot grill for a few minutes, until the almonds are crisp and golden and the meringue lightly browned. Serve at once.

Serves 5–6

MILK JELLY

50 g (2 oz) caster sugar
3 thin strips of lemon rind
568 ml (1 pint) milk
20 ml (4 level tsp) gelatine

1. Add the sugar and lemon rind to the milk and allow to infuse over a gentle heat for 10 minutes. Cool.
2. Soak the gelatine in 45 ml (3 tbsp) water in a small bowl. Dissolve by standing the bowl over a pan of gently simmering water. Add the cooled milk.
3. Pour into a 600-ml (1-pint) dampened mould and leave to set.
4. To serve, unmould on to a plate. Using the fingertips gently ease the jelly from the

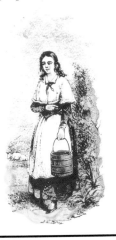

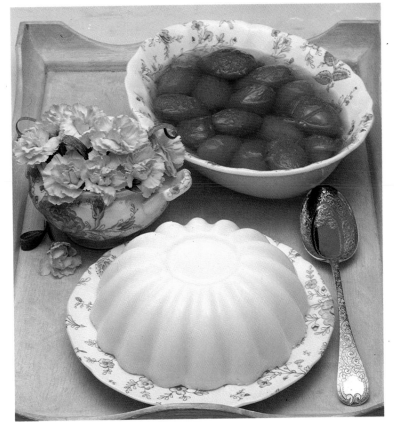

side of the mould. Dip the mould into a bowl of hot water for a few seconds. Place a serving plate upside down on top and invert the plate and mould. Using both hands carefully lift the mould from the jelly. Serve with stewed fruit.

Serves 4

Above:
MILK JELLY
Delicately flavoured with tangy lemon rind, a milk jelly looks beautiful when set in a mould, turned out, and served with a dish of piquant stewed fresh fruit, such as plums.

GINGER PINEAPPLE SUNDAE

50 g (2 oz) English butter
75 g (3 oz) ginger biscuits, crushed
50 g (2 oz) corn flakes, crushed
25 g (1 oz) walnuts, finely chopped
350 g (12 oz) canned pineapple, drained and chopped
15 ml (1 level tbsp) ginger marmalade
300 ml (½ pint) custard sauce (see page 153)
150 ml (5 fl oz) fresh double cream

1. Melt the butter and add the biscuit crumbs, corn flakes and walnuts. Mix together and allow to cool.
2. Reserving a little for decoration, add the pineapple with the marmalade to the cold custard sauce, then mix well.
3. Divide the custard equally between four individual glasses and form layers with the biscuit mixture, finishing with the custard. Whip the fresh cream until stiff. Decorate each with the fresh cream and reserved pineapple, then chill and serve.

Serves 4

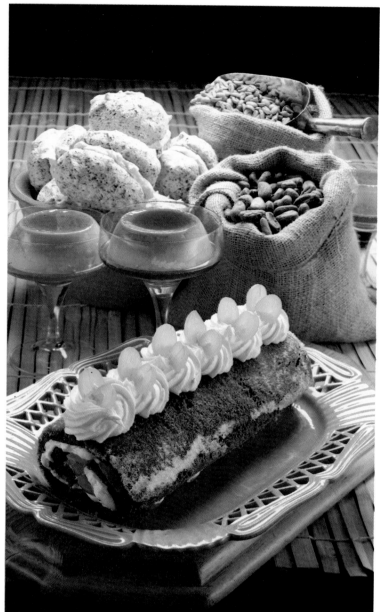

Above, from the top:
CHOCOLATE CHIP
MERINGUES, CRÈME
CARAMEL AU CAFÉ and
MOCHA ROULADE
The rich distinctive flavours of
chocolate and coffee are the
theme of these three tempting
desserts which taste as good as
they look.

The recipe for the Chocolate
Chip Meringue is given on page
236 and for the Mocha Roulade
on page 235.

Right:
CRÈME CARAMEL
Like many classic dishes, this
popular dessert relies on very
simple ingredients for its
delicious taste and tempting
appearance.

Variation

Individual custards are easier to turn out.
Divide the above mixture between six
150 ml ($\frac{1}{4}$-pint) caramel coated ramekin
dishes. Cook for about 45 minutes.
Serves 4

CRÈME CARAMEL AU CAFÉ

125 g (4$\frac{1}{2}$ oz) sugar
450 ml ($\frac{3}{4}$ pint) milk
15 ml (1 level tbsp) instant coffee powder
3 eggs, size 2
30 ml (2 tbsp) rum

1. Put 100 g (4 oz) sugar and 150 ml
($\frac{1}{4}$-pint) water into a small pan and heat
slowly until the sugar dissolves. Bring to the
boil and boil gently without stirring, until
golden.
2. Divide the caramel between four 200 ml
(7 fl oz) moulds. Stand these in a roasting
tin containing 2.5 cm (1 inch) water.
3. Warm the milk and dissolve the coffee in
it. Whisk the eggs with the remaining sugar
and rum until lightly stiff and pour over the
warm milk.
4. Strain into a jug and then divide between
the moulds.
5. Cover each mould with foil and bake in
the oven at 170°C (325°F) mark 3 for about
45 minutes until set.
6. Chill well (preferably overnight) before
turning out the caramels.
Serves 4

CRÈME CARAMEL

125 g (4$\frac{1}{2}$ oz) sugar
568 ml (1 pint) milk
4 eggs, beaten

1. Put 100 g (4 oz) sugar and 150 ml ($\frac{1}{4}$ pint)
water in a small pan and dissolve the sugar
slowly. Bring to the boil and boil gently
without stirring until it caramelises to a rich
golden brown colour.
2. Pour the caramel into a 15-cm (6-inch)
warm soufflé dish, turning the dish until the
bottom is completely covered.
3. Warm the milk, pour on to the lightly
whisked eggs and remaining sugar and
strain over the cooled caramel. Place the
dish in a shallow tin of water and bake in the
oven at 170°C (325°F) mark 3 for about
1 hour until set. Leave in the dish until quite
cold (preferably until the next day) before
turning out.

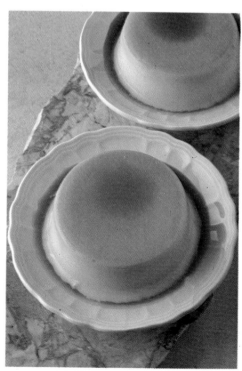

HOT PUDDINGS

COFFEE FUDGE PUDDING

225 g (8 oz) English butter

350 g (12 oz) soft brown sugar

2 eggs, beaten

90 ml (6 tbsp) coffee essence

225 g (8 oz) self-raising flour, sifted

50 g (2 oz) walnuts, chopped

568 ml (1 pint) milk

1. Whisk the butter and beat in 225g (8 oz) sugar. Gradually beat in the eggs with the coffee essence. Lightly beat in the flour with the walnuts, adding a little of the milk to give a soft dropping consistency.
2. Spoon into a 2.3-litre (4-pint) buttered ovenproof dish.
3. Blend together the remaining brown sugar and milk, pour evenly over the pudding mixture. Bake in the oven at 170°C (325°F) mark 3 for about 1 hour 25 minutes, until spongy to the touch. This pudding separates to give its own built-in sauce; also good served with chilled soured cream.

Serves 8

APPLE CRUNCH

450 g (1 lb) cooking apples, peeled, cored and sliced

25 g (1 oz) caster sugar

30 ml (2 tbsp) water

2.5 ml ($\frac{1}{2}$ level tsp) cinnamon (optional)

1 egg

30 ml (2 level tbsp) cornflour

15 ml (1 tbsp) golden syrup

300 ml ($\frac{1}{2}$ pint) milk

40 g ($1\frac{1}{2}$ oz) English butter

75 g (3 oz) rolled oats

40 g ($1\frac{1}{2}$ oz) brown sugar

slices of dessert apple to decorate

1. Gently cook the apples in the sugar and water until tender. Place in a $\frac{3}{4}$-litre (1-pint) ovenproof dish and sprinkle with cinnamon.
2. Beat the egg, cornflour and syrup together. Stir in the milk, then place in a pan and cook over a low heat, whisking continuously, until thickened. Cool slightly and pour over the apples.
3. Melt the butter in a pan, stir in the oats and sugar. Sprinkle over the custard. Bake in the oven at 180°C (350°F) mark 4 for 30 minutes. Serve hot, decorated with apple slices.

Variations
Use any fruit in season – gooseberries, rhubarb, pears or plums.

Serves 4

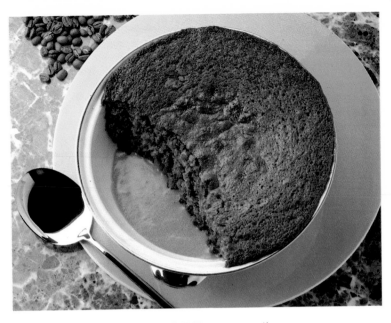

FRUIT CRUMBLE

50 g (2 oz) English butter

100 g (4 oz) flour

100 g (4 oz) caster sugar

450 g (1 lb) prepared fruit (apples, peaches, rhubarb, plums or gooseberries)

fresh double cream to serve

1. Rub the butter into the flour until the mixture resembles fine breadcrumbs, then stir in 50 g (2 oz) caster sugar.
2. Arrange half the prepared fruit in a 1.1-litre (2-pint) pie dish, sprinkle in about 50 g (2 oz) sugar, then top with the remaining fruit.
3. Spoon the crumble mixture over the fruit and lightly press it down.
4. Bake in the oven at 200°C (400°F) mark 6 for about 45 minutes, until the fruit is soft. Serve hot or cold with the fresh cream.

Serves 4

Above:
COFFEE FUDGE PUDDING
This delicious pudding is flavoured with coffee and walnuts and separates during baking to produce its own delectable sauce. Try it served with chilled soured cream.

Below:
FRUIT CRUMBLE
Using any prepared fruit, this good old-fashioned pudding is a firm favourite with all the family and can be served hot or cold with cool fresh cream.

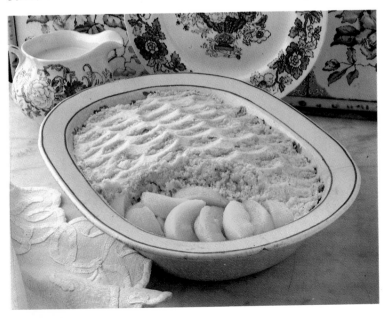

ORANGE PRINCESS

300 ml (½ pint) milk

1 orange

15 g (½ oz) English butter

75 g (3 oz) caster sugar

50 g (2 oz) fresh breadcrumbs

2 eggs, separated

glacé cherries, chopped, to decorate

1. Heat together the milk, orange rind and butter. Stir in 25 g (1 oz) sugar and the breadcrumbs. Add the egg yolks.
2. Pour into a buttered ¾-litre (1-pint) ovenproof dish. Bake in the oven at 170°C (325°F) mark 3 for 20 minutes. Remove from the oven and cover with layers of orange slices.
3. Whisk the egg whites until stiff then fold in the remaining 50 g (2 oz) sugar. Pile the meringue over the pudding.
4. Brown quickly in a hot oven, or under the grill, and decorate with cherries.
Serves 4

1. Whisk 150 g (5 oz) butter. Gradually stir in the sifted flour and salt; beat well after each addition. Add 45 ml (3 tbsp) cold water and mix thoroughly with the hands. Knead lightly with extra flour, as this pastry is sticky to handle. Chill.
2. Roll out the pastry and use to line a 23-cm (9-inch) ovenproof flan dish; flute the edge. Chill the case while preparing the filling.
3. Beat the eggs and milk together. Boil the sugar and syrup together in a saucepan for 3 minutes. Slowly pour on to the beaten eggs and stir in 50 g (2 oz) butter and vanilla flavouring.
4. Use half the nuts to cover the base of the pastry case, spoon the syrup mixture over and cover with the remaining nuts. Bake in the oven at 220°C (435°F) mark 7 for 10 minutes.
5. Reduce the heat to 170°C (325°F) mark 3 and cook for a further 45 minutes, until the filling is set. Serve warm or cold with the fresh cream.
Serves 6–8

PECAN PIE

200 g (7 oz) English butter

175 g (6 oz) flour

pinch of salt

3 eggs

15 ml (1 tbsp) milk

175 g (6 oz) demerara sugar

150 ml (¼ pint) maple or corn syrup

2.5 ml (½ tsp) vanilla flavouring

175 g (6 oz) pecan nuts, halved

fresh double cream to serve

Below:
PECAN PIE
This rich crunchy pie is a classic American version of our own old-fashioned treacle tart.

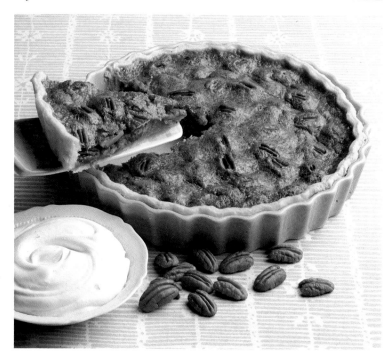

ALMOND PUDDING

100 g (4 oz) apricot jam

150 ml (5 fl oz) fresh single cream

150 ml (¼ pint) milk

25 g (1 oz) fresh breadcrumbs

50 g (2 oz) caster sugar

75 g (3 oz) ground almonds

rose or orange flower water

almond flavouring

2 eggs, plus 2 egg yolks

knob of English butter

150 ml (5 fl oz) fresh whipping cream

25 g (1 oz) flaked almonds, toasted

1. Put a layer of apricot jam into a buttered pie dish. Bring the fresh single cream and milk to boiling point, then pour on to the breadcrumbs in a bowl.
2. Leave to cool, then mix in the sugar, ground almonds and a little rose or orange flower water and almond flavouring.
3. Beat the eggs with the extra yolks and mix into the mixture. Pour into the dish.
4. Dot with the butter and bake in the oven at 150°C (300°F) mark 2 for 30 minutes. Whip the fresh cream until stiff. Serve the pudding hot with fresh cream and toasted flaked almonds.
Serves 4

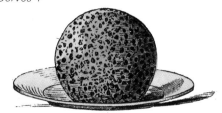

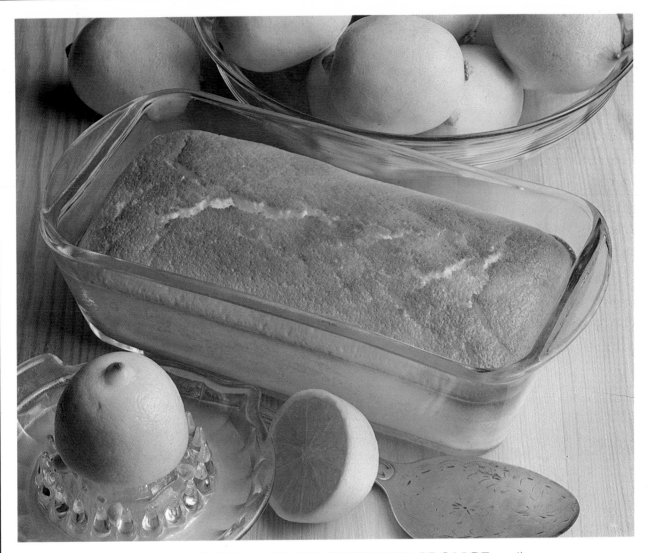

LEMON LAYER PUDDING

grated rind and juice of 1 lemon

50 g (2 oz) English butter

100 g (4 oz) sugar

2 eggs, separated

50 g (2 oz) self-raising flour

300 ml (½ pint) milk

1. Add the lemon rind to the butter and sugar and whisk the mixture until pale and fluffy. Add the egg yolks and flour and beat well. Stir in the milk and 30–45 ml (2–3 tbsp) lemon juice.
2. Whisk the egg whites until stiff, fold in and pour the mixture into a buttered ovenproof dish.
3. Stand in a shallow tin of water and cook in the oven at 200°C (400°F) mark 6 for about 45 minutes, until the top is set and spongy to the touch. This pudding will separate into a custard layer with a sponge topping.

Serves 4

RICH CUSTARD SPONGE

450 ml (¾ pint) milk

4 eggs, beaten

150 ml (5 fl oz) fresh double cream

50 g (2 oz) caster sugar

2.5 ml (½ tsp) vanilla flavouring

100 g (4 oz) trifle sponges

15 ml (1 level tbsp) currants

15 ml (1 level tbsp) sultanas

15 ml (1 level tbsp) raisins

2.5 ml (½ level tsp) grated nutmeg

fresh single cream to serve

1. Heat the milk in a saucepan; just before boiling, pour on to the beaten eggs, fresh double cream, sugar and vanilla flavouring.
2. Dip the sponges into the custard and use to line the sides only of a 1.1-litre (2-pint) ovenproof dish.
3. Place the dried fruit in the bottom of the dish and pour the rest of the custard over.
4. Sprinkle with nutmeg and bake in the oven at 150°C (300°F) mark 2 for about 1 hour until lightly set. Serve warm with the fresh cream.

Serves 6

Above:
LEMON LAYER
PUDDING
This light golden pudding tastes delicately of lemon, and during baking it gradually separates into a custard layer with a tempting sponge topping.
The dish this pudding is baked in should be placed in a shallow tin half-filled with warm water known as a bain-marie. A roasting tin is ideal for the purpose.

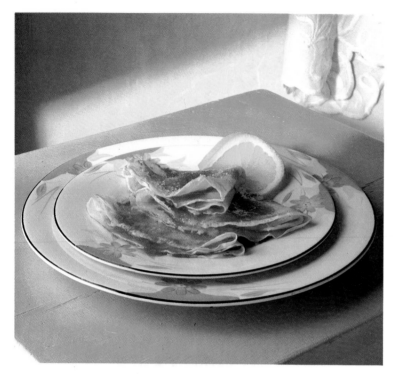

Above:
RUM BUTTER AND
ORANGE PANCAKES
A rich rum butter filling is the
hidden secret of these tempting
pancakes in which fresh orange
juice is used in the batter.

RUM BUTTER AND ORANGE PANCAKES

175 g (6 oz) English butter

175 g (6 oz) brown sugar

15 ml (1 tbsp) rum

225 g (8 oz) flour

2 eggs

450 ml (¾ pint) milk

150 ml (¼ pint) fresh orange juice

demerara sugar

12 orange slices, demerara sugar and fresh single cream to serve

1. Melt the butter and beat in the sugar and rum. Chill until needed.
2. Make pancake batter with the flour, eggs, milk and juice. (Follow the recipe on page 276.)
3. Cook twelve thin pancakes, keeping them warm in a low oven. Put a spoonful of chilled rum butter on to each and fold into triangles.
4. Serve with slices of orange, demerara sugar and the fresh cream.
Makes 12

CHERRY AND ALMOND PANCAKES

425-g (15-oz) can cherry pie filling

225-g (8-oz) can Morello cherries, pitted

15 ml (1 tbsp) kirsch or cherry brandy

8 pancakes (see page 276)

50 g (2 oz) flaked almonds, toasted

150 ml (¼ pint) fresh double cream

1. Heat the pie filling and cherries with the kirsch or cherry brandy.
2. Spread the mixture evenly over four pancakes, place on a large ovenproof plate or dish, cover with the four remaining pancakes and sprinkle the tops with flaked almonds.
3. Cover lightly with foil and bake in the oven at 180°C (350°F) mark 4 for 25–30 minutes. Serve the fresh cream separately.
Serves 4

APRICOT AND GINGER UPSIDE-DOWN PUDDING

60 ml (4 level tbsp) long grain rice

300 ml (½ pint) milk

150 g (5 oz) English butter

30 ml (2 tbsp) golden syrup

75 g (3 oz) demerara sugar

411-g (14½-oz) can apricot halves, drained

125 g (4 oz) soft brown sugar

2 eggs, separated

75 g (3 oz) self-raising flour

15 ml (3 level tsp) ground ginger

fresh single cream to serve

1. Simmer the rice in the milk in a covered pan for about 25 minutes, until tender and the milk is absorbed. Cool.
2. Melt 25 g (1 oz) butter with the syrup and demerara sugar. Spoon into a 18-cm (7-inch) square, base-lined tin. Arrange the apricots on the top.
3. Whisk the remaining butter until soft, gradually beat in the soft brown sugar, egg yolks and cool rice mixture.
4. Gently fold in the flour and ginger sifted together. Whisk the egg whites until stiff then fold into the mixture.
5. Spoon into the tin and bake in the oven at 180°C (350°F) mark 4 for about 55 minutes. Turn out and serve hot with the fresh cream.
Serves 6

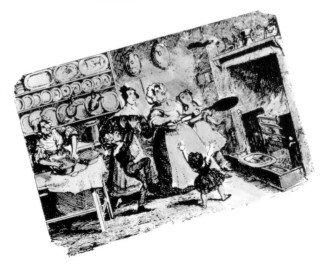

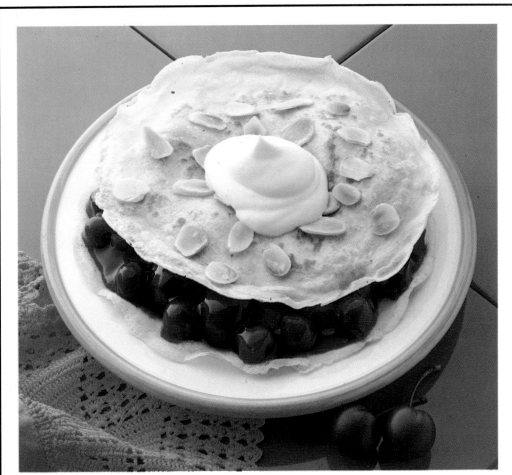

Left:
CHERRY AND ALMOND
PANCAKES
Spiked with cherry brandy or
kirsch, the luscious cherry filling
in these cream-topped pancakes
makes a sensational pudding
which is quick to prepare.

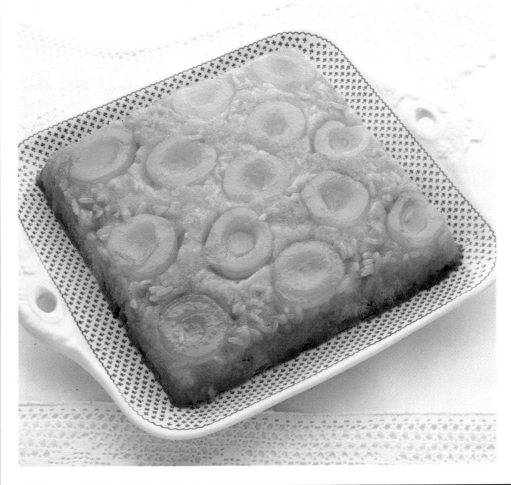

Left:
APRICOT AND GINGER
UPSIDE-DOWN
PUDDING
Topped with delicious apricot
halves, this rich baked dish with
a hint of ginger is a delicious
winter pudding, when served
with cold fresh cream.

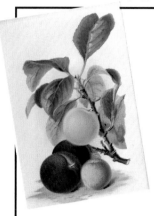

PLUM CRUNCH PUDDING

100 g (4 oz) flour

pinch of salt

1 egg

300 ml (½ pint) milk

50 g (2 oz) English butter

450 g (1 lb) cooking plums, halved and stoned

100 g (4 oz) caster sugar

5 ml (1 tsp) mixed spice

fresh single cream to serve

1. Sift the flour and salt into a bowl. Beat to a smooth batter with the egg and half the milk. Stir in remaining milk.
2. Put the butter into a 25 × 30 cm (10 × 12 inch) baking tin. Heat in the oven at 220°C (425°F) mark 7 for 1 minute.
3. Add the plums to the tin, sprinkle with sugar and spice and pour in batter.
4. Bake in the oven at 220°C (425°F) mark 7 for 30 minutes. Reduce temperature to 200°C (400°F) mark 6 for a further 15–20 minutes. Serve warm with the fresh cream.

Serves 6

MOULDED PINEAPPLE CONDÉ

45 ml (3 level tbsp) pudding rice

568 ml (1 pint) milk

150 g (5 oz) pineapple jam

432-g (15¼-oz) can pineapple pieces, with juice

10 ml (2 level tsp) gelatine

150 ml (5 fl oz) fresh double cream

10 ml (2 level tsp) arrowroot

15 ml (1 tbsp) lemon juice

1. Place the rice and milk in a small, heavy-based pan, simmer gently for about 35 minutes, until the milk is absorbed and rice tender. Stir in 30 g (1 oz) jam, cool.
2. Drain the pineapple, reserving the juices and chop roughly; stir into the rice mixture.
3. Soak the gelatine in 20 ml (4 tsp) water in a small bowl. Dissolve by standing the bowl in a pan of gently simmering water. Stir into the rice.
4. Whip the fresh cream until softly stiff and fold into the rice mixture. Spoon into a buttered 1-litre (1½-pint) fluted flan mould. Chill to set.
5. Mix the arrowroot with a little water to form a smooth paste. Warm the remaining jam with 120 ml (6 tbsp) pineapple juice until evenly blended. Stir in the arrowroot and cook until the mixture has thickened. Stir in the lemon juice and cool.

6. Turn out the rice mould, spoon over some sauce, serve rest separately. Best eaten on day of making.

Serves 6

BREAD AND BUTTER PUDDING

6 thin slices of white bread, crusts removed

50 g (2 oz) English butter

50 g (2 oz) currants or sultanas, or mixture

40 g (1½ oz) caster sugar

2 eggs

568 ml (1 pint) milk

1. Thickly spread bread slices with butter. Cut into fingers or small squares. Put half into a 1-litre (2-pint) buttered ovenproof dish. Sprinkle with all the fruit and half the sugar.
2. Top with the remaining bread, buttered side uppermost. Sprinkle with the rest of the sugar.
3. Beat the eggs and milk well together. Strain into dish over bread.
4. Leave to stand for 30 minutes, so that the bread absorbs some of the liquid. Bake in the oven at 170°C (325°F) mark 3 for 45 minutes–1 hour, until set and the top is crisp and golden.

Variation
Osbourne pudding
Use brown bread and butter, spread with marmalade. Omit the dried fruit.

Serves 4

APPLE FRITTERS

100 g (4 oz) flour

1.25 ml (¼ level tsp) salt

1 egg

15 g (½ oz) English butter, melted

150 ml (¼ pint) milk

3 cooking apples, peeled and cored

icing sugar

fresh single cream to serve

1. Sift the flour and salt into a bowl. Beat to a smooth batter with the egg, butter and milk.
2. Cut the apples into ½-cm (¼-inch) thick rings. Coat with batter. Fry in deep hot oil for 2–3 minutes, until golden.
3. Remove from pan. Drain on absorbent kitchen paper. Dredge with icing sugar. Serve with the fresh cream.

Serves 4

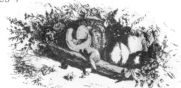

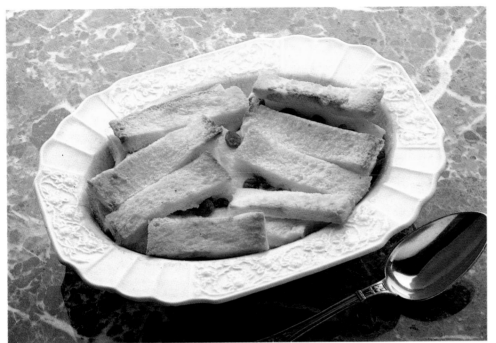

Left:
BREAD AND BUTTER
PUDDING
When properly made, using
thin slices of whole bread
lavishly spread with pure
English butter, this simple old-
fashioned pudding is a family
treat on a cold winter's day.

GOOSEBERRY PUDDING

175 g (7 oz) English butter
75 g (3 oz) soft brown sugar
25 g (1 oz) chopped nuts
350 g (12 oz) gooseberries, topped and tailed
100 g (4 oz) self-raising flour
1.25 ml (¼ level tsp) salt
100 g (4 oz) caster sugar
2 eggs, beaten

1. Melt 75 g (3 oz) butter in a pan, add the brown sugar, stir well, add the nuts.
2. Butter a deep ovenproof dish and pour in the mixture. Place the gooseberries in a layer on top.
3. Sieve the flour and the salt. Whisk the remaining 100 g (4 oz) butter with the caster sugar, add the eggs and flour gradually, stirring well.
4. Pour over the fruit and bake in the oven at 180°C (350°F) mark 4 for 35 minutes. When cooked, turn out on to a dish so that the gooseberries are on top.

Serves 4

APPLE FLAPJACK

900 g (2 lb) cooking apples, peeled, cored and sliced
65 g (2½ oz) sugar
150 g (5 oz) English butter
60 ml (4 level tbsp) golden syrup
225 g (8 oz) rolled oats
1.25 ml (¼ level tsp) salt
5 ml (1 level tsp) ground ginger
icing sugar and poached apple rings to decorate

1. Simmer the apples gently in a covered pan with 40 g (1½ oz) sugar, but no liquid, until pulpy. Cool slightly.
2. Butter and base-line an 18-cm (7-inch) round loose bottomed cake tin.
3. Heat the remaining sugar with the butter and syrup, until dissolved. Stir in the oats, salt and ginger.
4. Before it cools, line the base and sides with three-quarters of the flapjack mixture (up to 2.5 cm (1 inch) from rim).
5. Pour the apple pulp into the centre, cover with the remaining mixture pressing it down lightly.
6. Bake in the oven at 190°C (375°F) mark 5 for 35 minutes. Cool for 10 minutes before loosening edges and turning out. Serve warm, or well chilled, dredged with icing sugar and decorated with apple rings.

Serves 6 *(illustration on page 204)*

Below:
Sweet, crunchy apples are
among our most popular and
versatile fruits. They are
delicious when cooked with a
sprinkling of cinnamon or cloves
in hot pies and puddings; they
are good in sharp-tasting sauces
and stuffings for rich meats like
pork and, of course, they are
crushed and fermented to make
lusty English cider. Remember
too, that for a meal in a hurry,
a crisp shiny apple is a delicious
accompaniment to fine English
cheese.

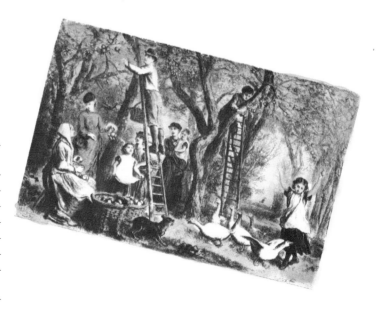

SWEET PASTRY PUDDINGS

SHORTCRUST PASTRY

225 g (8 oz) flour

pinch of salt

50 g (2 oz) English butter, cut into small pieces

50 g (2 oz) lard, cut into small pieces

1. Mix flour and salt together in a bowl.
2. Rub the butter and lard lightly into the flour between finger and thumb tips until the mixture resembles fine breadcrumbs.
3. Add 30–45 ml (2–3 tbsp) chilled water, sprinkling it evenly over the surface. Stir it in with a round-bladed knife until the mixture begins to stick together in large lumps.
4. Collect the dough mixture together to form a ball. Knead lightly for a few seconds to give a firm smooth dough. Do not over-handle the dough. The pastry can be used straight away, but it is better if allowed to 'rest' for about 30 minutes wrapped in foil or cling film in the refrigerator.
5. Roll out on a lightly floured work surface and use as required.

Quantity: For shortcrust pastry, the proportion of butter and lard to flour is half the quantity. Therefore, for a recipe using 100 g (4 oz) shortcrust pastry, use 100 g (4 oz) flour and 50 g (2 oz) butter and lard. Allow 5–7.5 ml (1-1½ tsp) water per 25 g (1 oz) flour.

SHORTCRUST PASTRY MADE IN A FOOD PROCESSOR

A food processor will make shortcrust pastry very quickly and gives good results. It is most important not to over-process the mixture as a food processor works in seconds not minutes. For even 'rubbing in', process by operating in short bursts rather than letting the machine run continuously. Make sure you know the capacity of your food processor and never overload the processor bowl. If making a large quantity of pastry, make it in two batches.

Mix the flour and salt together in the bowl of the food processor. Add the butter and lard to the flour. Fix the food processor lid and mix for a few seconds until the mixture resembles fine breadcrumbs. Add about 30 ml (2 tbsp) water and switch on until the mixture forms a smooth dough. Roll out as for shortcrust pastry.

SHORTCRUST PASTRY MADE IN A MIXER

A mixer will make excellent shortcrust pastry in a very short time. It is important to remember, however, that the machine works quickly and efficiently, so never let it over-mix as the resulting pastry will be disappointing. As the hands do not touch the pastry, it remains cool, thus improving the end result.

Place the flour and salt in the mixer bowl. Add the butter and lard to the flour. Switch on to minimum speed until the ingredients are incorporated. Gradually increase the mixer speed as the butter and lard breaks up until the mixture resembles fine breadcrumbs. Switch off the mixer and quickly sprinkle 45 ml (3 tbsp) water on top of the mixture. Incorporate this on medium speed and switch off the machine as soon as the mixture forms a compact dough. Roll out as for shortcrust pastry.

RICH SHORTCRUST PASTRY

225 g (8 oz) flour

pinch of salt

125 g (4 oz) English butter, cut into small pieces

45–60 ml (3–4 tbsp) cold milk

1. Mix the flour and salt together in a bowl.
2. Rub the butter into the flour until the mixture resembles fine breadcrumbs.
3. Sprinkle the milk over the crumbs. Mix with a round-bladed knife until the mixture begins to stick together.
4. Collect together to form a ball. Knead lightly until smooth.
5. Do not use immediately, leave covered in the refrigerator for at least 30 minutes.
6. Roll out on a lightly floured work surface and use as required.

PÂTE BRISÉE

This is a very rich shortcrust pastry suitable for quiches and tarts. It is light and crisp, and should be handled as lightly as possible. The proportion of fat to flour is very high, and the pastry is consequently rather fragile.

175 g (6 oz) flour

pinch of salt

pinch of icing sugar

125 g (4 oz) English butter, cut into small pieces

1. Sift the flour on to a work surface together with the salt and icing sugar. Cut the butter into the flour with a palette knife then rub in with the fingertips until the mixture resembles fine breadcrumbs.
2. Sprinkle with a little chilled water, then gather together into a ball.
3. Sprinkle a little flour on to the work surface and, using the heel of your hand, quickly spread the dough away from you on to the floured board. This will ensure that

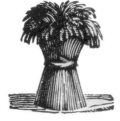

the butter is evenly distributed. This whole operation should be done as quickly and lightly as possible. Gather up into a ball again and leave in the refrigerator to rest for at least 1 hour.

4. Leave the dough at room temperature for a little while before rolling out, so that it becomes malleable again. If it is very hard at first, hit it with a rolling pin, but do not knead again.

CINNAMON AND RAISIN FLANS

125 g (4 oz) English butter, cut into small pieces

225 g (8 oz) wholemeal flour

175 g (6 oz) caster sugar

about 90 ml (6 tbsp) milk to bind

2 eggs

25 g (1 oz) plain flour

1.25 ml ($\frac{1}{4}$ level tsp) ground cinnamon

142 g (5 oz) natural yogurt

50 g (2 oz) seedless or muscatel raisins

1. Rub the butter into the wholemeal flour, stir in 50 g (2 oz) sugar and add enough cold milk to form a dough.

2. Roll out the pastry and use to line six 10-cm (4-inch) flan dishes or tins. Bake blind in the oven at 200°C (400°F) mark 6 for about 15 minutes until set.

3. Whisk together the eggs and remaining sugar until really thick and fluffy.

4. Sift together the flour and cinnamon, fold into egg mixture with the yogurt. Pour into

pastry shells, and return to the oven at 180°C (350°F) mark 4 for 10 minutes.

5. Remove dishes from the oven and sprinkle the raisins over the top of each one. Return the flans to the oven for 15–20 minutes until browned. Serve warm or cold on day of making.

Serves 6   (illustration on page 204)

ALMOND CUSTARD TARTS

125 g (4 oz) English butter, cut into small pieces

225 g (8 oz) flour

200 ml (7 fl oz) milk, plus about 45 ml (3 tbsp) to bind

2 eggs

50 g (2 oz) caster sugar

1.25 ml ($\frac{1}{4}$ tsp) ratafia flavouring

flaked almonds, toasted

1. Rub the butter into the flour. Bind to a firm dough with about 45 ml (3 tbsp) milk.

2. Butter ten 7.5-cm (3-inch) fluted brioche tins and place on a baking sheet. Roll out the pastry thinly and use to line the tins. Chill for 20 minutes. Bake blind in the oven at 200°C (400°F) mark 6 for 15 minutes.

3. Whisk together the milk, eggs, caster sugar and ratafia flavourng. Pour into the pastry cases. Scatter toasted almonds on top. Reduce oven to 180°C (350°F) mark 4 and bake for a further 15–20 minutes until just set. Leave to cool before serving.

Makes 10

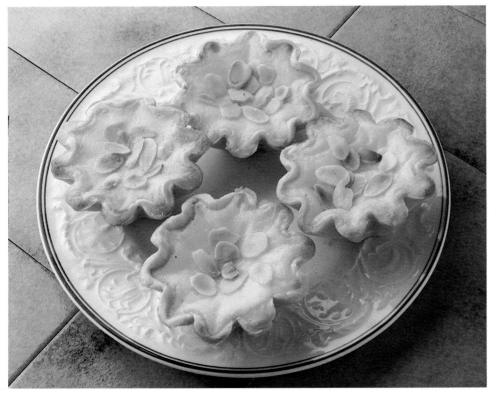

Left:
ALMOND CUSTARD TARTS
These melt-in-the-mouth tarts, richly scented with the taste of almonds, are a delicious pudding when served with a cold, fresh cream, or they are equally good for tea.

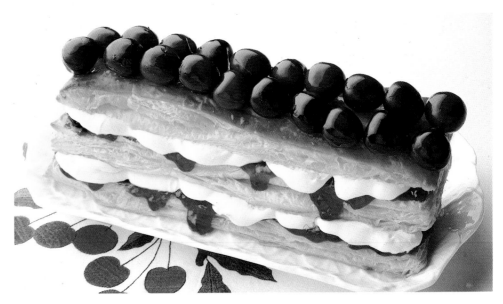

CHERRY MILLE-FEUILLES

212-g (7-oz) packet frozen puff pastry,
thawed

100 g (4 oz) black cherry jam

150 ml (5 fl oz) fresh double cream

175 g (6 oz) red cherries

1. Roll out the pastry to a 23-cm (10-inch) square, trim edge and cut into three strips. Place on baking sheets, prick well all over.
2. Bake in the oven at 220°C (425°F) mark 7 for about 12 minutes, until well browned; turn the pastry strips over and return to the oven for a few minutes to dry out. Cool on a wire rack.
3. Spread half the jam over two of the pastry slices. Whip the fresh cream until softly stiff. Spread a layer of fresh cream over the jam. Place the pastry slices on top of each other and cover with the plain pastry slice.
4. Warm the remaining jam and brush a thin covering over the top of the mille-feuilles.
5. Halve and stone the cherries and arrange over the jam, glaze with remaining jam.
6. Chill for at least 2 hours before slicing and serving in wedges.
Serves 4

CITRUS APPLE FLAN

175 g (6 oz) flour

pinch of salt

175 g (6 oz) English butter

75 g (3 oz) caster sugar

3 egg yolks

3 medium thin-skinned oranges

900 g (2 lb) cooking apples, peeled, cored
and roughly chopped

45 ml (3 level tbsp) granulated sugar

60 ml (4 tbsp) thick-cut orange marmalade

fresh whipping or single cream to serve

1. Sift the flour and salt on to a work surface. Make a well in the centre and place in it 125 g (4 oz) softened butter, caster sugar and egg yolks. Work the ingredients together with the fingertips of one hand until smooth. Gradually draw in the flour, with the help of a palette knife; knead lightly until smooth.
2. Chill, covered, for 30 minutes, then roll out and use to line a 20.5-cm (8-inch) flan ring. Bake blind in the oven at 200°C (400°F) mark 6 for 10–15 minutes. Leave to cool.
3. Add grated orange rind to apples in pan with remaining butter, sugar and half the marmalade. Cover and cook gently for about 15 minutes, until fruit is soft. Open-boil to a thick pulp, stirring frequently. Cool.
4. Remove remaining rind and pith from the oranges and thinly slice the flesh. Fill the flan case with the apple purée. Arrange the orange slices on top.
5. Heat the remaining marmalade with 15 ml (1 tbsp) water and sieve. Brush over the orange slices. Serve cold with the fresh cream.
Serves 6

APRICOT BORDELAISE FLAN

175 g (6 oz) shortcrust pastry (see page 230)

2 egg yolks

50 g (2 oz) caster sugar

25 g (1 oz) flour

300 ml (½ pint) milk

kirsch or almond flavouring

25 g (1 oz) English butter

15 ml (1 level tbsp) crushed macaroons

225 g (8 oz) canned apricots, drained

25 g (1 oz) flaked almonds

icing sugar

1. Roll out the pastry and use to line a 20-cm (8-inch) flan dish or ring placed on a baking sheet. Bake blind in the oven at 200°C (400°F) mark 6 for 10–15 minutes

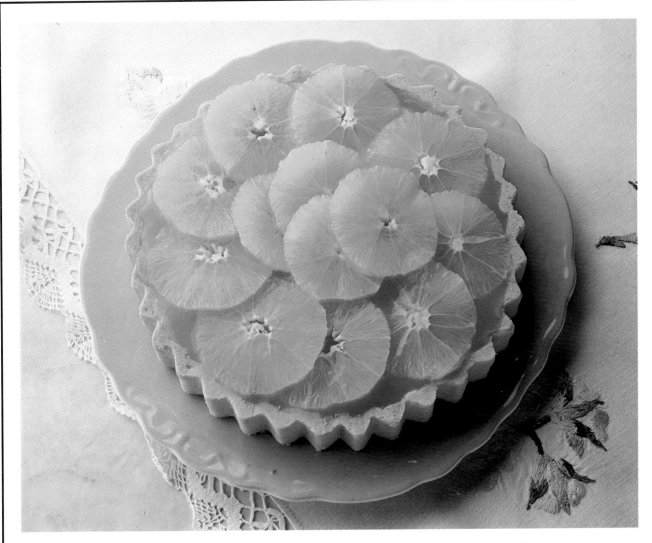

until set. Remove the baking beans, return to the oven and bake for a further 15 minutes until firm and golden brown.

2. Whisk the egg yolks and caster sugar until light in colour; whisk in the flour and milk. Pour into a saucepan and bring to the boil stirring continuously. Flavour with kirsch or almond flavouring. Stir in the butter and macaroons.

3. Place a layer of the egg yolk mixture in the flan case, cover with apricots, then top with another layer of mixture.

4. Sprinkle with flaked almonds, then cover thickly with icing sugar and brown under a hot grill.

Serves 4

WELSH AMBER PUDDING

2 eggs, plus 2 egg yolks
75 g (3 oz) sugar
grated rind of $\frac{1}{2}$ lemon
30 ml (2 level tbsp) fine-cut marmalade
100 g (4 oz) English butter, melted
175 g (6 oz) shortcrust pastry (see page 230)

1. Beat together the eggs, egg yolks, sugar, grated lemon rind and marmalade. Whisk in the melted butter.

2. Roll out the pastry and use to line a 15-cm (7-inch) tart tin. Bake blind in the oven at 200°C (400°F) mark 6 for 10–15 minutes until set.

3. Pour in the egg mixture and bake at 190°C (375°F) mark 5 for a further 20 minutes.

Serves 6

Above:
CITRUS APPLE FLAN
A zesty swirl of carefully sliced orange rings is the finishing touch to this mouthwatering flan which combines apples and oranges in a crunchy sweet-pastry case.

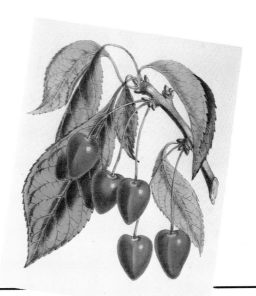

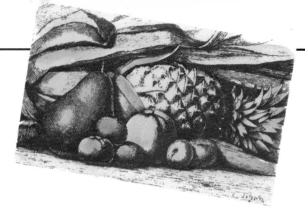

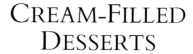

CREAM-FILLED DESSERTS

CHOUX CREAM PUFFS

175 g (6 oz) English butter, cut into pieces

200 g (7½ oz) flour

6 eggs, beaten

900 ml (1½ pints) fresh whipping cream

icing sugar

450 g (1 lb) plain chocolate

75 g (3 oz) caster sugar

1. Place the butter in a medium saucepan with 400 ml (¾ pint) water. Heat gently until the butter melts then bring to a fast boil.
2. Immediately remove from the heat and beat in the sifted flour until the mixture leaves the sides of the pan. Allow to cool.
3. Gradually beat in the eggs, keeping the mixture stiff.
4. Using a piping bag and plain nozzle, pipe into forty rings on dampened baking sheets; allow room to spread.
5. Bake in the oven at 200°C (400°F) mark 6 for about 30 minutes until well risen and crisp. Split open and cool on wire racks.
6. Whip the fresh cream until stiff. Fill the buns with the fresh cream and dust with icing sugar. Chill for 1 hour.
7. Put broken chocolate in a saucepan and warm gently with the caster sugar and 600 ml (1 pint) water until dissolved. Simmer gently in an open pan until the sauce reduces and thickens slightly. Serve in a sauce boat or jug.

Serves 20 buffet portions

Opposite, top:
PAVLOVA
This classic light-as-air meringue, topped with fresh whipped cream and decorated with the fruit of your choice, was named in honour of Anna Pavlova, the ballerina.

Opposite, bottom:
CHOUX CREAM PUFFS
These mouthwatering pastries are split open, filled with fresh whipped cream and served with a warm, luscious chocolate sauce.

Below:
APPLE AND BLACKBERRY TART
Apples and blackberries are two delicious fruits which are traditionally cooked together in old-fashioned tarts and pies. Topped with a delicious creamy swirl, this lovely pudding, with a hint of cinnamon, makes a mouthwatering end to a late summer or early autumn meal.

APPLE AND BLACKBERRY TART

100 g (4 oz) shortcrust pastry (see page 230)

450 g (1 lb) cooking apples, peeled, cored and sliced

50 g (2 oz) English butter

1 egg, separated

50 g (2 oz) brown sugar

25 g (1 oz) sultanas

225 g (8 oz) blackberries, or 200-g (7-oz) can blackberries, drained

2.5 ml (½ level tsp) ground cinnamon

150 ml (5 fl oz) fresh double cream

1. Roll out the pastry and use to line a 20.5-cm (8-inch) flan ring. Arrange the apples in the flan case.
2. Melt the butter, remove from heat and cool. Beat in the egg yolk and add the sugar, sultanas, blackberries, cinnamon and butter. Mix well together and place in the flan case.
3. Bake in the oven at 200°C (400°F) mark 6 for 30–35 minutes. Allow to cool.
4. Whip the fresh cream until softly stiff. Whip the egg white until stiff and fold into the fresh cream. Pile on top of tart and serve.

Serves 6

PAVLOVA

3 egg whites

a pinch of salt

250 g (9 oz) caster sugar

5 ml (1 tsp) vanilla flavouring

5 ml (1 tsp) vinegar

300 ml (10 fl oz) fresh double cream, fresh strawberries, raspberries, kiwi fruit or canned passion fruit, drained to decorate

1. Draw a 23-cm (9-inch) circle on non-stick paper and place on a baking sheet.
2. Whisk the egg whites with the salt until very stiff, then gradually whisk in the sugar. Beat until it forms stiff peaks again. Fold in the vanilla flavouring and vinegar.
3. Spread the meringue mixture over the circle and bake in the oven at 140°C (275°F) mark 1 for about 1 hour until firm.
4. Leave to cool. Then carefully remove the paper and place the Pavlova on a plate. Whip the fresh cream until stiff then pile on to the meringue and decorate with the fruit.

Serves 4

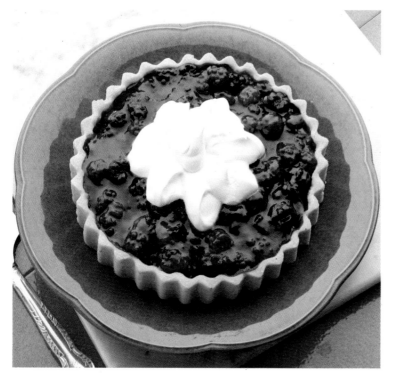

PEACH AND HAZELNUT GÂTEAU

3 eggs
175 g (6 oz) caster sugar
finely grated rind and juice of 1 lemon
75 g (3 oz) flour
75 g (3 oz) ground hazelnuts, toasted
700 g (1½ lb) medium peaches
300 ml (5 fl oz) fresh whipping cream

1. Butter and base-line a 23-cm (9-inch) round cake tin, Dust with sugar and flour.
2. Place the eggs, 125 g (4 oz) sugar and lemon rind in a large deep bowl. Whisk vigorously until very thick and light.
3. Fold the sifted flour lightly through the mixture with 50 g (2 oz) hazelnuts; spoon into prepared tin.
4. Bake in the oven at 180°C (350°F) mark 4 for about 35 minutes, until firm to the touch. Turn out and cool on a wire rack.
5. Make a sugar syrup from the remaining sugar, 300 ml (½ pint) water and 30 ml (2 tbsp) lemon juice. Reserve two peaches, poach remaining skinned, sliced peaches until tender, drain.
6. Whip the fresh cream until softly stiff. Split the gâteau into three, layer with the fresh whipped cream and peaches; chill. To serve, decorate with peaches and nuts.
Serves 8

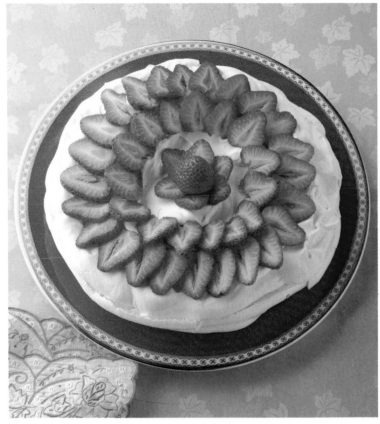

MOCHA ROULADE

15 ml (3 level tsp) instant coffee powder
100 g (4 oz) plain chocolate
4 eggs, size 2, separated
100 g (4 oz) caster sugar
300 ml (10 fl oz) fresh double cream, whipped
175 g (6 oz) white grapes, halved and seeded

1. In a small bowl, blend the coffee to a smooth paste with 15 ml (1 tbsp) water. Break up the chocolate, put into the bowl and melt over a pan of hot water. Cool.
2. Cut a 30.5-cm (12-inch) square of non-stick paper, fold up 2.5 cm (1 inch) all round. Snip into corners, secure edges with paperclips to form a free-standing paper case. Place on a baking sheet.
3. Whisk the yolks and sugar until thick then stir in the cool coffee chocolate. Whisk the egg whites until stiff and fold into the mixture. Spread into the paper case.
4. Bake in the oven at 180°C (350°F) mark 4 for about 15 minutes, until firm.
5. Turn the roulade out on sugared greaseproof. Place another sheet of greaseproof on top and roll up. Leave to cool.
6. When cold unroll and remove paper. Spread the roulade with cream and grapes (reserve some for decoration).
7. Roll up using the sugared paper. Decorate with piped cream and grapes.
Serves 6–8   (illustration on page 222)

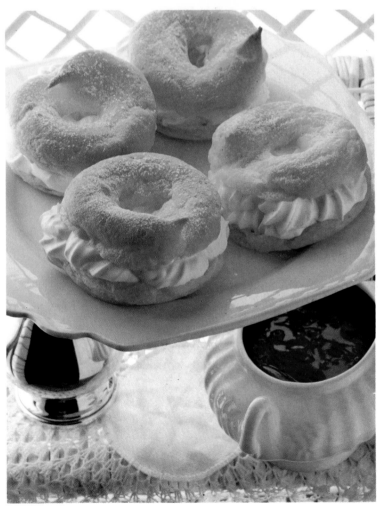

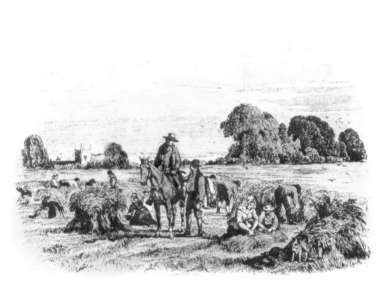

heat and stir in the flour and ginger sifted together.
2. Finely grate the rind of half the lemon into the pan, stir into the mixture with the brandy.
3. Place twelve 15 ml (table-spoonfuls) on to baking sheets lined with non-stick paper, allowing them plenty of room to spread.
4. Bake in the oven at 180°C (350°F) mark 4 for 8–10 minutes, until golden. Cool slightly then slide off the paper on to cooling racks.
5. Whip the fresh cream until stiff and use to sandwich together three ginger crisps along with sliced strawberries. Reserve four whole strawberries for decoration. Repeat twice.
6. Chill the ginger crisps for at least 1 hour and decorate just before serving.
Serves 4

CHOCOLATE CHIP MERINGUES

125 g (4 oz) plain chocolate cake covering

4 egg whites

225 g (8 oz) caster sugar

300 ml ($\frac{1}{2}$ pint) fresh double or whipping cream

1. Finely grate the chocolate through a mouli grater.
2. Whisk the egg whites until stiff but not dry in appearance. Whisk in 20 ml (4 level tsp) caster sugar, keeping the mixture stiff. Fold in the remaining sugar with the grated chocolate.
3. Spoon out into twelve meringues on to a non-stick paper-lined baking sheet, allowing them room to spread.
4. Bake in the oven at 130°C (250°F) mark $\frac{1}{2}$ for about 1$\frac{1}{2}$ hours, until dry. Peel off the paper and cool on a wire rack. Store if wished in an airtight container.
5. To serve, whip the fresh cream until softly stiff and use to sandwich together the meringues.
Serves 6   (illustration on page 222)

STRAWBERRY GINGER CRISPS

50 g (2 oz) golden syrup

50 g (2 oz) caster sugar

50 g (2 oz) English butter

50 g (2 oz) flour

2.5 ml ($\frac{1}{2}$ level tsp) ground ginger

1 lemon

5 ml (1 tsp) brandy

300 ml (10 fl oz) fresh whipping cream

225 g (8 oz) strawberries, hulled

1. Warm the syrup, sugar and butter together in a pan until dissolved. Remove from the

RED CURRANT GRIESTORTE

3 eggs, size 2, separated

125 g (4 oz) caster sugar

grated rind and juice of $\frac{1}{2}$ lemon

50 g (2 oz) fine semolina

15 ml (1 level tbsp) ground almonds

175 ml (6 fl oz) fresh double cream

15 ml (1 tbsp) milk

125 g (4 oz) red currants

icing sugar

1. Butter and line a 20.5 × 30.5 cm (8 × 12 inch) swiss-roll tin with non-stick paper to extend above the sides. Butter the paper, sprinkle with caster sugar and a dusting of flour.
2. Whisk the egg yolks with the sugar until thick and pale. Whisk in the lemon juice. Stir in the rind, semolina and almonds mixed together. Whisk the egg whites until stiff; fold the egg yolk mixture through the whites.
3. Turn into the tin, level surface and bake in the oven at 180°C (350°F) mark 4 for about 30 minutes, until puffed and pale gold.
4. Turn carefully on to a sheet of non-stick

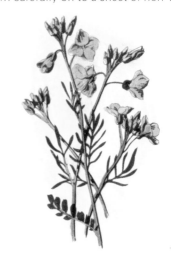

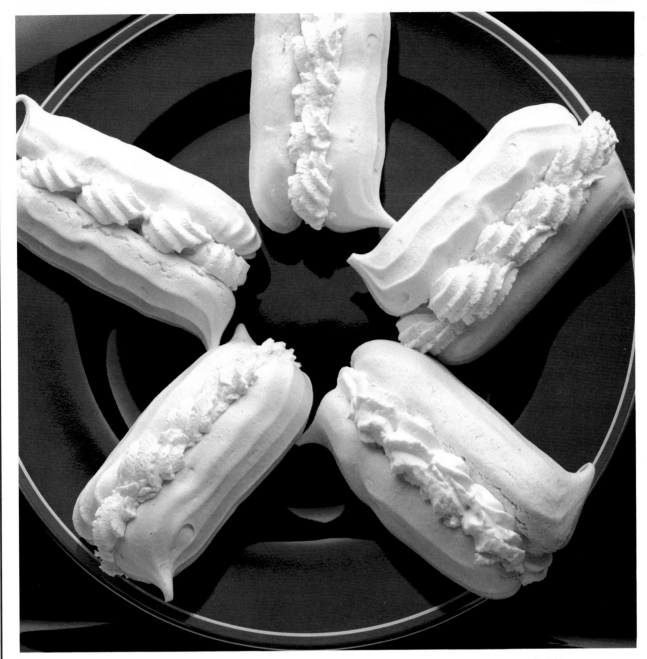

paper dusted with caster sugar. Trim long edges, roll up loosely with paper inside. Cool on a wire rack.

5. To finish, whisk together the fresh cream and milk until softly stiff. Unroll the Griestorte – don't worry if it cracks a little – spread over the fresh cream, but not quite to the edges, sprinkle with red currants reserving a few on the stem for decoration. Roll up, pressing lightly into shape. Dust with icing sugar and decorate with the reserved red currants. Eat the same day.

Serves 6   (illustration on page 206)

CREAM MERINGUES

2 egg whites
125 g (4 oz) caster sugar
150 ml (5 fl oz) fresh double cream

1. Line two baking sheets with non-stick baking paper.

2. Whisk the egg whites until stiff. Add the caster sugar a tablespoon at a time, whisking well for about 1 minute after each addition.

3. Pipe or spoon 10–12 rounds or oblongs of the meringue on to the non-stick paper. Bake in the oven at 110°C (225°F) mark $\frac{1}{4}$ for about 2–3 hours, changing the position of the trays half way through the cooking. Cool on a wire rack.

4. Whip the fresh cream until stiff and use to sandwich together the meringue shells.

Serves 5–6

Above:
CREAM MERINGUES
The secret of these delicious melt-in-the-mouth meringues, sandwiched lavishly with fresh cream, is to let them 'dry out' rather than bake, in a very slow oven.

Historians of cookery say that meringues were invented in 1720 by a Swiss pastry-cook called Gasparini. They have been a popular sweet for royalty for centuries and legend has it that Marie-Antoinette, the doomed Queen of France, used to make them herself.

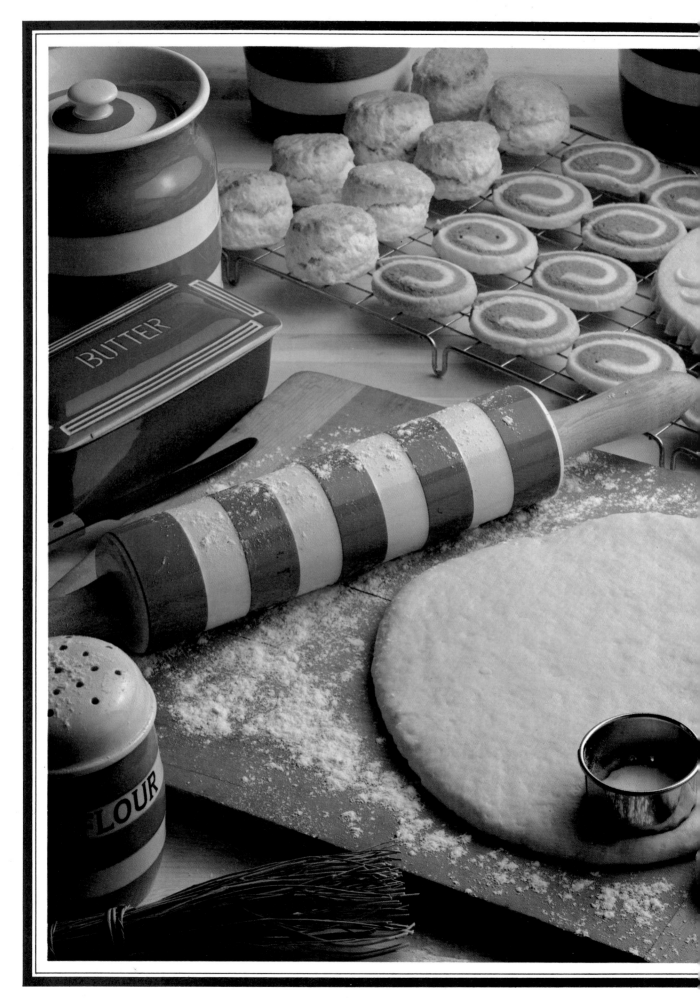

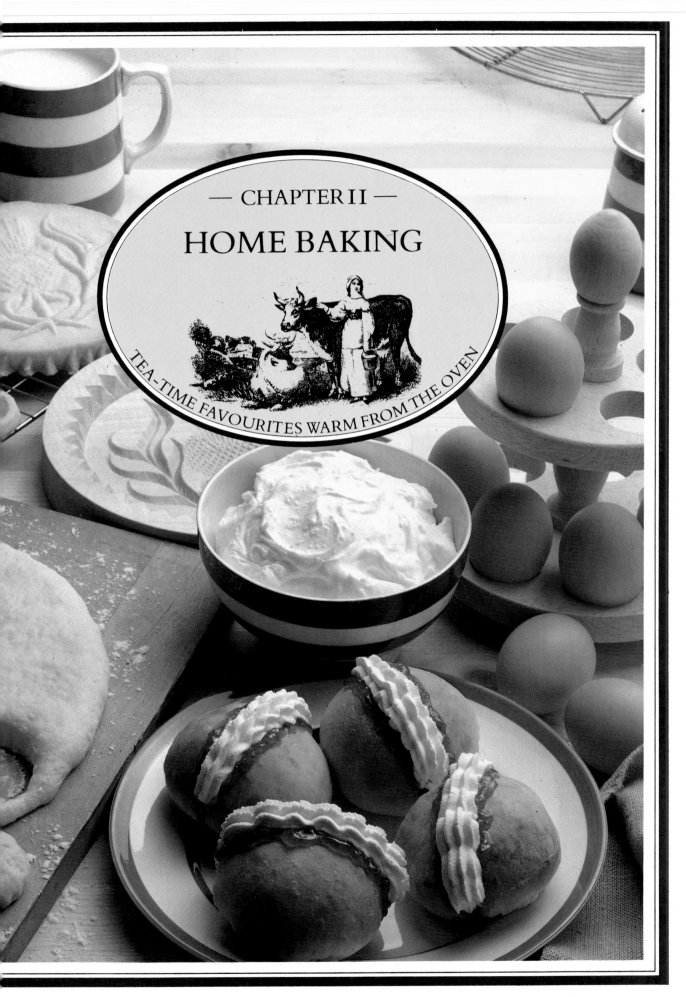

— CHAPTER II —

HOME BAKING

TEA-TIME FAVOURITES WARM FROM THE OVEN

ome baking isn't a thing of the past. Far from it. Our traditional teatime favourites with regional and local specialities: the fancy teabreads, fat scones, plain and fruited, gingerbread, parkin, sponges inches high and miraculously risen, the layer cakes, Dundee cakes, rich fruit loaves, the beautifully iced and decorated special occasion cakes, the rock buns, jam tarts, brandysnaps, Shrewsbury biscuits. They're all a part of our history and heritage – English home baking at its best.

Afternoon tea, between 4 and 5, was always an elegant affair with beautiful china, silver tea service, pretty linen – and food to match: light feathery sponges, tiny cakes, dainty biscuits, all rich, exquisite and delightful to look at.

High tea was and is something else, a far more substantial and homely meal with sturdy, farmhouse tradition behind it. It's eaten later in the evening, around 5 or 6 and is always a grand spread, with bread, cheese, a hot or cold savoury, plate tarts, scones, homemade jam and good English butter, spice loaf, cut-and-come-again cake, all set out together. You are expected to do justice to it and to be ready for a bit of supper at bedtime into the bargain.

High tea, fed by all the wonderful regional recipes of the country that go back through generations of loving and inspired farmhouse baking and relying on butter, fresh cream, milk and eggs from the farmhouse dairy – this is something uniquely English.

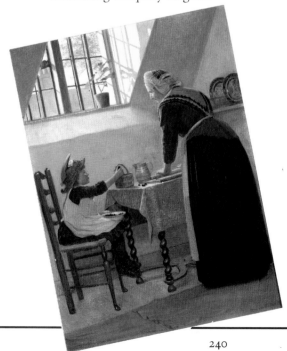

TRADITIONAL FAVOURITES

ORANGE AND RAISIN DROP SCONES

225 g (8 oz) self-raising flour
1.25 ml ($\frac{1}{4}$ level tsp) salt
60 ml (4 level tbsp) caster sugar
2.5 ml ($\frac{1}{2}$ level tsp) baking powder
finely grated rind and juice of 1 orange
2 eggs
300 ml ($\frac{1}{2}$ pint) milk
15 g ($\frac{1}{2}$ oz) English butter, melted
75 g (3 oz) raisins

1. Sift together the flour, salt, sugar and baking powder into a bowl. Add the grated orange rind.
2. Gradually beat in the eggs, milk and melted butter. Sir in 30 ml (2 tbsp) orange juice and the raisins.
3. Lightly butter and heat a large griddle iron, or heavy frying pan. Drop small rounds of scone mixture from a tablespoon into pan.
4. Cook over a moderate heat until bubbles show on the scone surface. Carefully turn over with a knife and cook for a further 2 minutes. Repeat until all the mixture is used up. Keep scones warm in a folded tea-towel. Serve warm or cold with butter, on day of making.
Makes about 24

DEVONSHIRE SPLITS

450 g (1 lb) flour
2.5 ml ($\frac{1}{2}$ level tsp) salt
15 g ($\frac{1}{2}$ oz) fresh yeast, or 7.5 g ($\frac{1}{4}$ oz) dried yeast
150 ml ($\frac{1}{4}$ pint) tepid milk
5 ml (1 level tsp) caster sugar
25 g (1 oz) butter
strawberry or raspberry jam and 150 ml (5 fl oz) fresh double cream to serve

1. Sieve the flour and salt into a bowl.
2. Blend the fresh yeast with a little of the milk and the sugar. If using dried yeast, spinkle it into a little of the milk and the sugar and leave in a warm place for 15 minutes until frothy.
3. Melt the butter in the remaining milk and 150 ml ($\frac{1}{4}$ pint) of lukewarm water.
4. Make a well in the centre of the flour and add the dissolved yeast and the melted butter mixture. Mix to a dough. Leave to prove in a warm place for 1 hour.
5. Divide mixture into 12 pieces and knead each into a ball. Flatten into a round 1-cm ($\frac{1}{2}$-inch) thick. Place on a buttered and floured baking sheet and leave to prove for 20 minutes in a warm place.

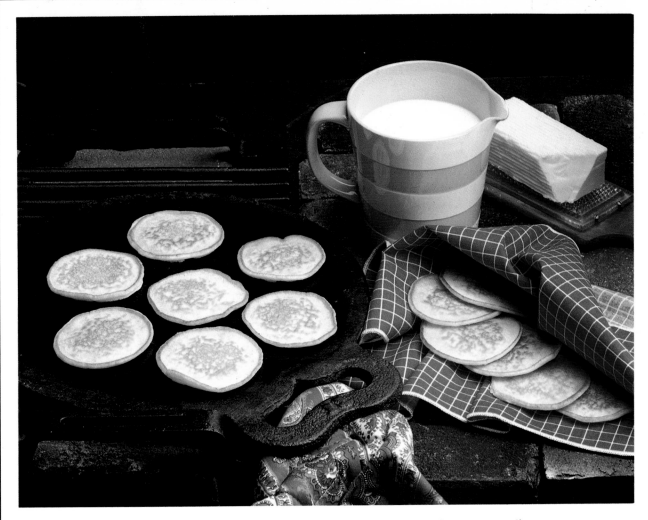

6. Brush with milk and bake in the oven at 230°C (450°F) mark 8 for 15 minutes. Cut through and spread with jam. Whip the fresh cream until stiff and pipe inside the splits. Serve warm.

Serves 12

YOGURT SCONES

5 ml (1 level tsp) baking powder

1.25 ml ($\frac{1}{4}$ level tsp) bicarbonate of soda

450 g (1 lb) flour

10 ml (2 level tsp) salt

15 ml (1 level tbsp) sugar

300 g (10 oz) natural yogurt

1. Sift the baking powder, bicarbonate of soda, flour, salt and sugar into a bowl.
2. Stir in the natural yogurt and about 150 ml ($\frac{1}{4}$ pint) water and bind to a smooth, soft but manageable dough. Knead dough lightly.
3. Shape into a 15-cm (6-inch) round. Make two or three slashes across the top. Place on a buttered baking sheet and bake in the oven at 190°C (375°F) mark 5 for about 40 minutes until the base sounds hollow when tapped. Cut into wedges for serving.

Serves 8

DROP SCONES

225 g (8 oz) self-raising flour

2.5 ml ($\frac{1}{2}$ level tsp) salt

15 ml (1 level tbsp) caster sugar

1 egg

300 ml ($\frac{1}{2}$ pint) milk

25–50 g (1–2 oz) English butter, melted

1. Sift flour and salt into bowl. Add sugar then mix to a smooth batter with the egg and half the milk. Stir in the remaining milk.
2. Lightly brush a large griddle iron, or heavy frying pan with melted butter and heat. Drop small rounds of scone mixture (about twelve in all), from a tablespoon, into pan. Cook over a moderate heat until bubbles show on the scone surface. Carefully turn over with knife and cook for further 2 minutes. Repeat until all the mixture is used up. Keep scones warm in a folded tea-towel.
3. Serve immediately with butter and jam, golden syrup or honey.

Makes about 24

Above:
DROP SCONES
These warm tea-time treats get their name from the fact that spoonfuls of the mixture are dropped on to a hot, lightly greased griddle or heavy frying pan to let them cook.

A griddle (or girdle) is a traditional way of cooking a wide variety of simple scones and bread in Scotland, the North of England and Ulster.

Opposite:
CHERRY SCONES
A scrumptious tea-time treat. Glacé cherries and crunchy wheatgerm are mixed into the scone mixture which is then cut into crescent shapes.

WELSH CAKES

225 g (8 oz) flour

2.5 ml (½ level tsp) baking powder

pinch of salt

75 g (3 oz) English butter

75 g (3 oz) sugar

50 g (2 oz) currants or sultanas

2.5 ml (½ level tsp) mixed spice (optional)

1 egg, beaten

milk to mix

1. Sieve the flour, baking powder and salt together into a bowl.
2. Rub in the butter and the remaining dry ingredients.
3. Stir in the egg, then add enough milk to make a firm dough.
4. Roll out the dough to 1–2 cm ($\frac{1}{4}$–$\frac{1}{2}$ inch) thick, cut it in to 8-cm (3-inch) rounds and cook on a hot buttered griddle iron or in a heavy frying pan for about 10 minutes, turning when the underside is brown. Serve warm with butter and honey.

Makes about 10

TEA-TIME SCONES

350 g (12 oz) self-raising flour

5 ml (1 level tsp) salt

10 ml (2 level tsp) baking powder

30 ml (2 level tbsp) caster sugar

75 g (3 oz) English butter

175 ml (6 fl oz) milk

150 ml (5 fl oz) fresh double cream

1. Sift together the flour, salt and baking powder into a bowl and add the sugar and butter. Rub in the butter until the mixture resembles fine breadcrumbs. Gradually mix in the milk to make a dough.
2. Knead the dough on a lightly floured work surface until smooth.
3. Roll out the dough to about 1 cm ($\frac{1}{2}$ inch) thick, then cut out 5-cm (2-inch) rounds with a plain or fluted cutter, kneading and rerolling the dough until it is all used up.
4. Arrange scones on baking sheets then brush tops with milk. Bake in the oven at 230°C (450°F) mark 8 for 10–12 minutes, until well risen with lightly golden tops.
5. Whip the fresh cream until stiff. Split the scones and fill with butter, strawberry jam and fresh cream.

Makes 18–24

HOT PEACH SCONE

125 g (4 oz) self-raising flour

2.5 ml (½ level tsp) mixed spice

25 g (1 oz) English butter

10 ml (2 level tsp) caster sugar

about 60 ml (4 tbsp) milk

410-g (14½-oz) can sliced peaches

142 ml (5 fl oz) soured cream

15 ml (1 level tbsp) demerara sugar

1. Sift the flour and spice together into a bowl and rub in the butter until mixture resembles fine breadcrumbs. Stir in the sugar and mix to a soft dough with the milk.
2. Pat out on a buttered baking tray to an 18-cm (7-inch) round; crimp the edges. Arrange the drained peaches spirally on top. Spread the soured cream over the fruit and sprinkle with sugar.
3. Bake at 220°C (425°F) mark 7 for about 25 minutes. Serve in wedges, straight from the oven.

Serves 4

CHERRY SCONES

50 g (2 oz) English butter

225 g (8 oz) self-raising flour

25 g (1 oz) caster sugar

50 g (2 oz) glacé cherries, roughly chopped

25 g (1 oz) crunchy wheatgerm

about 150 ml (¼ pint) milk

1. Rub the butter into the flour in a bowl until the mixture resembles fine breadcrumbs; stir in the caster sugar.
2. Stir the cherries into the flour mixture until evenly distributed then add the wheatgerm.
3. Mix to a soft dough with about 150 ml (¼ pint) milk, kneading lightly until just smooth.
4. Roll out the dough on a lightly floured work surface to about a 2-cm ($\frac{3}{4}$-inch) thickness. Stamp out crescent shapes using a 6.5-cm (2½-inch) fluted cutter, kneading and rerolling the dough until it is all used up.
5. Place the scones on a preheated baking sheet, brush tops with milk and bake in the oven at 230°C (450°F) mark 8 for 10–12 minutes; cool on a wire rack.
6. Serve immediately, split and spread with butter.

Makes about 14

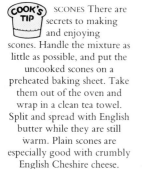

COOK'S TIP SCONES There are secrets to making and enjoying scones. Handle the mixture as little as possible, and put the uncooked scones on a preheated baking sheet. Take them out of the oven and wrap in a clean tea towel. Split and spread with English butter while they are still warm. Plain scones are especially good with crumbly English Cheshire cheese.

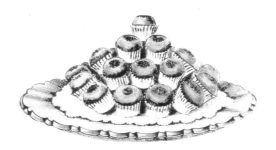

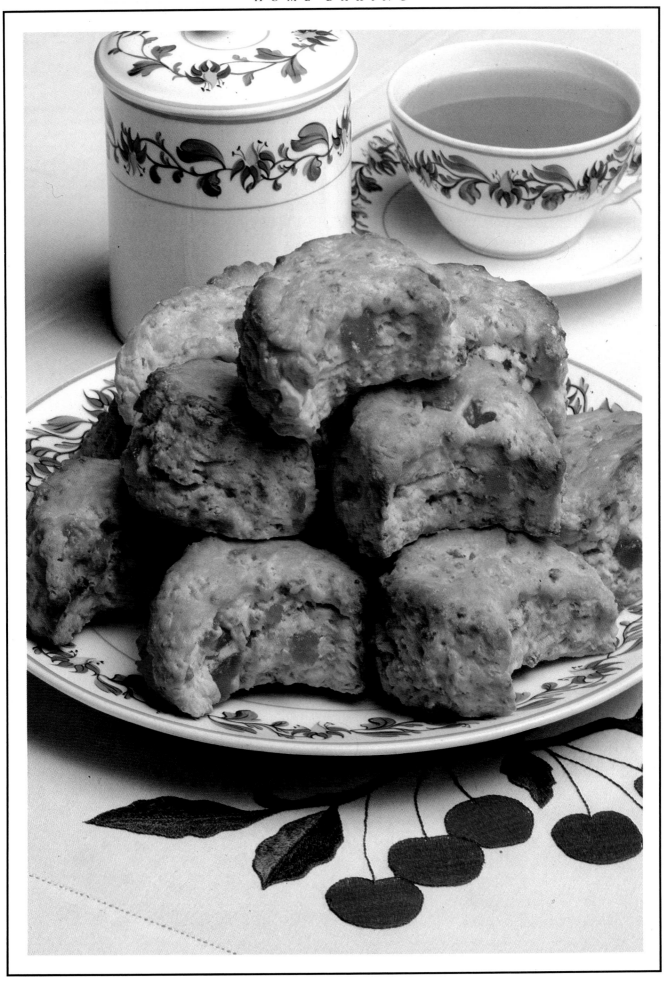

MAKING CROISSANTS

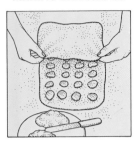

1 Adding the butter and folding the dough

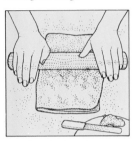

2 Rolling the dough

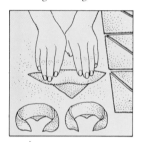

3 Shaping the croissants

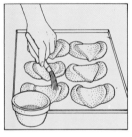

4 Brushing with egg glaze

NORFOLK SCONE

450 g (1 lb) self-raising flour
5 ml (1 level tsp) salt
150 g (5 oz) English butter
2 eggs, beaten
175 ml (6 fl oz) milk
125 g (4 oz) currants
2.5 ml ($\frac{1}{2}$ level tsp) grated nutmeg
75 g (3 oz) soft brown sugar
25 g (1 oz) demerara sugar

1. Sift together the flour and salt into a bowl. Rub in 100 g (4 oz) butter until the mixture resembles fine breadcrumbs. Mix to a soft dough with eggs and milk; divide in half.
2. Lightly knead each piece on a floured work surface, then roll out into 20-cm (8-inch) rounds about 2 cm ($\frac{3}{4}$ inch) thick.
3. Place one round on a buttered baking sheet, then spread remaining butter over dough. Mix together the currants, nutmeg and soft sugar; spoon evenly over butter. Top with the second round of dough; press down lightly. Cut into eight wedges through the top layer only. Brush with milk, sprinkle with demerara sugar. Bake in the oven at 200°C (400°F) mark 6 for about 35–40 minutes. Serve immediately with butter.
Serves 8

SYRUP OAT SCONES

350 g (12 oz) self-raising flour
15 ml (3 level tsp) baking powder
5 ml (1 level tsp) ground ginger
75 g (3 oz) English butter
50 g (2 oz) porridge oats
60 ml (4 level tbsp) golden syrup
200 ml (7 fl oz) milk, at room temperature

1. Sift the flour with the baking powder and ground ginger into a large bowl. Rub in the butter until the mixture resembles fine breadcrumbs. Stir in the oats.
2. Warm the syrup gently and add to the milk. Mix the dry ingredients to a soft dough with the syrup and milk, adding more milk if necessary.
3. Roll out 1 cm ($\frac{1}{2}$ inch) thick on a floured work surface. Divide into 5-cm (2-inch) triangles, kneading and rerolling the dough until it is all used up.
4. Place the scones on buttered preheated baking trays. Glaze with milk and bake in the oven at 230°C (450°F) mark 8 for 10–12 minutes. Serve immediately.
Makes about 20

CROISSANTS

25 g (1 oz) fresh yeast, or 15 g ($\frac{1}{2}$ oz) dried yeast and pinch of sugar
225 ml (8 fl oz) tepid water
2 eggs
450 g (1 lb) strong plain flour
10 ml (2 level tsp) salt
25 g (1 oz) lard
225 g (8 oz) English butter
2.5 ml ($\frac{1}{2}$ level tsp) caster sugar

1. Blend the fresh yeast with the tepid water. If using dried yeast sprinkle it on to the water and sugar and leave in a warm place for 15 minutes until frothy.
2. Whisk one egg into yeast liquid. Sift flour and salt into a large bowl, rub in lard. Make a well in centre, pour in yeast liquid. Mix and then beat in flour until bowl is left clean. Turn on to a lightly floured work surface, knead well for about 10 minutes until dough is firm and elastic.
3. Roll out dough on clean, dry floured work surface to an oblong about 51 × 20.5 cm (20 × 8 inches), keeping edges as square as possible.
4. Soften butter slightly and divide into three. Dot one portion over the top two-thirds of the dough but clear of the edge. Turn up bottom third of dough over half the butter, then fold down remainder. Seal edges with rolling pin. Turn dough so that the fold is on the right.
5. Press dough lightly at intervals along its length, then roll out to an oblong again. Repeat twice, rolling and folding with other portions of butter. Rest dough in refrigerator for 30 minutes, loosely covered with oiled cling film. Repeat rolling three more times, cover, chill for 1 hour.
6. Roll out dough to an oblong about 48 × 33 cm (19 × 13 inches), lay a piece of oiled cling film over the top and leave to rest for 10 minutes. Trim off 1 cm ($\frac{1}{2}$ inch) all round and cut the dough in half lengthwise, then cut each half into three squares. Halve each square, making 12 triangles.
7. Beat remaining egg, 15 ml (1 tbsp) water and sugar together for the glaze and brush it

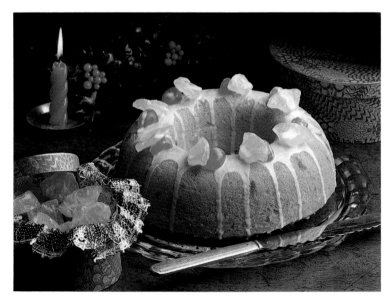

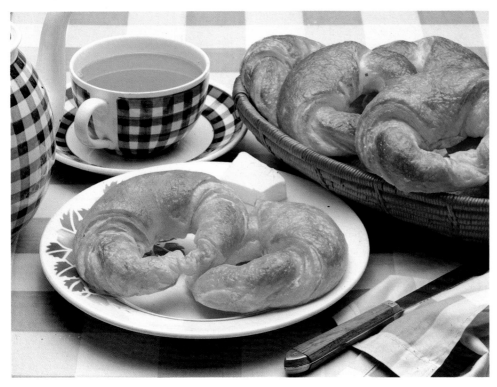

Left:
CROISSANTS
*A breakfast of hot buttery
croissants, eaten plain or with
jam, accompanied by a cup of
fragrant freshly made coffee, is
one of the best reasons there is
for getting up.*

over the triangles. Roll each triangle up from long edge finishing with tip underneath. Curve into crescents and place, spaced apart, on unbuttered baking sheets, allowing room to spread. Cover loosely with oiled cling film.

8. Leave croissants at room temperature for about 30 minutes, then brush with more glaze. Bake in preheated oven at 220°C (425°F) mark 7 for about 15 minutes, until crisp and well browned. Allow to cool on wire racks.

Makes 12

LARGE CAKES

PINEAPPLE AND CHERRY RING

175 g (6 oz) English butter

175 g (6 oz) caster sugar

2 eggs, beaten

225 g (8 oz) self-raising flour, sifted

45 ml (3 tbsp) milk

65 g (2½ oz) glacé cherries, quartered

25 g (1 oz) glacé pineapple, chopped

white glacé icing (see page 265), glacé pineapple, quartered, and glacé cherries to decorate

1. Butter and line a ring mould.
2. Whisk together butter and sugar in a bowl until pale and fluffy. Beat in the eggs, a little at a time, beating well after each addition, and add 15 ml (1 level tbsp) flour with last amount of egg. Fold the remaining flour into the mixture, then add milk, cherries and pineapple.
3. Turn mixture into the prepared tin and bake in the oven at 180°C (350°F) mark 4 for 55–60 minutes. Turn out and cool on a wire tray.
4. Decorate with glacé icing. Spread a layer on top of ring, and decorate with the pineapple and cherries, then trickle remaining icing over fruit, letting some run down the sides.

Serves 6

STICKY GINGERBREAD

225 g (8 oz) molasses

300 ml (½ pint) milk

10 ml (2 tsp) lemon juice

100 g (4 oz) lard

25 ml (1½ level tbsp) ground ginger

5 ml (1 level tsp) bicarbonate of soda

350 g (12 oz) flour

1. Butter and line an 18-cm (7-inch) square cake tin.
2. Put the molasses, milk, lemon juice, lard and ginger in a saucepan and stir until melted. Remove from the heat and beat for 10 minutes.
3. Dissolve the soda in a little boiling water and mix it in. Add the flour, gradually making a stiff batter.
4. Pour the mixture into the prepared tin. Bake in the oven at 180°C (350°F) mark 4 for about 1 hour, until lightly browned, covering loosely with foil if the top gets too brown.

Serves 12

Opposite:
*PINEAPPLE AND
CHERRY RING*
*This elegant cake, dripping with
glacé icing and decorated with
cherries and pineapple, is perfect
for a special occasion.*

8. Whip the fresh cream until stiff. Place one cake on a serving plate, cover with the whipped fresh cream, and top with the second cake. Dust the top of the cake with icing sugar and serve.

Serves 6–8

HAMPTON COURT TART

212-g (7-oz) packet frozen puff pastry, thawed

50 g (2 oz) English butter

225 g (8 oz) cottage cheese

50 g (2 oz) ground rice

125 g (4 oz) caster sugar

50 g (2 oz) sultanas

grated rind and juice of 1 large lemon

150 ml (5 fl oz) fresh single cream

2 eggs, separated

1. Roll out the pastry and use it to line a 20.5-cm (8-inch) flan dish or tin placed on a baking sheet. Prick the base with a fork.
2. Melt the butter in a large saucepan. Remove pan from heat and cool a little, then add the cottage cheese, ground rice, sugar, sultanas, lemon rind and juice, fresh single cream and egg yolks. Stir together.
3. Whisk the egg whites until stiff and gently fold them into the mixture in the pan.
4. Turn the mixture into the pastry case, bake in the oven at 190°C (375°F) mark 5 for about 40 minutes, until the top is golden brown and the pastry cooked. Serve hot or cold.

Serves 6–8

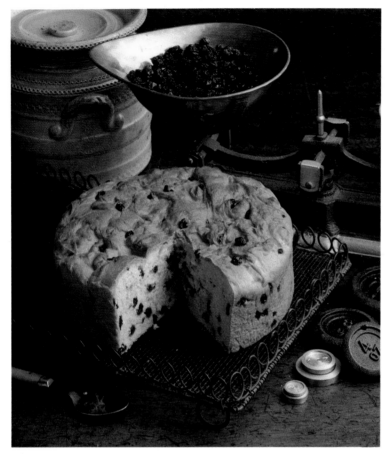

Above:
SAFFRON CAKE
The dried stigma of a purple-flowering crocus, saffron was one of the currencies of the medieval world. The Arabs introduced it to Spain and from there it reached Cornwall, where this cake is believed to originate. (Saffron crocuses were grown commercially in Stratton in north Cornwall until the beginning of this century.) Saffron is indispensable in this lovely golden cake as it adds flavour as well as colour.

LEMON SYRUP CAKE

175 g (6 oz) English butter

175 g (6 oz) caster sugar

finely grated rind and juice of 1½ lemons

3 eggs, beaten

175 g (6 oz) self-raising flour

75 g (3 oz) icing sugar

300 ml (10 fl oz) fresh double cream

icing sugar

1. Butter and line the base of two 20.5-cm (8-inch) sandwich tins.
2. Whisk the butter and sugar together in a bowl until pale and fluffy, then beat in the grated lemon rind. Gradually add the beaten eggs and beat well. Sift the flour and gently fold it into the cake mixture.
3. Divide the mixture between the two tins, and smooth surface. Bake in the oven at 180°C (350°F) mark 4 for about 25 minutes, until well risen and firm to the touch.
4. Leave the cakes to cool slightly in the tins, then turn out and stand one cake on top of the other on a plate.
5. Pierce through both layers of cake with a skewer.
6. Put the lemon juice and icing sugar in a pan over a gentle heat, stir until the sugar dissolves, then bring almost to boiling point.
7. Slowly pour the hot syrup all over the top of the cakes allowing time for it to be absorbed. Cover with cling film and leave for 1 hour.

SAFFRON CAKE

pinch of saffron strands

25 g (1 oz) fresh yeast, or 15 g (½ oz) dried yeast and a pinch of sugar

150 ml (¼ pint) tepid milk

450 g (1 lb) strong plain flour

5 ml (1 level tsp) salt

100 g (4 oz) English butter

175 g (6 oz) currants

grated rind of ½ lemon

25 g (1 oz) caster sugar

1. Soak the saffron in 150 ml (¼ pint) boiling water overnight.
2. Butter a 20.5-cm (8-inch) round cake tin. Blend the fresh yeast with the milk. If using dried yeast, sprinkle it into the milk and sugar and leave in a warm place for 15 minutes until frothy.
3. Mix the flour and salt together in a bowl and rub in the butter until the mixture resembles fine breadcrumbs. Stir in the currants, lemon rind and sugar.
4. Strain the saffron infusion into a pan and warm slightly; pour into the other

ingredients, add the milk and yeast mixture and beat well. Turn the dough into the tin, cover with a clean cloth and leave in a warm place to rise for about 1 hour until nearly to the top of the tin.
5. Bake in the oven at 200°C (400°F) mark 6, for 30 minutes, reduce to 180°C (350°F) mark 4, and bake for a further 30 minutes. Do not open the oven door during cooking. Turn out and cool on a wire rack.
Serves 8

VICTORIA SANDWICH CAKE

Use this recipe for making the cake for the base of a trifle.

175 g (6 oz) English butter
175 g (6 oz) caster sugar
3 eggs, beaten
175 g (6 oz) self-raising flour
30 ml (2 level tbsp) jam
caster sugar to dredge

1. Butter two 18-cm (7-inch) sandwich tins and line the base of each with a round of buttered greaseproof paper.
2. Beat the butter and sugar together until pale and fluffy. Add the eggs a little at a time, beating well after each addition. Fold in half the flour, using a metal spoon, then fold in the rest.
3. Place half the mixture in each tin and level with a knife. Bake in the oven at 190°C (375°F) mark 5 for about 20 minutes, until they are well risen, firm to the touch and beginning to shrink away from the sides of the tins. Turn out and cool on a wire rack.
4. When the cakes are cool, sandwich them together with jam and sprinkle the top with caster sugar.

Variations
Chocolate
Replace 45 ml (3 level tbsp) flour by 45 ml (3 level tbsp) cocoa powder. Sandwich cakes together with vanilla or chocolate butter frosting (see pages 264–5). For a moister cake blend the cocoa with water to give a thick paste then beat into the beaten butter, sugar and egg mixture.

Orange or lemon
Add the finely grated rind of one orange or lemon to the mixture. Sandwich the cakes together with orange or lemon butter frosting (see page 265). Use some of the juice from the fruit to make glacé icing (see page 265).

Coffee
Add 10 ml (2 level tsp) instant coffee powder, dissolved in a little warm water, to the butter and sugar with the egg. Or use 10 ml (2 tsp) coffee essence.

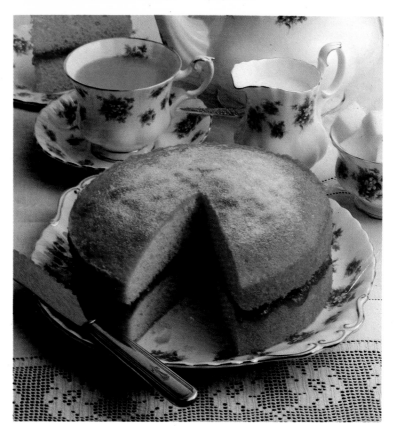

Pineapple
Sandwich the cakes together with butter frosting (see page 264), but replace the milk in the frosting with pineapple juice and decorate the cake with glacé pineapple.
Serves 6–8

Above:
VICTORIA SANDWICH CAKE
Named after Queen Victoria, this famous cake is made of melt-in-the-mouth sponge, sandwiched together with jam and dredged in icing sugar. It's light as a feather!

PARKIN

2.5 ml ($\frac{1}{2}$ level tsp) bicarbonate of soda
300 ml ($\frac{1}{2}$ pint) milk
225 g (8 oz) treacle
225 g (8 oz) golden syrup
100 g (4 oz) English butter
450 g (1 lb) flour
350 g (12 oz) medium oatmeal
5 ml (1 level tsp) salt
50 g (2 oz) sugar
5 ml (1 level tsp) ground ginger
1 egg, beaten

1. Butter a 23-cm (9-inch) square cake tin.
2. Dissolve the soda in the milk. Melt the treacle, syrup and butter together.
3. Mix all the dry ingredients together, pour in the melted butter mixture, stir well, add the egg and milk; stir well. Turn into the prepared tin.
4. Bake in the oven at 180°C (350°F) mark 4 for 1$\frac{1}{2}$–2 hours. Turn out of the tin when cold.
Serves about 16

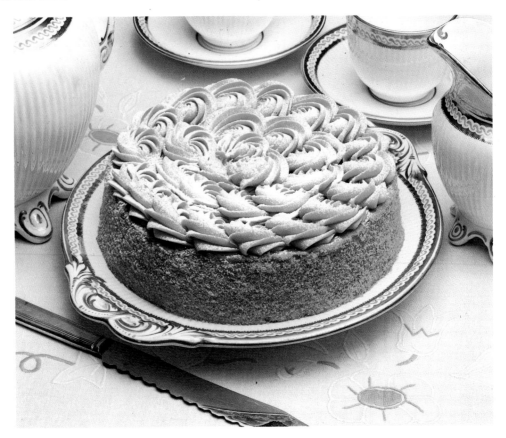

ICING AND DECORATING A CAKE

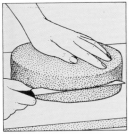

1 Splitting the cake

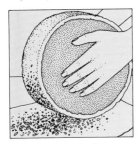

2 Rolling the iced cake in nuts

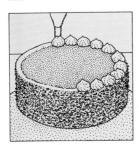

3 Decorating the cake with rosettes

COFFEE PRALINE GÂTEAU

150 g (6 oz) caster sugar

75 g (3 oz) blanched almonds

3 eggs

75 g (3 oz) flour

75 g (3 oz) English butter, melted

15 ml (1 tbsp) coffee essence

butter cream (see page 265)

icing sugar

1. Prepare the praline: heat 75 g (3 oz) sugar with the nuts until the sugar caramelises. Turn out on to an oiled baking sheet, cool. When cold, grind through a mouli grater.
2. Butter and base-line a 20.5-cm (8-inch) round cake tin. Dust with a little sugar and flour.
3. Whisk the eggs in a bowl with the remaining sugar until really thick. Lightly fold in the sifted flour with 60 ml (4 level tbsp) praline followed by the cool but still flowing butter.
4. Turn the mixture into prepared tin. Bake in the oven at 180°C (350°F) mark 4 for about 25 minutes, until light golden and shrunken away from the tin. Turn out on to a wire rack to cool.
5. Beat the coffee essence and the remaining praline into half the butter cream.
6. Split the cake and sandwich sparingly with the praline butter cream. Spread the rest round the edges. Pipe the plain butter cream in whirls on un-iced top. Dust the whole with icing sugar.

Serves 6–8

COFFEE FUDGE SANDWICH

175 g (6 oz) English butter

175 g (6 oz) soft brown sugar

3 eggs

30 ml (2 tbsp) coffee essence

175 g (6 oz) self-raising flour

fudge frosting (see page 265)

1. Butter and base-line a 20.5-cm (8-inch) round cake tin.
2. Whisk the butter and sugar together in a bowl until pale and fluffy. Gradually beat in the eggs and coffee essence. Fold in the flour.
3. Turn into the prepared tin and bake in the oven at 180°C (350°F) mark 4 for about 40 minutes. Turn out on to a wire rack to cool.
4. Split the cake and sandwich with half the fudge frosting. Spread and swirl the remainder over the top.

Serves 6–8

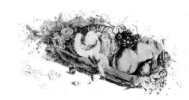

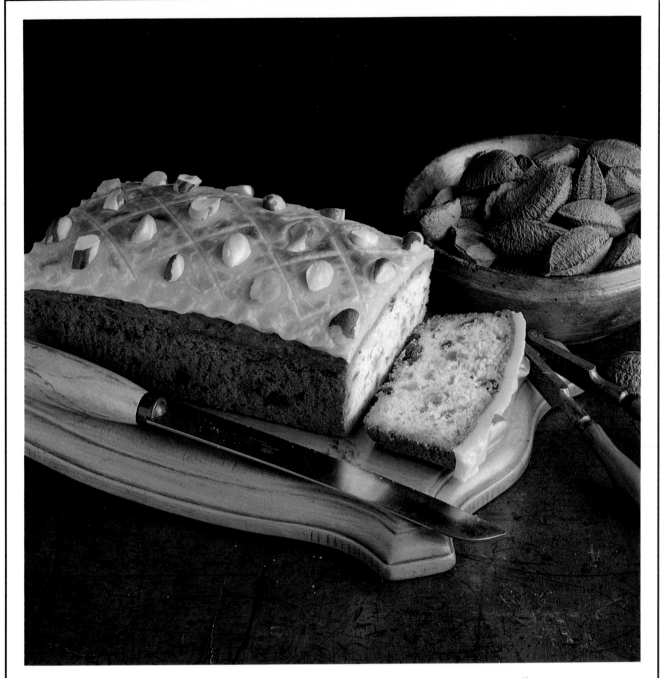

FRUIT BRAZIL BUTTER CAKE

175 g (6 oz) English butter
175 g (6 oz) caster sugar
3 eggs, size 2, beaten
50 g (2 oz) candied lemon peel, finely chopped
125 g (4 oz) dried apricots, cut into small pieces
125 g (4 oz) sultanas
125 g (4 oz) Brazil nuts, roughly chopped
125 g (4 oz) plain flour
125 g (4 oz) self-raising flour
apricot jam, sieved and melted
225 g (8 oz) bought marzipan and Brazil nuts to decorate

1. Line a 900 g (2 lb) loaf tin with buttered greaseproof paper.
2. Whisk the butter and sugar together in a bowl until pale and fluffy. Gradually add the eggs, beating all the time.
3. Mix lemon peel, apricots, sultanas and nuts together.
4. Sift the plain and self-raising flours and fold into the whisked mixture, then add the fruit and nuts. Spoon into the prepared tin.
5. Bake in the oven at 180°C (350°F) mark 4 for about 1¼ hours (cover if the top is becoming too brown). Cool a little then turn out on to a wire rack.
6. Brush the top of the cake with apricot glaze, then cover with rolled-out marzipan. Crimp the edges and cut a diamond pattern. Place a sliced nut in each square. Grill cake until evenly browned.

Serves 6–8

Above:
FRUIT BRAZIL BUTTER CAKE
English butter, fresh eggs, candied lemon peel, dried apricots are superb ingredients indeed. When you add that most exotic nut, the Brazil, and some marzipan, the result cannot fail to be a delicious success.

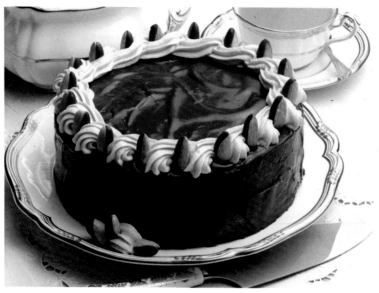

Above:
CHOCOLATE FUDGE CAKE
This enticing chocolate treat is as welcome at an afternoon tea party as at a child's birthday. But whenever it's served there is no doubt it will be the talking point.

Below:
LIGHT CHRISTMAS CAKE
An ideal cake to make for Christmas. The addition of lemon and orange peel gives it a welcome zesty taste. It is equally delicious plain or iced.

CHOCOLATE FUDGE CAKE

325 g (12 oz) plain chocolate cake covering
275 g (10 oz) English butter
175 g (6 oz) caster sugar
4 eggs, size 2, beaten
175 g (6 oz) self-raising flour
50 g (2 oz) ground rice
10 ml (2 tsp) vanilla flavouring
100 g (4 oz) icing sugar, sifted
10–15 ml (2–3 tsp) coffee essence
toasted almonds half dipped in melted chocolate to decorate

1. Line a 23-cm (9-inch) round cake tin with buttered greaseproof paper.
2. Warm half the cake covering in a bowl over a pan of hot water. Whisk 225 g (8 oz) butter and caster sugar together in a bowl until pale and fluffy then gradually beat in eggs, keeping mixture stiff. Lightly beat in the flour with ground rice, vanilla and cool, but still liquid, chocolate cake covering.

3. Turn the mixture into cake tin. Bake in the oven at 180°C (350°F) mark 4 for about $1\frac{1}{4}$ hours. Cool in the tin 30 minutes before turning out.
4. Melt the remaining chocolate cake covering and use to coat the top and sides.
5. Whisk the remaining butter in a bowl, beat in icing sugar and essence. Pipe around cake top using 1-cm ($\frac{1}{2}$-inch) large star nozzle.
6. Decorate with chocolate toasted almonds.
Serves 6–8

LIGHT CHRISTMAS CAKE

125 g (4 oz) glacé cherries
50 g (2 oz) glacé pineapple
225 g (8 oz) currants
225 g (8 oz) sultanas
125 g (4 oz) chopped mixed peel
125 g (4 oz) plain flour
225 g (8 oz) English butter
finely grated rind of 1 lemon
finely grated rind of 1 orange
225 g (8 oz) soft brown sugar
50 g (2 oz) ground almonds
4 eggs, beaten
100 g (4 oz) self-raising flour
30 ml (2 tbsp) lemon juice
45 ml (3 tbsp) brandy
apricot jam, sieved and melted, 550 g ($1\frac{1}{4}$ lb) marzipan and 700 g ($1\frac{1}{2}$ lb) royal icing (see page 265)

1. Butter and line a 20.5-cm (8-inch) round cake tin.
2. Quarter the cherries, wash if syrupy and dry well. Cut the pineapple into small cubes and mix all the fruit well together with 45 ml (3 level tbsp) plain flour.
3. Whisk the butter, add the lemon and orange rind, the sugar and continue to whisk until pale and fluffy. Stir in the almonds. Beat in the eggs little by little and lastly fold in the remaining sifted flours, fruit, strained lemon juice and brandy.
4. Turn into the prepared tin. Bake in the oven at 170°C (325°F) mark 3 for about $2\frac{1}{2}$–3 hours, covering loosely with foil if the top gets too brown. Cool in the tin.
5. Store the cake in an airtight tin for at least 1 month before brushing with apricot glaze and covering with marzipan. Leave to dry then decorate with royal icing.
Serves 24–30

MARMALADE SPICE CAKE

175 g (6 oz) English butter
120 ml (8 level tbsp) golden syrup
2 eggs, size 2, beaten
150 g (5 oz) medium-cut orange marmalade, chopped
350 g (12 oz) self-raising flour
5 ml (1 level tsp) baking powder

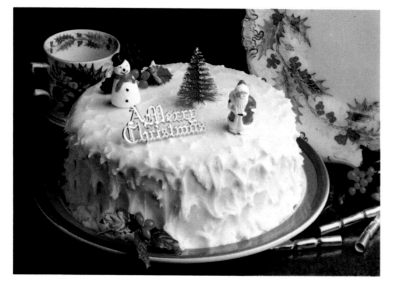

5 ml (1 level tsp) grated nutmeg

5 ml (1 level tsp) ground cinnamon

1.25 ml ($\frac{1}{4}$ level tsp) ground cloves

about 150 ml ($\frac{1}{4}$ pint) milk

50 g (2 oz) corn flakes

1. Butter and base-line a 20.5-cm (8-inch) square cake tin.
2. In a large bowl beat the butter – which should be at room temperature – with 90 ml (6 level tbsp) golden syrup until well mixed. Gradually beat in the eggs, keeping the mixture stiff.
3. Stir half the chopped marmalade into the cake mixture. Mix in the flour sifted with the baking powder and spices, adding sufficient milk to make a fairly stiff consistency.
4. Turn the mixture into prepared cake tin and level the surface.
5. Crush the corn flakes and mix with the remaining syrup and chopped marmalade. Carefully spread over the cake mixture.
6. Bake in the oven at 180°C (350°F) mark 4 for about 1 hour. Turn out and cool on a wire rack.

Serves 6–8

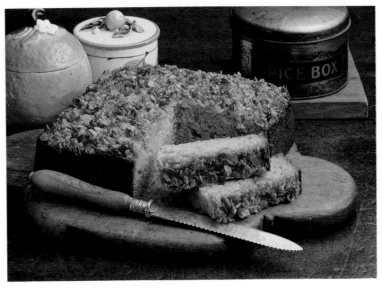

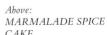

TODDY CAKE

225 g (8 oz) English butter

175 g (6 oz) soft brown sugar

1 lemon

3 eggs, beaten

175 g (6 oz) self-raising flour, sifted

60 ml (4 tbsp) whisky

30 ml (2 level tbsp) thick honey

175 g (6 oz) icing sugar, sifted

a few walnut halves

1. Butter and base-line two 18-cm (7-inch) straight-sided sandwich tins.
2. Whisk 175 g (6 oz) butter, add sugar and finely grate in the lemon rind. Continue to whisk until pale and fluffy. Gradually beat in the eggs, keeping the mixture stiff.
3. Fold in half the sifted flour, then the whisky and lastly the remaining flour. Spoon into prepared tins.
4. Bake in the oven at 190°C (375°F) mark 5 for 20–25 minutes, turn out and cool on a wire rack.
5. Whisk the remaining butter with the honey and gradually work in the icing sugar and 15 ml (1 tbsp) lemon juice.
6. Sandwich the cake together with half the butter cream and swirl the rest over the top. Decorate with walnuts.

Serves 6–8

Above:
MARMALADE SPICE CAKE
A slice of this sharp spicy cake, topped with a marmalade and corn flake mixture, makes an extra-hearty snack.

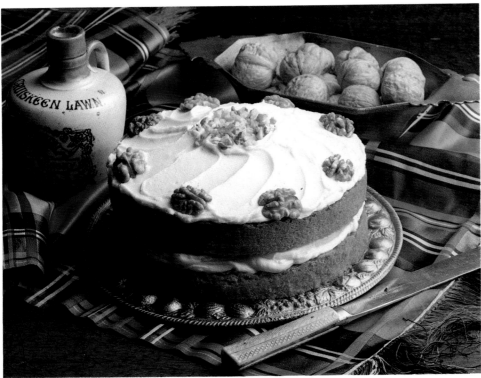

Left:
TODDY CAKE
A generous dash of whisky, tangy lemon butter cream and fresh walnut halves lift this cake out of the ordinary.

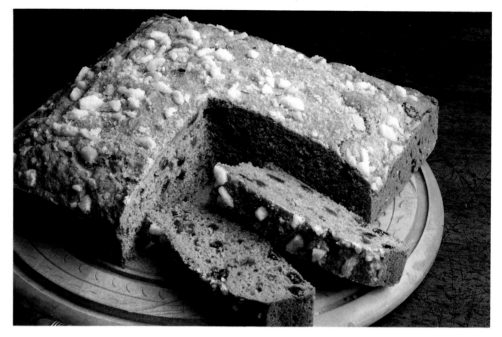

Right:
FARMHOUSE SULTANA
CAKE
A favourite cake of young and old. The sultanas grown in Turkey and Greece are still superior to new seedless varieties; those from Izmir in Turkey are reputed to be the best you can get. Choose dullish, dry-looking sultanas, rather than shiny ones which have been coated in mineral oil.

FARMHOUSE SULTANA CAKE

225 g (8 oz) plain flour
10 ml (2 level tsp) mixed spice
5 ml (1 level tsp) bicarbonate of soda
225 g (8 oz) plain wholemeal flour
175 g (6 oz) English butter
225 g (8 oz) soft brown sugar
225 g (8 oz) sultanas
1 egg, beaten
about 300 ml (½ pint) milk
10 sugar cubes

1. Butter and base-line a 20.5-cm (8-inch) square cake tin.
2. Sift the plain flour with the spice and soda into a large mixing bowl; stir in the wholemeal flour.
3. Rub in the butter until the mixture resembles fine breadcrumbs and stir in the sugar and sultanas.
4. Make a well in the centre of the dry ingredients and add the egg and milk. Beat gently until well mixed and of a soft dropping consistency adding more milk if necessary. Turn into the prepared tin.
5. Roughly crush the sugar cubes with the end of a rolling pin and scatter over the cake.
6. Bake in the oven at 170°C (325°F) mark 3 for about 1 hour 40 minutes until cooked. (When tested with a fine skewer, no traces of moist cake should remain.) Turn out and cool on a wire rack.

Serves 16–20

DARK CHOCOLATE SWIRL CAKE

175 g (6 oz) English butter
175 g (6 oz) caster sugar
2 eggs, beaten
60 ml (4 level tbsp) cocoa powder
175 ml (6 fl oz) milk
5 ml (1 tsp) vanilla flavouring
225 g (8 oz) flour
7.5 ml (1½ level tsp) bicarbonate of soda
pinch of salt
1 square bakers' unsweetened chocolate, melted
125 g (4 oz) icing sugar
50 g (2 oz) plain chocolate cake covering, melted

1. Butter and base-line two straight-sided 19-cm (7½-inch) sandwich tins.
2. Whisk 125 g (4 oz) butter until soft and gradually work in the sugar. Continue until pale and fluffy, then gradually beat in the eggs.
3. Blend the cocoa with 90 ml (6 tbsp) milk to a smooth paste. Stir in the remaining milk and the vanilla.
4. Sift flour with the bicarbonate and salt and gradually beat into the butter mixture, alternating with cocoa liquid.
5. Spoon the mixture into prepared tins. Swirl the unsweetened chocolate around the top of one cake.
6. Bake in the oven at 180°C (350°F) mark 4 for about 30 minutes. Leave to cool in tins before turning out.
7. Whisk the remaining butter, sift in the icing sugar and continue to beat well. Work in the cake covering. Use to sandwich the cakes together.

Serves 6–8

BAKING CAKES When cooked, small cakes should be well risen, golden brown in colour and firm to the touch – both on top and underneath – and they should begin to shrink from the sides of the tin on being taken out of the oven.

Larger cakes present more difficulty, especially for beginners, although the oven heat and time of cooking give a reasonable indication, but the following tests are a guide:

★ Press the centre top of the cake very lightly with the finger-tip. The cake should be spongy and should give only very slightly to pressure, then rise again immediately, retaining no impression.

★ In the case of a fruit cake lift it out gently from the oven and 'listen' to it. A continued sizzling sound indicates that the cake is not cooked through.

★ Insert a hot skewer or knitting needle (never a cold knife) in the centre of the cake. It should come out perfectly clean.

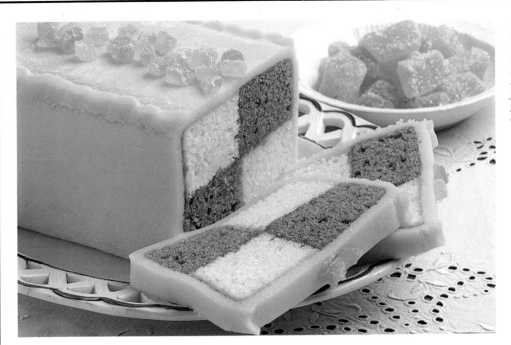

Left:
COFFEE BATTENBERG
*A magical cake straight out of
Alice in Wonderland,
Battenberg is one of those treats
children and adults alike never
forget. In this one the contrast of
plain cake with coffee is as
dramatic to look at as it is to eat.*

COFFEE BATTENBERG

175 g (6 oz) English butter

175 g (6 oz) caster sugar

3 eggs, beaten

175 g (6 oz) self-raising flour

20 ml (4 tsp) coffee essence

15 ml (1 tbsp) milk

150 ml (10 level tbsp) ginger marmalade or apricot jam

450 g (1 lb) bought marzipan

crystallised ginger, roughly chopped, to decorate (optional)

1. Butter a 20.5-cm (8-inch) square cake tin. Divide the tin in half by making a pleat, the height of the tin, in the centre of a piece of foil. Use the foil to base-line the tin, sliding a piece of cardboard inside the pleat to support it.
2. Whisk the butter and sugar together in a bowl and gradually beat in the eggs, keeping the mixture fairly stiff. Lightly beat in the flour.
3. Divide the mixture in half and fold the coffee essence into one portion and the milk into the other.
4. Spoon one flavour into each side of the tin and bake in the oven at 190°C (375°F) mark 5 for about 30 minutes. Turn out and cool on a wire rack.
5. Trim each piece of cake and divide in half lengthwise. Sandwich together alternately with half the marmalade or jam.
6. Cut out a sheet of non-stick paper to exactly cover the cake, leaving the ends bare, and roll out the marzipan on top to just fit it. Spread the remaining jam over the marzipan and wrap closely around the Battenberg. Remove the paper. Pinch the top edges and press the roughly chopped ginger into the paste.

Serves 6–8

GINGER RAISIN CAKE

225 g (8 oz) treacle

75 g (3 oz) sugar

225 g (8 oz) flour

5 ml (1 level tsp) bicarbonate of soda

15 ml (3 level tsp) ground ginger

125 g (4 oz) English butter

225 g (8 oz) raisins

1 egg, size 2

30 ml (2 tbsp) lemon juice

150 ml ($\frac{1}{4}$ pint) milk

1. Butter and base-line an 18-cm (7-inch) round cake tin.
2. Warm the treacle and sugar gently to liquify the treacle and dissolve the sugar; cool.
3. Sift the flour with the bicarbonate of soda and ground ginger into a bowl. Rub in the butter and mix in the raisins.
4. Make a well in the centre of the dry ingredients and add the cooled treacle, egg, lemon juice and milk. Beat well to thoroughly mix.
5. Pour into prepared cake tin and bake in the oven at 170°C (325°F) mark 3 for about 1$\frac{1}{4}$ hours. Test with a fine skewer which should come out clean when the cake is cooked.
6. Cool in the tin for 15 minutes, before turning out on to a wire rack.
7. When cold wrap and store in an airtight container for at least 2 days before eating.

Serves 6–8

COOK'S TIP ALL ABOUT FLOUR

There are two main types of flour available – high-gluten (strong) and low-gluten (weak or soft).

Strong flour is usually used for breads and other yeasted goods which need to have a large volume and a light open texture; it is also best for puff pastry, batters and steamed puddings.

A soft starchy flour is ideal for cakes, biscuits and shortcrust pastry, where a smaller rise and a closer, finer texture is required. Such a flour absorbs fat well and produces a light, soft texture.

Self-raising flour is popular because it eliminates errors, ensuring a happy balance of rising agents, which are evenly blended throughout the flour. If you only have plain flour, use 225 g (8 oz) flour and 12.5 ml (2½ level tsp) baking powder to replace self-raising.

PLUM AND ALMOND TORTE

125 g (4 oz) shortcrust pastry (see page 230)

125 g (4 oz) English butter

125 g (4 oz) caster sugar

1 egg, separated, plus 1 egg yolk

25 g (1 oz) ground almonds

2.5 ml (½ tsp) almond flavouring

125 g (4 oz) self-raising flour

30 ml (2 tbsp) lemon juice

30 ml (2 tbsp) milk

90 ml (6 level tbsp) plum jam

25 g (1 oz) flaked almonds

1. Butter and base-line a 21.5-cm (8½-inch) straight-sided sandwich tin. Roll out the pastry and use to line the tin, prick well with a fork. Bake blind in the oven at 200°C (400°F) mark 6 for 10–15 minutes until just set.

2. Whisk the butter and sugar until pale and fluffy. Gradually beat in the egg yolks one by one, and stir in ground almonds and flavouring.

3. Fold in the flour, lemon juice and milk. Whisk one egg white and gently mix into the mixture.

4. Spread the jam over the pastry base. Spoon over the cake mixture, level and sprinkle with flaked almonds.

5. Bake in the oven at 180°C (350°F) mark 4 until golden brown and firm to the touch, about 30 minutes. Cool in the tin.

Serves 12

MANDARIN ALMOND FLAN

175 g (6 oz) shortcrust pastry (see page 230)

125 g (4 oz) English butter

125 g (4 oz) caster sugar

1 egg, separated, plus 1 egg yolk

25 g (1 oz) ground almonds

25 g (1 oz) desiccated coconut

2.5 ml (½ tsp) almond flavouring

75 g (3 oz) self-raising flour

30 ml (2 tbsp) milk

175 g (6 oz) apricot jam

312-g (11-oz) can mandarins, drained, to decorate

1. Roll out the pastry and use to line a 21.5-cm (8½-inch) fluted flan dish or ring placed on a baking sheet. Bake blind in the oven at 200°C (400°F) mark 6 for 10–15 minutes until set but not brown.

2. Whisk the butter until soft then add sugar and continue to whisk until pale and fluffy. Beat in the egg yolks with the ground almonds, coconut and almond flavouring. Fold in the flour and milk. Whisk the egg white until stiff, then fold into the mixture.

3. Spread 125 g (4 oz) jam over the pastry case and top with the almond mixture.

4. Bake in the oven at 180°C (350°F) mark 4 for about 35 minutes, slide on to a plate and cool.

5. Glaze the flan with remaining warmed jam and decorate with mandarins.

Serves 8

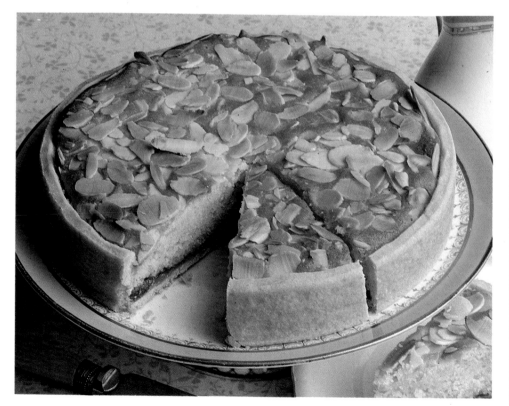

Right:
PLUM AND ALMOND TORTE
This torte is a filling flavoursome finale to a light lunch. Or serve it with steaming coffee in the middle of the afternoon.

ORANGE MADEIRA

175 g (6 oz) English butter

175 g (6 oz) caster sugar

3 eggs, beaten

100 g (4 oz) plain flour

150 g (5 oz) self-raising flour

1 orange

25 g (1 oz) sugar cubes

1. Butter and base-line an 18-cm (7-inch) round deep cake tin.
2. Whisk the butter and caster sugar together in a bowl until pale and fluffy.
3. Gradually beat in the eggs. Fold in the plain flour and self-raising flour, sifted together.
4. Grate in the orange rind and fold in with 30 ml (2 tbsp) orange juice. Spoon into the prepared tin. Smooth the surface with a palette knife.
5. Roughly crush the cube sugar with the end of a rolling pin, then sprinkle evenly over the cake surface.
6. Bake in the oven at 170°C (325°F) mark 3 for about 1¼ hours until firm to the touch. Turn out on to a wire rack to cool.

Serves 8

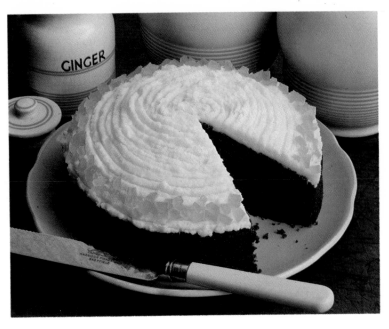

DARK GINGER CAKE

175 g (6 oz) treacle

40 g (1½ oz) demerara sugar

75 g (3 oz) English butter

175 g (6 oz) flour

10 ml (2 level tsp) ground ginger

5 ml (1 level tsp) mixed spice

2.5 ml (½ level tsp) bicarbonate of soda

2 eggs, beaten

100 ml (4 fl oz) milk

butter frosting (see page 264) and 50 g (2 oz) stem ginger, drained and finely chopped, to decorate

1. Butter and base-line an 18-cm (7-inch) round deep cake tin.
2. Gently heat the treacle, sugar and butter until melted and well mixed.
3. Sift the flour, spices and bicarbonate of soda together into a bowl.
4. Make a well in the centre of the dry ingredients and pour in the treacle mixture with the eggs and milk. Beat well with a wooden spoon until smooth.
5. Pour into the prepared tin and bake in the oven at 170°C (325°F) mark 3 for about 1¼ hours. Turn out on to a wire rack to cool. Store in an airtight container for 24 hours before eating.
6. Decorate the cake with butter frosting and stem ginger.

Serves 8–10

APRICOT AND CINNAMON CAKE

225 g (8 oz) self-raising flour

10 ml (2 level tsp) ground cinnamon

125 g (4 oz) English butter

150 g (5 oz) soft brown sugar

125–175 g (4–6 oz) dried apricots, chopped

15 ml (1 tbsp) honey

45 ml (3 tbsp) milk

2 eggs, beaten

runny honey to glaze

1. Butter and base-line an 18-cm (7-inch) round deep cake tin.
2. Combine the flour and cinnamon in a bowl. Rub in the butter until the mixture resembles fine breadcrumbs.
3. Stir in the sugar and dried apricots. Mix the honey and milk together and add to dry ingredients with the eggs. Mix well together and spoon into the prepared tin.
4. Bake in the oven at 170°C (325°F) mark 3 for about 1 hour 20 minutes until firm to the touch. Cool slightly, turn out on to a wire rack.
5. While still warm brush the top of the cake with runny honey; glaze again while cooling.

Serves 6–8

Above:
DARK GINGER CAKE
Like all gingerbread, this rich spicy cake should be stored for a little while to let the sharp mellowness of the ginger mature. Traditionally, in parts of Devon, gingerbread was served at fairs accompanied by spiced ale.

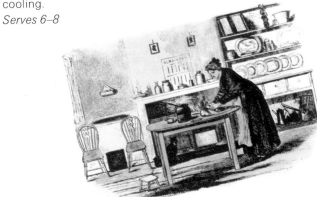

BALMORAL ALMOND CAKE

175 g (6 oz) English butter
125 g (4 oz) caster sugar
almond flavouring
2 eggs, beaten
50 g (2 oz) ground almonds
125 g (4 oz) self-raising flour
30 ml (2 tbsp) milk
125 g (4 oz) icing sugar
toasted flaked almonds to decorate

1. Butter a 900-ml (1½-pint) ribbed Balmoral cake tin or loaf tin.
2. Whisk 125 g (4 oz) butter and the caster sugar together in a bowl until pale and fluffy. Add a few drops of almond flavouring. Beat in the eggs a little at a time. Fold in the ground almonds and flour with the milk.
3. Spoon into the prepared tin. Bake in the oven at 170°C (325°F) mark 3 for 45–50 minutes, until firm to the touch.
4. Turn out on to a wire rack to cool. Whisk remaining butter and icing sugar together and flavour with almond flavouring. Pipe down the centre of the cake, decorate with the almonds and dust lightly with icing sugar.

Serves 6–8

CHERRY AND COCONUT CAKE

250 g (9 oz) self-raising flour
1.25 ml (¼ level tsp) salt
125 g (4 oz) English butter
75 g (3 oz) desiccated coconut
125 g (4 oz) caster sugar
125 g (4 oz) glacé cherries, finely chopped
2 eggs, beaten
225 ml (8 fl oz) milk
25 g (1 oz) shredded coconut

1. Butter and base-line a rectangular cake tin with funnelled ends or a 1.3-litre (2¼-pint) loaf tin. Dust with flour.
2. In a bowl combine the flour and salt. Rub in the butter. Stir in the coconut, sugar and cherries.
3. Whisk together the eggs and milk and beat into the other ingredients.
4. Spoon the mixture into the prepared tin, levelling the top and scatter over the shredded coconut.
5. Bake in the oven at 180°C (350°F) mark 4 for about 1½ hours. Cover with foil after 40 minutes.
6. Turn out on to a wire rack and leave to cool.

Serves 6–8

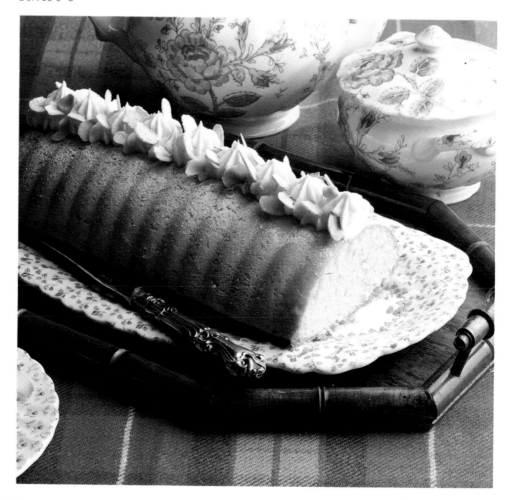

Right:
BALMORAL ALMOND CAKE
The almond tree was important enough to be mentioned in the Book of Genesis. The nuts are used in many parts of the world for sweets and cakes and even – in the Middle East especially – for savoury dishes. This subtle cake shows them off to perfection.

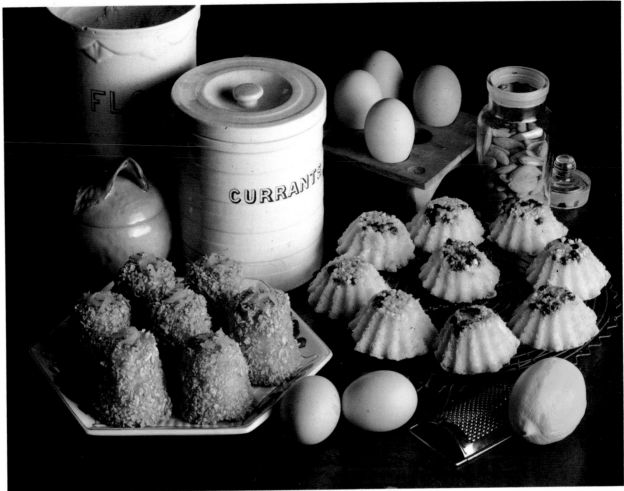

SMALL CAKES

UPSIDE-DOWN CURRENT BUNS

30 ml (2 level tbsp) currants

30 ml (2 level tbsp) chopped almonds

150 g (5 oz) English butter

150 g (5 oz) caster sugar

2 eggs

2.5 ml ($\frac{1}{2}$ tsp) vanilla flavouring

grated rind of 1 lemon

100 g (4 oz) flour

1. Butter fifteen individual brioche moulds and divide the currants and almonds between the bases.
2. Whisk the butter and sugar together in a bowl until pale and fluffy. Gradually beat in the eggs, vanilla and grated lemon rind. Sift over the flour and fold in.
3. Divide the mixture evenly between the tins and level with a knife.
4. Bake in the oven at 190°C (375°F) mark 5 for 25–30 minutes. Ease out of the tins immediately and cool on a wire rack.

Makes 15

ORANGE AND CARAWAY CASTLES

75 g (3 oz) English butter

50 g (2 oz) caster sugar

125 g (4 oz) marmalade

1 orange

2 eggs, beaten

125 g (4 oz) self-raising flour

pinch of salt

2.5–5 ml ($\frac{1}{2}$–1 level tsp) caraway seeds

25 g (1 oz) breakfast cereal, crushed

1. Butter ten dariole moulds.
2. Whisk the butter and sugar together in a bowl until pale and fluffy. Beat in 25 g (1 oz) marmalade and the grated rind of the orange. Gradually beat in the eggs.
3. Sift together the flour and salt and gently fold into the mixture with the caraway seeds.
4. Divide the mixture between the prepared moulds, placed on a baking sheet. Bake in the oven at 170°C (325°F) mark 3 for about 25 minutes.
5. Sieve the remaining marmalade, reserving the shreds. Heat the marmalade gently and use to glaze the sides of each cake. Roll the cakes in the crushed cereal. Decorate with reserved marmalade shreds.

Makes 10

Above:
ORANGE CARAWAY CASTLES (left) and UPSIDE-DOWN CURRANT BUNS
Two excellent small cakes which can be made in a few minutes, look scrumptious and taste it too!

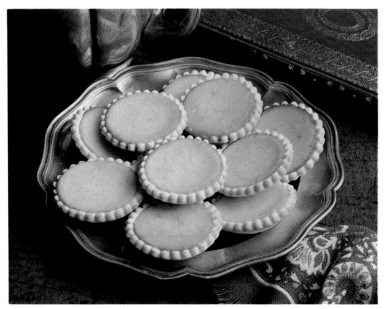

Above:
MAIDS OF HONOUR
These delicious tartlets are reputed to have been invented by a baker in Richmond, conveniently near Henry VIII's palace. The king was very fond of them and tradition has it that the cakes are named after the ladies-in-waiting who carried them back to the palace.

DATE AND HONEY BARS

175 g (6 oz) dates, stoned and chopped

45 ml (3 level tbsp) thick honey

30 ml (2 tbsp) lemon juice

10 ml (2 level tsp) plain flour

125 g (4 oz) self-raising flour

125 g (4 oz) demerara sugar

150 g (5 oz) rolled oats

175 g (6 oz) English butter, melted

1. Butter and base-line an 18-cm (7-inch) square tin which is 2.5 cm (1 inch) deep.
2. Place the dates in a pan with the honey, strained lemon juice, plain flour and 120 ml (8 tbsp) water. Bring slowly to the boil, stirring, and cook gently for 3–4 minutes. Turn out and cool.
3. Mix the self-raising flour, sugar, oats and melted butter together and spread half over the base of the tin, pressing down well.
4. Spread the date mixture over the top, and finish with remaining crumble mixture pressing evenly all over the surface.
5. Bake in the oven at 190°C (375°F) mark 5 for about 25 minutes, until golden; cool in the tin for at least 30 minutes.
6. Cut into bars and ease out of the tin.

Makes about 18

MAIDS OF HONOUR

150 ml (¼ pint) milk

25 g (1 oz) cake crumbs

50 g (2 oz) English butter, cut into small pieces

25 g (1 oz) caster sugar

40 g (1½ oz) ground almonds

1 egg, beaten

grated rind of 1 lemon

few drops of almond flavouring

175 g (6 oz) shortcrust pastry (see page 230)

raspberry jam

1. Heat milk in a saucepan to almost boiling point, then stir in cake crumbs, butter, sugar, ground almonds, egg, lemon rind and almond flavouring. Stir well and leave to stand for about 5 minutes.
2. Meanwhile roll out the pastry and cut fifteen rounds using a fluted 6.5-cm (3-inch) cutter. Place in buttered patty tins and spread jam in the base of each. Divide the filling equally among them.
3. Bake in the oven at 220°C (425°F) mark 7 for 15–20 minutes, until firm and golden.

Makes 15

BISCUITS AND COOKIES

LEMON BISCUITS

225 g (8 oz) self-raising flour

pinch of salt

150 g (6 oz) English butter

100 g (4 oz) caster or icing sugar, sifted

5 ml (1 level tsp) finely grated lemon rind

beaten egg to mix

1. Sift flour and salt into a bowl, then rub in butter until mixture resembles fine breadcrumbs. Add sugar and lemon rind, and mix to very stiff dough with beaten egg.
2. Turn out on to lightly floured work surface. Knead gently until smooth. Wrap in cling film or foil. Chill in the refrigerator for 30 minutes.
3. Roll the dough out fairly thinly. Cut into about thirty rounds with a 5-cm (2-inch) plain or fluted biscuit cutter.
4. Place on buttered baking trays. Prick biscuits well with fork.
5. Bake in the oven at 180°C (350°F) mark 4 for about 12–15 minutes, until pale golden. Leave on trays for 2–3 minutes, then cool on a wire rack. Store in an airtight tin.

Makes about 30

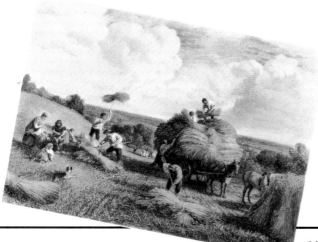

STRAWBERRY SHORTCAKE

450–700 g (1–1½ lb) strawberries

225 g (8 oz) plain flour

15 ml (3 level tsp) baking powder

1.25 ml (¼ level tsp) salt

50 g (2 oz) caster sugar

125 g (4 oz) English butter

175 ml (6 fl oz) milk

150 ml (5 fl oz) fresh double cream

icing sugar

1. Reserve six whole strawberries and mash the rest (with a little sugar if liked) in a bowl. Leave to stand for 1 hour.
2. Grease two 20-cm (8-inch) sandwich tins.
3. Sift the flour, baking powder and salt into a bowl. Stir in the caster sugar and rub in 75 g (3 oz) butter to give a coarse oatmeal consistency. Stir in the milk and mix until just blended.
4. Divide the dough between the two tins, spread level then dot with the remaining butter.
5. Bake in the oven at 230°C (450°F) mark 8 for about 12 minutes, until well risen, golden and firm to the touch. Turn out and cool on a cake rack.
6. Whip the fresh cream until stiff. Place one shortcake upside down on a serving plate; cover with a thick layer of whipped fresh cream then the crushed strawberries. Top with the other layer of shortcake, the right side up.
7. Dust top with icing sugar and then pipe six rosettes with remaining whipped fresh cream and decorate each with a strawberry.

Serves 6

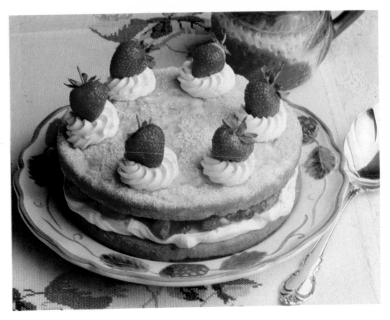

DIGESTIVE BISCUITS

100 g (4 oz) English butter

350 g (12 oz) wholemeal flour

pinch of salt

pinch of bicarbonate of soda

5 ml (1 tsp) milk

1 egg, beaten

50 g (2 oz) sugar

1. Rub the butter well into the flour and salt until the mixture resembles breadcrumbs. Mix the bicarbonate of soda in the milk, add to the egg and sugar and mix well with the dry ingredients.
2. Gradually pour in 150 ml (¼ pint) cold water, mixing quickly and roll out on a floured work surface.
3. Cut into rounds, prick all over with a fork and bake in the oven at 180°C (350°F) mark 4 for 25 minutes.

Makes about 30

Above:
STRAWBERRY
SHORTCAKE
What could be more summery than fresh strawberries and cream sandwiched between crisp golden buttery shortcake? It is perfect eaten outdoors under a hot shimmering sun, but very good, too, any time of the year.

Below:
JUMBLES
These melt-in-the-mouth biscuits are pretty to look at and delicately flavoured with almonds and lemon.

JUMBLES

150 g (5 oz) English butter

150 g (5 oz) sugar

1 egg

300 g (10 oz) self-raising flour

5 ml (1 level tsp) grated lemon rind

50 g (2 oz) ground almonds

1. Whisk the butter and sugar together in a bowl until pale and fluffy, add half the egg, stir in the sieved flour, the lemon rind, almonds and the rest of the egg.
2. Form the mixture into rolls the thickness of a finger, shape each into an 'S', and place on a buttered baking sheet. Bake in the oven at 180°C (350°F) mark 4 for 10 minutes.

Makes about 18

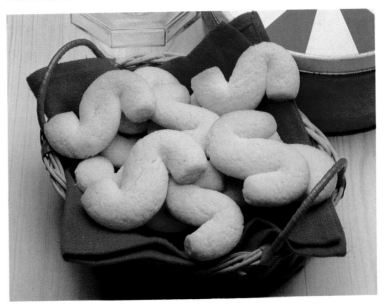

REFRIGERATOR COOKIES are a marvellous standby. They are also very easy to mix, take only few minutes to prepare and can literally be baked to order! Make a mixture from:

225 g (8 oz) plain flour
5 ml (1 level tsp) baking powder
100 g (4 oz) English butter
175 g (6 oz) caster sugar
5 ml (1 level tsp) vanilla flavouring
1 egg, beaten

1. Sift flour and baking powder into a bowl.
2. Rub in the butter. Add sugar.
3. Add vanilla and egg and mix to a dough.
4. Shape into a long roll about 5-cm (2-inch) diameter and wrap in foil.
5. Refrigerate overnight.

SHAPING AND BAKING
Cut as many cookies as required. The remainder of the roll can be returned to the refrigerator and stored for up to a week.
1. Slice the roll very thinly and place cookies well apart on a buttered baking tray.
2. Bake in the oven at 190°C (375°F) mark 5 for 10–12 minutes until golden brown.
3. Cool on a wire rack. Store in an airtight tin.
Makes 50–60.

VARIATIONS
Walnut: add 50 g (2 oz) very finely chopped walnuts with the sugar.
Coconut: add 50 g (2 oz) desiccated coconut with the sugar.
Sultana: add 50 g (2 oz) very finely chopped sultanas with the sugar.
Chocolate: add 50 g (2 oz) very finely grated plain chocolate with the sugar.
Spicy: omit the vanilla and add 10 ml (2 level tsp) mixed spice with the flour.
Lemon: omit the vanilla and add the finely grated rind of 1 lemon with the sugar.
Ginger: omit the vanilla and add 7.5 ml (1½ level tsp) ground ginger with the flour.
Cherry: add 50 g (2 oz) very finely chopped glacé cherries with the sugar.
Orange: omit the vanilla and add the finely grated rind of 1 orange with the sugar.

SHORTBREAD

150 g (5 oz) plain flour
45 ml (3 level tbsp) rice flour
50 g (2 oz) caster sugar
100 g (4 oz) English butter

1. Sift the flours into a bowl and add the sugar. Work in the butter with your fingertips – keep it in one piece and gradually work in the dry ingredients.
2. Knead well and pack into a floured shortbread mould or an 18-cm (7-inch) sandwich tin. If using a mould turn out on to the baking sheet and prick well.
3. Bake in the oven at 170°C (325°F) mark 3 for about 45 minutes, until firm and golden. If using a sandwich tin, cool slightly before turning out. When cool, dredge with sugar. Serve cut into wedges.

Variation
The rice flour is a traditional ingredient of shortbread, but it can be omitted, in which case use 175 g (6 oz) plain flour.
Makes 6–8

CHOCOLATE VIENNESE FINGERS

125 g (4 oz) English butter
25 g (1 oz) icing sugar plus a little to dredge
25 g (1 oz) plain chocolate, melted
125 g (4 oz) flour
1.25 ml (¼ level tsp) baking powder
15 ml (1 level tbsp) drinking chocolate powder
vanilla flavouring

1. Beat the butter until smooth then beat in the icing sugar and the cooled, but still liquid, chocolate.
2. Sift the flour, baking powder and drinking chocolate. Beat well, adding a few drops of vanilla.
3. With a medium star nozzle pipe out finger shapes about 7.5 cm (3 inch) long on to buttered baking sheets, spaced apart.
4. Bake at 190°C (375°F) mark 5 for 15–20 minutes. Cool on a wire rack. Dredge half with icing sugar before serving.
Makes about 18

MADELEINE COOKIES

150 g (5 oz) self-raising flour
50 g (2 oz) fine semolina
50 g (2 oz) cornflour
225 g (8 oz) English butter
75 g (3 oz) icing sugar plus icing sugar to dredge
125 g (4 oz) plain chocolate, melted

1. Butter eighteen madeleine moulds.
2. Into a bowl sift the flour, semolina and cornflour. Whisk the butter and icing sugar together until pale and fluffy. Stir in the flour mixture using a fork to form a soft paste.
3. Press a little of the mixture into each mould and smooth off the top. Bake in the oven at 180°C (350°F) mark 4 for 15–20 minutes. Leave to cool a little in the tins before gently easing out. When cold dredge with icing sugar and dip ends in melted chocolate.
Makes 18

NUT BUTTER BISCUITS

50 g (2 oz) English butter
25 g (1 oz) caster sugar
75 g (3 oz) flour
25 g (1 oz) mixed almonds, walnuts and hazelnuts, ground or very finely chopped
150 g (5 oz) coffee butter frosting (see page 265) (optional)
chopped nuts to decorate

1. Whisk the butter in a bowl until soft, but not oily. Add the caster sugar and beat again. Use a fork to stir in the flour and the nuts.
2. Turn out on to a lightly floured work surface and knead lightly into a ball.
3. Roll out thinly between sheets of non-stick paper and stamp out twelve rounds using a plain or fluted 6.5-cm (2½-inch) cutter, kneading and rerolling until all the dough is used up.
4. Place the rounds on buttered baking sheets. Bake in the oven at 170°C (325°F) mark 3 for 20–25 minutes, until slightly coloured. Cool on a wire rack. Decorate with coffee butter frosting if liked and sprinkle with chopped nuts.
Makes about 12

GRANTHAM GINGERBREADS

100 g (4 oz) English butter
350 g (12 oz) caster sugar
1 egg, beaten
250 g (9 oz) self-raising flour
5 ml (1 level tsp) ground ginger

1. Whisk the butter and sugar together in a bowl until pale and fluffy. Gradually beat in the egg.
2. Sift the flour and ginger into the mixture and work in with a fork until a fairly firm dough is obtained.
3. Roll the dough into small balls about the size of a walnut and put them on buttered baking sheets, spaced apart.
4. Bake in the oven at 150°C (300°F) mark 2 for 40–45 minutes until crisp, well risen, hollow and very lightly browned.
Makes 30

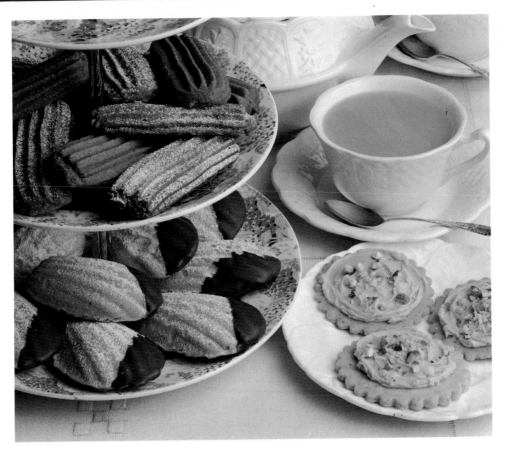

Left:
Clockwise from top:
CHOCOLATE VIENNESE
FINGERS, NUT BUTTER
BISCUITS and
MADELEINE COOKIES
Fresh butter is the essential
ingredient in these three
excellent varieties of biscuit.

GOOSNARGH CAKES

175 g (6 oz) English butter

225 g (8 oz) flour

40 g (1½ oz) caster sugar

2.5 ml (½ level tsp) caraway or coriander
    seeds

1. Rub the butter into the flour until it starts to bind together. Pat out into a shallow base-lined 30.5×18 cm (11×7 inch) tin.
2. Dredge liberally with the sugar combined with caraway and coriander seeds.
3. Leave overnight in a cool place, then bake in the oven at 180°C (350°F) mark 4 for about 20 minutes. Cut into fingers and cool in the tin. Leave for a day before eating.

Makes about 30

PINWHEEL COOKIES

100 g (4 oz) English butter, softened

50 g (2 oz) caster sugar

50 g (2 oz) cornflour

100 g (4 oz) flour

finely grated rind of ½ lemon

15 ml (1 tbsp) lemon juice

15 ml (1 tbsp) coffee essence

milk

1. Whisk half of the butter and half the sugar together in a bowl until pale and fluffy. Gradually work in half the flours with the lemon rind and juice. Knead well with

hands, wrap in cling film and chill in the refrigerator for at least 30 minutes.
2. Whisk the remaining butter and sugar together as before. Add the remaining flours and coffee essence. Knead, wrap and chill as above.
3. Roll out both pieces of dough to oblongs 25.5×18 cm (10×7 inches). Brush a little milk over one layer and top with second piece of dough. Roll up from the narrow edge; wrap in cling film and chill for 30 minutes.
4. Cut the roll into eighteen slices and place on buttered baking sheets. Bake at 180°C (350°F) mark 4 for about 20 minutes. Cool on wire racks.

Makes 18

Below:
GRANTHAM
GINGERBREADS
How these crisp, pale, spicy
cookies got their name is a
mystery, since they are biscuits
rather than what we know as
gingerbread. In the Norfolk fens
they are called White Buttons
and are sometimes rolled in
sugar after they have been
cooked.

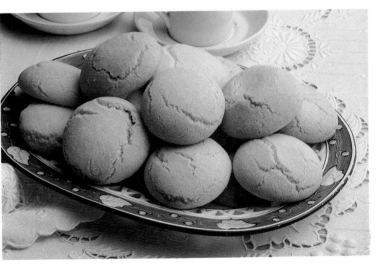

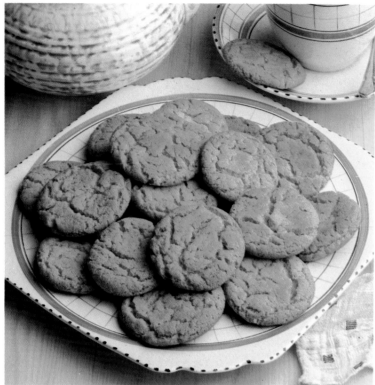

1. Sift the flour with the salt, baking powder and bicarbonate of soda, ginger and mixed spice. Rub in the butter and add the sugar.
2. Warm the syrup and add it to the other ingredients; mix well to a fairly stiff consistency.
3. Roll into small balls and place them 10 cm (4 inch) apart on two buttered baking sheets. Bake in the oven at 200°C (400°F) mark 6 for about 8 minutes.
Makes 24

BAKED CHEESECAKES

BAKED FRUIT CHEESECAKE

175 g (6 oz) self-raising flour

50 g (2 oz) cornflour

175 g (6 oz) English butter, softened

50 g (2 oz) icing sugar

grated nutmeg

3 eggs, separated

225 g (8 oz) full fat soft cheese

50 g (2 oz) caster sugar

grated rind of 1 lemon

142 ml (5 fl oz) soured cream

25 g (1 oz) chopped mixed peel

50 g (2 oz) seedless raisins

1. Butter and line a 20.5-cm (8-inch) square cake tin.
2. Sift the flour and cornflour together into a bowl. Lightly rub in the butter then sift in the icing sugar and add a generous pinch of nutmeg. Mix well, then bind mixture together with one egg yolk using a knife. Knead lightly.
3. Use half of the pastry to base-line tin. Bake blind in the oven at 200°C (400°F) mark 6 for 10 minutes.
4. Soften the cheese, add the caster sugar and lemon rind. Fold in remaining egg yolks, soured cream and grated nutmeg.
5. Whisk the whites until stiff and fold into the cheese mixture. Sprinkle on peel and raisins. Pour the mixture into the pastry base; roll out remaining pastry to fit the tin and place on top of filling, do not press down.
6. Bake in the oven at 180°C (350°F) mark 4 for 40–45 minutes until firm. Cool in the tin, turn out, cut into nine squares, dust with icing sugar.
Serves 9

Above:
CORNISH FAIRINGS
From late medieval times gingerbreads were sold at fairs all over England. It became traditional in the Cornish market town of Launceston to buy these sweet gingery nibbles at the annual ' maid-hiring' fair. They keep very well in an airtight tin.

OAT CRUNCHIES

25 g (1 oz) plain flour

5 ml (1 level tsp) baking powder

2.5 ml (½ level tsp) salt

175 g (6 oz) wholemeal flour

25 g (1 oz) medium oatmeal

75 g (3 oz) English butter

75 g (3 oz) sugar

about 75 ml (5 tbsp) milk

1. Sift plain flour, baking powder and salt into a bowl. Add the wholemeal flour and oatmeal. Rub in butter, add sugar, then mix to a firm dough with the milk.
2. Roll out on floured work surface until 0.5 cm (¼ inch) thick. Cut into squares.
3. Place on buttered baking tray. Brush with milk. Bake in the oven at 200°C (400°F) mark 6 for about 10 minutes, until just golden.
4. Cool and store in an airtight container.
Makes 16

Opposite:
BAKED FRUIT CHEESECAKE
This classic sweet has a long history: cheesecakes were as popular in medieval times as they are today. The account books of the Countess of Leicester, for example, are dated 1265 and detail the large quantities of soft cheese she bought for tarts. This luscious fruit cheesecake really is in a fine English tradition.

CORNISH FAIRINGS

100 g (4 oz) flour

pinch of salt

5 ml (1 level tsp) baking powder

5 ml (1 level tsp) bicarbonate of soda

5 ml (1 level tsp) ground ginger

2.5 ml (½ level tsp) mixed spice

50 g (2 oz) English butter

50 g (2 oz) sugar

45 ml (3 tbsp) golden syrup

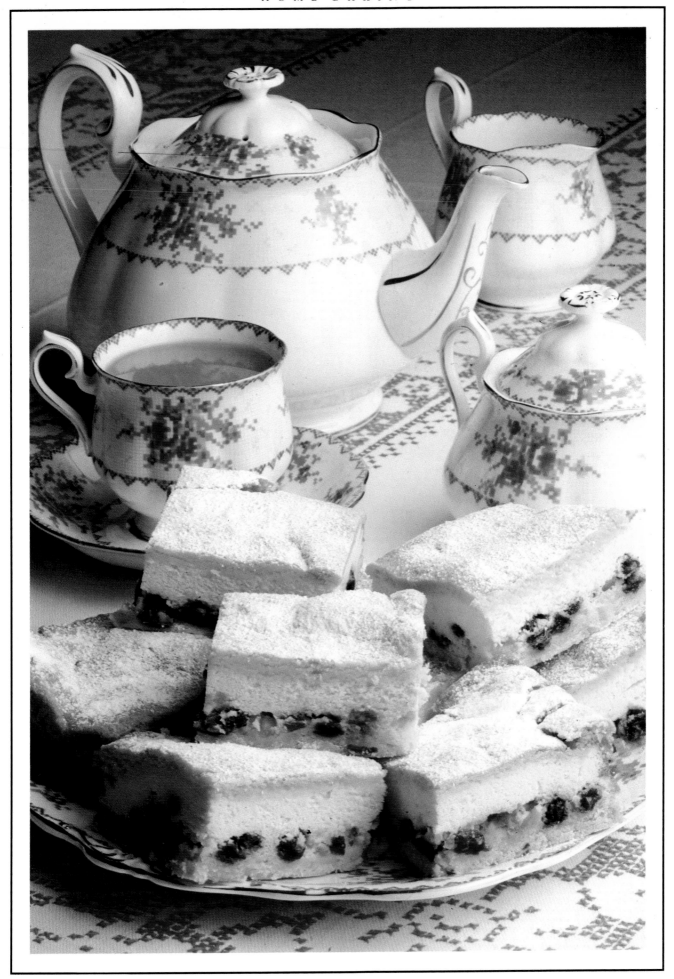

BAKED RUM AND RAISIN CHEESECAKE

75 g (3 oz) raisins

75 ml (5 tbsp) rum

225 g (8 oz) self-raising flour

5 ml (1 level tsp) bicarbonate of soda

5 ml (1 level tsp) cream of tartar

75 g (3 oz) English butter

grated rind of 1 lemon

142 ml (5 fl oz) soured cream

125 g (4 oz) cottage cheese

125 g (4 oz) full fat soft cheese

2 eggs, separated

50 g (2 oz) caster sugar

150 ml (5 fl oz) fresh double cream

1. Put the raisins and rum in a saucepan and bring to the boil. Remove from the heat and leave to cool.
2. Sift the flour, bicarbonate of soda and cream of tartar into a bowl, then rub in the butter. Add the lemon rind. Bind to a smooth dough with the soured cream.
3. Butter a 25.5-cm (10-inch) flan dish and line with the dough.
4. Beat together the cottage and full fat soft cheeses, then stir in the rum and raisins.
5. Whisk the egg yolks and caster sugar together in a bowl until pale and fluffy. Still whisking, add the fresh cream, and continue until mixture is stiff. Fold into rum and raisin mixture.
6. Whisk the egg whites until stiff then fold into the mixture. Pour into the prepared pastry case and bake in the oven at 180°C (350°F) mark 4 for about 1 hour. Turn off heat and leave to cool in oven for 15 minutes. Serve warm or cold.
Serves 8

COOK'S TIP CHEESECAKES The first recorded cheesecakes, dating back to the thirteenth century, used cottage cheese, which was pounded in a mortar then mixed with egg yolks, ginger, cinnamon and sugar, for a tart filling. Two centuries later cheese tarts were still popular but other ingredients were being added – eggs, dried fruit, lemons, butter, milk and almonds – and sometimes savoury tarts were made. Many of the cheesecakes popular today, made from full fat soft cheese on a biscuit-crust base, are American in origin: folklore there has it that the best cheesecakes in America are those from New York.

CUSTARD CREAM CHEESECAKE

175 g (6 oz) rich shortcrust pastry (see page 230)

100 g (4 oz) full fat soft cheese

100 g (4 oz) caster sugar

3 eggs, beaten

450 ml (¾ pint) milk

2.5 ml (½ tsp) vanilla flavouring

150 ml (5 fl oz) fresh double cream

15 ml (1 tbsp) rum

25 g (1 oz) sultanas

grated nutmeg

1. Roll out the pastry and use to line a 23-cm (9-inch) flan dish or tin placed on a baking sheet.
2. Whisk the cheese and sugar together in a bowl, then beat in the eggs.

3. Warm the milk and gradually beat it into the mixture, then mix in vanilla, fresh cream and rum.
4. Sprinkle sultanas over the pastry base and spoon filling over. Sprinkle with a little nutmeg.
5. Bake in the oven at 200°C (400°F) mark 6 for 10 minutes then at 180°C (350°F) mark 4 for about 40 minutes, until set.
6. Cool, then refrigerate before serving.
Serves 6–8

YORKSHIRE CHEESECAKE

150 g (6 oz) English butter

25 g (1 oz) lard

200 g (7 oz) flour

1 egg

150 ml (¼ pint) milk

225 g (8 oz) cottage cheese, sieved

40 g (1½ oz) caster sugar

30 ml (2 level tbsp) raisins

grated rind of ½ lemon

1. Butter a deep 20.5-cm (8-inch) flan dish or ring placed on a buttered baking sheet.
2. Make pastry by rubbing 100 g (4 oz) butter and the lard into the flour until the mixture resembles fine breadcrumbs. Mix to a smooth dough with 30–45 ml (2–3 tbsp) cold water. Roll out the pastry and use to line the dish or ring. Chill while making the filling.
3. Whisk the egg in the milk, then mix into the cottage cheese with the sugar. Whisk until the mixture is smooth. Melt the remaining butter and stir into the mixture with the raisins and lemon rind. Turn the mixture into the pastry case.
4. Bake in the oven at 190°C (375°F) mark 5 for about 30 minutes, until the pastry is cooked and the filling is just set. Serve warm or cold.
Serves 6

ICINGS AND FROSTINGS

BUTTER FROSTING

225 g (8 oz) icing sugar

100 g (4 oz) English butter

vanilla flavouring (or other flavouring)

15–30 ml (1–2 tbsp) milk

1. Sift the icing sugar into a bowl. Whisk the butter until soft and gradually beat in the icing sugar, adding a few drops of flavouring and the milk.

Sufficient to coat the sides of a 20.5-cm (8-inch) cake and provide a topping or a filling.

Variations

Orange or lemon butter frosting
Omit the vanilla and add a little finely grated orange or lemon rind and a little of the juice, beating well to avoid curdling the mixture.

Walnut butter frosting
Stir 30 ml (2 level tbsp) finely chopped walnuts into the butter frosting.

Almond butter frosting
Stir 30 ml (2 level tbsp) very finely chopped toasted almonds into the butter frosting.

Coffee butter frosting
Omit the vanilla and flavour with 10 ml (2 level tsp) instant coffee powder dissolved in some of the liquid, heated. Alternatively, use 15 ml (1 tbsp) coffee essence to replace an equal amount of the liquid.

Chocolate butter frosting
Flavour either by adding 25–40 g (1–1½ oz) melted plain chocolate, omitting 15 ml (1 tbsp) liquid; or by adding 15 ml (1 level tbsp) cocoa powder dissolved in a little hot water (this should be cooled before adding to the mixture).

Mocha butter frosting
Dissolve 5 ml (1 level tsp) cocoa powder and 10 ml (2 level tsp) instant coffee powder in a little warm liquid taken from the measured amount. Cool before adding to the mixture.

FUDGE FROSTING

50 g (2 oz) English butter
125 g (4 oz) soft brown sugar
45 ml (3 tbsp) coffee essence
30 ml (2 tbsp) fresh single cream
200 g (7 oz) icing sugar, sifted

1. Place the butter, brown sugar, coffee essence and fresh cream in a saucepan.
2. Place over a low heat until the sugar dissolves. Bring to the boil and boil briskly for 3 minutes.
3. Remove from the heat and gradually stir in the icing sugar. Beat until smooth using a wooden spoon and continue to beat for about 2 minutes until the icing is thick enough to spread. Use immediately, spreading with a wet palette knife.

Variation
Chocolate fudge frosting
Omit the coffee essence and add 75 g (3 oz) plain chocolate, broken, with the butter, sugar and fresh cream in the pan.
Sufficient to fill and cover top of a 20.5-cm (8-inch) cake.

WHIPPED CREAM FROSTING

150 ml (5 fl oz) fresh whipping cream
15 ml (1 level tbsp) caster sugar

1. Whip the cream until softly stiff. Gently fold in the sugar. Use immediately.

BUTTER CREAM (CRÈME AU BEURRE)

2 egg yolks
75 g (3 oz) caster sugar
175 g (6 oz) English butter

1. Beat the egg yolks in a deep bowl.
2. Place the sugar and 60 ml (4 tbsp) water in a pan, heat to dissolve sugar without boiling. Then bring to the boil and boil steadily for 2–3 minutes to reach 107°C (225°F) (use a sugar thermometer).
3. Pour the syrup on to the yolks in a steady stream, whisking all the time. Continue whisking until thick, cold and mousse-like.
4. Whisk the butter until pale and fluffy. Beat in the egg syrup gradually. Flavour to taste with melted chocolate, coffee essence, praline, orange or lemon zest.

GLACÉ ICING

The quantities given make sufficient to cover the top of an 18-cm (7-inch) cake or up to eighteen small cakes. To cover the top of a 20.5-cm (8-inch) cake, increase the quantities to 175 g (6 oz) icing sugar and use 30 ml (2 tbsp) warm water. This will give a 175 g (6 oz) quantity of icing.

100 g (4 oz) icing sugar
edible food colouring (optional)

1. Sift the icing sugar into a bowl (add a few drops of flavouring, if you wish) and gradually add 15 ml (1 tbsp) warm water. The icing should be thick enough to coat the back of a spoon. If necessary add more water or sugar to adjust the consistency. Add colouring, if liked, and use at once.

ROYAL ICING

4 egg whites
900 g (2 lb) icing
15 ml (1 tbsp) lemon juice
10 ml (2 level tsp) glycerine

1. Whisk the egg whites in a bowl until slightly frothy.
2. Sift and stir in about a quarter of the icing sugar with a wooden spoon. Continue adding more sugar gradually, beating well after each addition, until about three quarters of the sugar has been added. Beat in the lemon juice and continue beating for about 10 minutes until the icing is smooth and meringue-like. Beat in the remaining sugar until the required consistency is achieved, depending on how the icing will be used.
3. Finally, stir in the glycerine to prevent the icing becoming hard.
Makes about 900 g (2 lb)

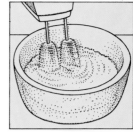

1 Beating the egg yolks

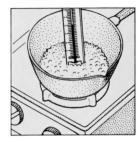

2 Boiling the sugar syrup

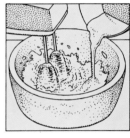

3 Whisking syrup into the mixture

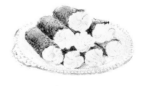

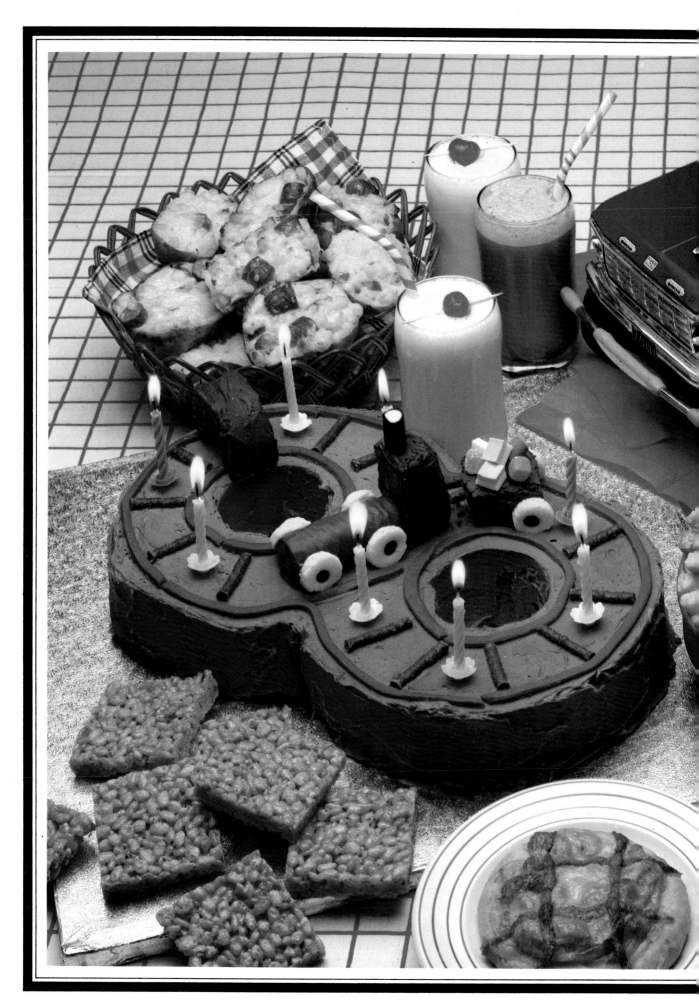

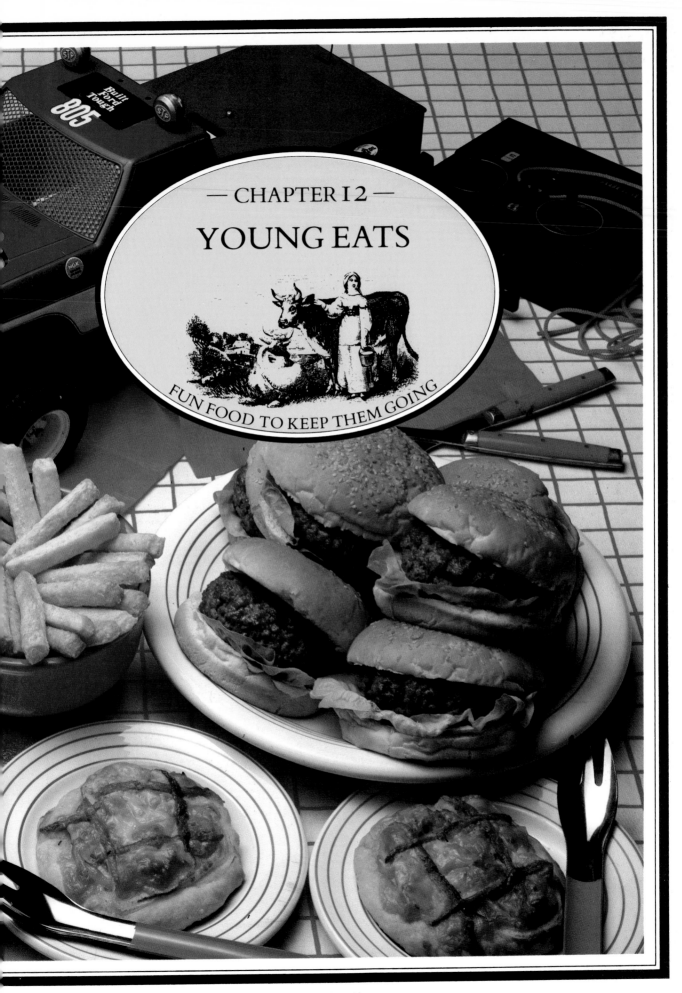

— CHAPTER 12 —

YOUNG EATS

FUN FOOD TO KEEP THEM GOING

Children love fun food, informal food, snacks, treats and things made specially for them. At the same time they're active, hungry and growing so they need good food that will provide nourishment to keep them healthy, strong and full of energy.

Snack food doesn't have to be junk food and it can meet all the demands of time, money and convenience. Turn the children's tastes to your own advantage: if snacks, burgers and pizzas are what they like then that's what to give them, as long as the basic ingredients are well balanced. You can include plenty of protein by relying on dairy products, especially milk and cheese. These together with bread and potatoes are nourishing, good value for money and easily transformed into something substantial but not fussy.

Term time is one time when a busy parent has to produce satisfying interesting packed lunches and then instant fillers the minute the children are through the door at tea time; the holidays are another.

'What's for tea? I'm starving.' Food for this end of the day has to be fast as well as filling so you need a flexible repertoire of quickly-prepared dishes.

Throwing a party needn't throw you. All the favourites like burgers, pizzas and pancakes make fantastic party food especially with teenagers who prefer casual, spur-of-the-moment type eats.

BURGERS AND DECKERS

BEEFBURGERS

450 g (1 lb) lean minced beef
50 g (2 oz) fresh breadcrumbs
60 ml (4 tbsp) milk
1 small onion, skinned and finely grated
2.5 ml (½ level tsp) prepared mustard
5 ml (1 tsp) Worcestershire sauce
salt and freshly ground pepper
40 g (1½ oz) English butter
buns and lettuce to serve

1. Combine all the ingredients, except the butter, and divide into eight equal-sized pieces. Shape each into a 1-cm (½-inch) thick cake.
2. Heat the butter in a frying pan. Add the burgers, three or four at a time and fry briskly for 1 minute on each side.
3. Reduce heat and cook more slowly for a further 6–8 minutes, turning twice. Keep hot while cooking remaining burgers. Serve in a lettuce-lined bun.

Variations
Cheese Burger: When the burger is cooked, place a slice of English Cheddar cheese over the top and grill until the cheese is bubbling.
Grated Cheese and Mayonnaise Topped Burger: Mix together 50 g (2 oz) grated English Cheddar cheese, and 30 ml (2 tbsp) mayonnaise; use to top the burger.
Cheese Tiered Special Burger: Use two burgers inside the bun, with a slice of English Cheddar cheese between the two and crumbled Blue Stilton cheese on the top. Serve with relishes.
Serves 4

DANISH FRITTER CAKES

225 g (8 oz) stewing beef
225 g (8 oz) pie pork
75 g (3 oz) onions, skinned
100 g (4 oz) flour
salt and freshly ground pepper
1 egg, beaten
300 ml (½ pint) milk
oil for frying

1. Mince the beef, pork and onions together and place in a bowl.
2. Sift the flour and seasoning into another bowl. Gradually blend in the egg and milk to make a smooth batter.
3. Stir the meat mixture into the batter and leave aside for about 30 minutes.
4. Slowly heat ½ cm (¼ inch) of oil in a frying pan.

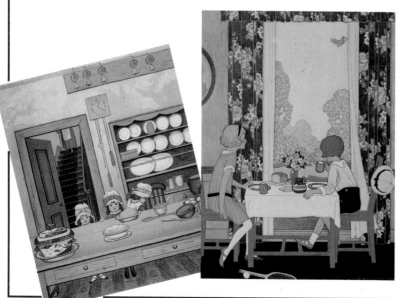

5. Spoon rounded tablespoonfuls of the mixture into the pan. Lower the heat and fry for about 15 minutes, turning from time to time, until the batter is crisp and the meat cooked through. Serve immediately.
Makes about 24

CHEESY SQUARES

4 slices of bread, crusts removed

100 g (4 oz) English butter

175 g (6 oz) English Cheddar cheese, sliced

2 eggs, beaten

salt and freshly ground pepper

pinch of mustard powder

1. Spread the slices of bread on one side with half the butter. Using slices of cheese, make up sandwiches, then cut each sandwich into four squares.
2. Beat together the eggs, salt, freshly ground pepper and mustard in a shallow dish. Dip in each sandwich to thoroughly coat.
3. Melt the remaining butter in a frying pan. Fry the sandwiches for about 5 minutes on each side, until golden and crispy on the outside. Drain well and keep hot. Serve with fried bacon and tomatoes.

Variation
Cheesemen: Make up the sandwiches as above, but cut out 'cheesemen' shapes using a gingerbread man cutter. Cook as above, then garnish with sultanas for eyes and strips of tomatoes for the mouth.
Serves 4

WELSH RAREBIT

4 slices of thick bread, crusts removed

50 g (2 oz) English butter

225 g (8 oz) English Cheddar cheese, grated

150 ml ($\frac{1}{4}$ pint) beer or stout

2.5 ml ($\frac{1}{2}$ level tsp) paprika

5 ml (1 level tsp) mustard powder

2 egg yolks, beaten

1. Toast the bread and keep warm.
2. Melt the butter in a double saucepan or over a very low heat; add the cheese, stir, then add the beer or stout slowly, stirring all the time until smooth.
3. Add the paprika, mustard and eggs. Keep stirring until warm throughout then pour over the toast and serve. (Do not let the mixture boil or bubble or it will become stringy and lumpy.)
Serves 4

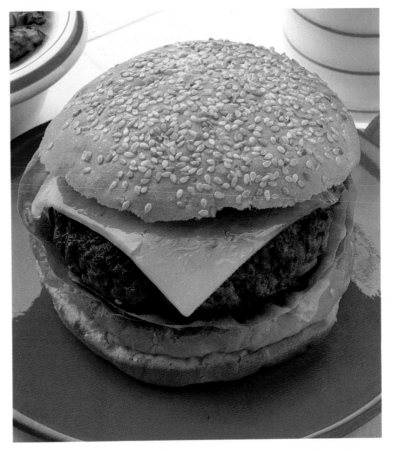

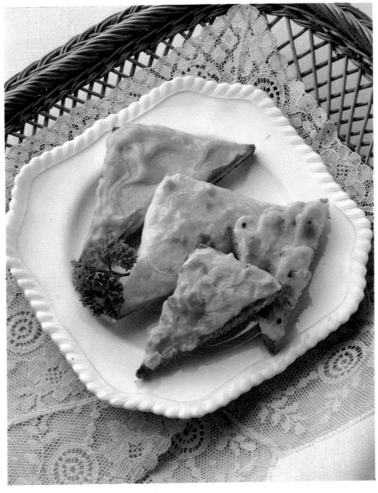

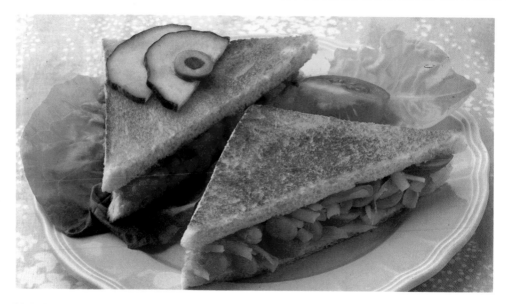

Right:
GRATED CHEESE AND
RELISH SANDWICH (left)
and CHEESE, BEAN AND
FRANKFURTER
SANDWICH
Hearty sandwiches are perfect
lunch-time fare. They are also
excellent with steaming soup for
a filling supper.

Opposite, top:
COX'S CHEESE 'N' NUT
TOASTIES
Cheese, apples and walnuts
have always been eaten together.
Try this deliciously different
way of combining them.

Opposite, below:
GOLDEN BAKED
POTATOES
Potatoes baked in the oven are
all-in-one meals which taste
wonderful.

Variations

Onion Rarebit: Toast one side of the bread only. Add 30 ml (2 tbsp) fresh breadcrumbs to the cheese mixture and replace the beer with cider. Thinly slice two medium onions and place on the untoasted side. Spread over the cheese mixture and grill until bubbling.
Serves 4

Cotswold Rarebit: Replace the English Cheddar with Cotswold cheese and use brown bread for toast. Toast one side of the bread only. Spread over the cheese mixture and grill until bubbling.
Serves 4

Cheese and Onion Crisp: Omit the cheese mixture. Toast one side of the bread only and butter with English butter. Thinly slice two medium onions and place on the untoasted side. Sprinkle with salt and crumble over 125 g (4 oz) Lancashire cheese and grill until bubbling.
Serves 4

TOASTED SANDWICHES

Peanut Butter Special Sandwich: Butter four slices of granary bread with 120 ml (8 level tbsp) crunchy peanut butter. Add 100 g (4 oz) grated English Cheddar cheese and $\frac{1}{4}$ of a sliced cucumber. Toast both sides of sandwich.
Serves 2

Grated Cheese and Relish Sandwich: Mix together 100 g (4 oz) grated English Cheddar cheese, 60 ml (4 level tbsp) hamburger relish and seasoning. Spread over two slices of bread and top with another two slices. Toast both sides of sandwich.
Serves 2

Cheese, Beans and Frankfurter Sandwich: Mix together 75 g (3 oz) grated English Cheddar or Cheshire cheese, four sliced frankfurters and a 219-g (7¾-oz) can of baked beans. Use to fill eight slices of toast.
Serves 4

FRIED CHEESE SLICES

2 rashers of bacon
2 slices of bread
50 g (2 oz) English butter
2 slices of mature English Cheddar cheese

1. Grill the bacon until crisp, crumble and set aside.
2. In a frying pan, fry the slices of bread in the butter on one side until golden.
3. Turn the slices over and lay the cheese on top. Cover the pan and cook gently until the cheese melts.
4. Just before serving, sprinkle with the bacon.
Serves 1–2

COX'S CHEESE 'N' NUT TOASTIES

3 Cox's apples
juice of $\frac{1}{2}$ lemon
225 g (8 oz) English Cheddar cheese, grated
Worcestershire sauce
4 slices of bread
50 g (2 oz) English butter
25 g (1 oz) walnuts, chopped

1. Core the apples and cut one apple into eight thin rings, then dip in lemon juice. Peel and grate the other two apples into a bowl.
2. Mix the cheese and grated apple with a few drops of Worcestershire sauce.
3. Toast the bread then butter one side. Spread the cheese mixture on the toast and sprinkle with chopped nuts. Grill for 3–4 minutes until golden brown. Garnish each piece of toast with two apple rings.
Serves 4

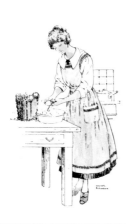

POTATO SPECIALS

GOLDEN BAKED POTATOES

4 potatoes, scrubbed and pricked

25 g (1 oz) English butter

125 g (4 oz) onion, skinned and finely chopped

60 ml (4 tbsp) milk

125 g (4 oz) English Cheddar cheese, grated

salt and freshly ground pepper

Worcestershire sauce

1. Bake each potato in its jacket in the oven at 200°C (400°F) mark 6 for about 1¼–1½ hours, until just tender.

2. Halve the potatoes and scoop out the insides, leaving a thin shell. Mash the potato flesh.

3. Heat the butter in a frying pan and lightly brown the onion, then add the milk and heat gently.

4. Beat this mixture into the mashed potato with half the cheese, the seasoning and a few drops of Worcestershire sauce.

5. Pile the mixture back into the potato shells, scatter over remaining grated cheese.

6. Return to the oven for about 20 minutes, until golden. Serve immediately.

Serves 8

Variation

Hot Dog Tatties: Use 6 large potatoes and cook in the same way. Halve and scoop out to leave a thin shell. Mash the potato and combine with the contents of a 113-g (4-oz) can hot dog sausages, sliced, a 198-g (7-oz) can sweetcorn, drained, 142 ml (5 fl oz) soured cream and seasoning. Fill the potato shells and arrange in a shallow ovenproof dish. Sprinkle over 50 g (2 oz) grated English Cheddar cheese and return to the oven at 220°C (425°F) mark 7 for 20 minutes.

Serves 6

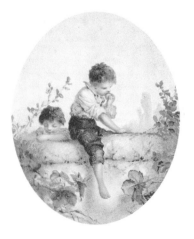

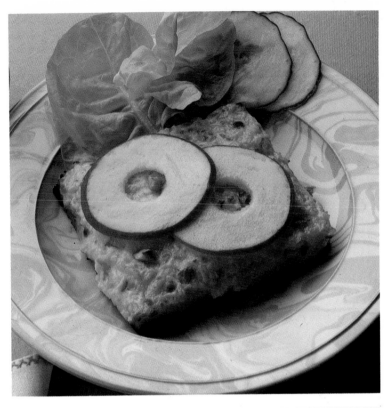

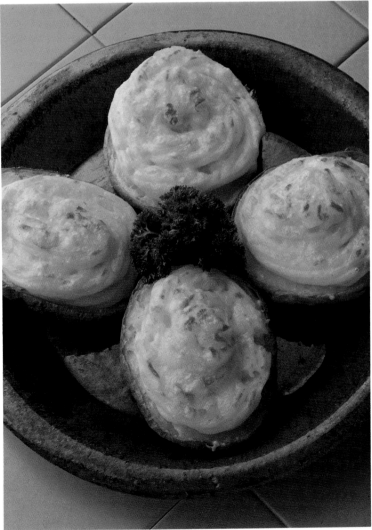

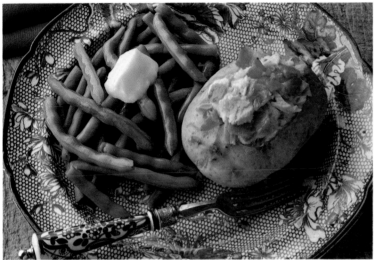

Above:
BAKED TUNA STUFFED POTATO
These extra-special baked potatoes are stuffed with tangy tuna and soured cream and topped with crisp bacon.

Below:
CHICKEN AND SWEETCORN POTATO CAKES
What an exciting change from ordinary potato cakes! Chicken and sweetcorn give a wonderful lift to a useful standby.

BAKED TUNA STUFFED POTATOES

4 large potatoes, scrubbed and pricked
198-g (7-oz) can tuna, flaked
25 g (1 oz) English butter
142 ml (5 fl oz) soured cream
salt and freshly ground pepper
125 g (4 oz) streaky bacon, chopped

1. Bake the potatoes in the oven at 180°C (350°F) mark 4 for 1½–2 hours, until just tender.
2. Slice the tops off the potatoes and scoop out the flesh, leaving a thin shell.
3. Mash the potato flesh, then stir in the tuna with its oil, the butter, soured cream and seasoning.
4. Spoon the tuna mixture back into the potato shells and mark the surface with a knife.
5. Place the bacon on top of the potatoes.
6. Place the potatoes in a shallow ovenproof dish and return to the oven at 220°C (425°F) mark 7 for 20–25 minutes. Serve with freshly cooked green beans or a green bean salad.
Serves 4

CHEESE AND POTATO EGGS

450 g (1 lb) potatoes, peeled
25 g (1 oz) English butter
100 g (4 oz) English Cheddar cheese, grated
15 ml (1 tbsp) chopped fresh chives
salt and freshly ground pepper
4 eggs, hard-boiled
1 egg, beaten
75 g (3 oz) fresh breadrumbs
vegetable oil for frying

1. Boil the potatoes in a saucepan of fast boiling salted water until tender, then mash.
2. Mix the potatoes with the butter, cheese, chives and seasoning and beat until smooth. Turn on to a floured work surface and divide into four pieces.
3. Place one hard-boiled egg in the centre of each piece and mould round the egg to completely cover, sealing all the edges well.
4. Brush with the beaten egg and coat in the breadcrumbs. Chill in the refrigerator for 30 minutes to firm.
5. Deep fry the potato balls in hot fat until crisp and golden. Drain on absorbent kitchen paper and serve hot with barbecue sauce (see page 151).
Serves 4

CHICKEN AND SWEETCORN POTATO CAKES

200 ml (7 fl oz) milk
2 eggs
125 g (4 oz) flour
salt and freshly ground pepper
450 g (1 lb) potatoes, peeled and coarsely grated
225 g (8 oz) onion, skinned and thinly sliced
225 g (8 oz) cooked chicken, finely chopped
198-g (7-oz) can sweetcorn, drained
English butter and vegetable oil for frying

1. Whisk the milk and eggs together, then beat in the flour and a pinch of salt, until smooth. Chill in the refrigerator.
2. Blanch the potato and onion together in a pan of boiling salted water for 2–3 minutes. Drain well and press out as much liquid as possible.
3. Stir the chicken into the batter with the sweetcorn, potato and onion, and add seasoning to taste.
4. Heat 0.5 cm (¼ inch) butter and oil in a frying pan. Spoon heaped tablespoonfuls of the mixture into the pan, flatten and fry for

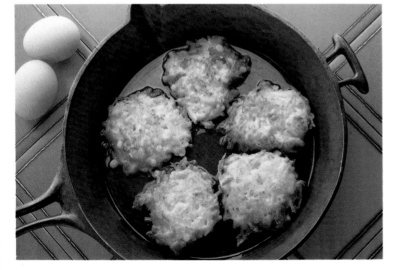

about 4 minutes on each side. Drain well and keep warm, uncovered, in a low oven. Repeat until all the mixture is used. Serve hot.
Makes 12

QUICK SAVOURIES AND SNACKS

TOAD IN THE HOLE

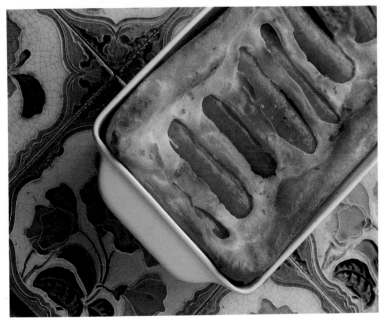

100 g (4 oz) flour

pinch of salt

1 egg

300 ml ($\frac{1}{2}$ pint) milk

15 ml (1 level tbsp) English butter, melted

450 g (1 lb) pork sausages

1. Sift the flour and salt into a bowl. Beat to a smooth batter with the egg, half the milk and the melted butter. Stir in the remaining milk.
2. Arrange the sausages in a small shallow baking tin and bake in the oven at 220°C (425°F) mark 7 for 10 minutes.
3. Remove from oven, pour the batter over the sausages and bake for a further 30 minutes.
4. Reduce temperature to 200°C (400°F) mark 6 and bake for a further 15–20 minutes. Serve immediately.

Variation
Pickle Popovers: Using the same batter and omitting the sausages, cook in twelve buttered patty tins. When cooked, put a little pickle in the centre of each and serve immediately.
Serves 4

QUICK PIZZA

225 g (8 oz) self-raising flour

2.5 ml ($\frac{1}{2}$ level tsp) salt

65 g (2$\frac{1}{2}$ oz) English butter

150 ml ($\frac{1}{4}$ pint) milk

1 large onion, skinned and sliced

3 large tomatoes, peeled and thinly sliced, or 200-g (7-oz) can tomatoes, drained and mashed

salt and freshly ground pepper

2.5 ml ($\frac{1}{2}$ tsp) dried mixed herbs

175 g (6 oz) English Cheddar cheese, thinly sliced

2 rashers of streaky bacon, cut into narrow strips

1. Sift the flour and salt into a bowl, then rub in 50 g (2 oz) of butter until the mixture resembles fine breadcrumbs. Add the milk and mix to a soft dough.
2. Turn on to a floured work surface. Knead until smooth. Roll out to one large or four individual circles, 1-cm ($\frac{1}{2}$-inch) thick. Place on a buttered baking tray.
3. In a frying pan, fry the onion in the remaining butter. Place on the pizza base and top with the tomato slices, seasoning, mixed herbs and cheese. Decorate with the bacon strips, arranged in a pattern.
4. Bake in the oven at 220°C (425°F) mark 7 for 20–25 minutes, until cooked and golden. Serve hot.

Variation
Make the lattice with canned sardines, drained anchovies or sausages sliced lengthways.
Serves 4

Above:
TOAD IN THE HOLE
In Norfolk this old-time favourite is known as Pudding-pye-doll. It is simply delicious for lunch and tea and – needless to say – children love it.

Below:
QUICK PIZZA
The Italians are experts at making wholesome welcoming food in a flash. And pizzas must be one of their most successful and scrumptious dishes.

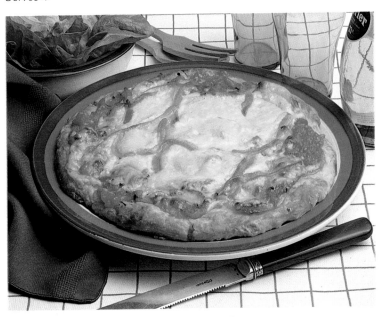

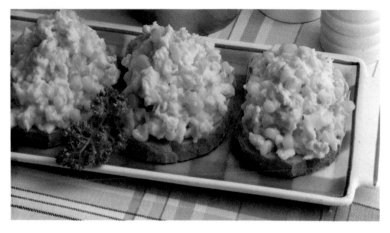

Above:
CORN AND HAM
SCRAMBLE
When properly made, scrambled eggs are a delicious and satisfying light meal at almost any time of the day, particularly when served on rounds of lovely hot buttered toast.

This tasty version of scrambled eggs made with fresh cream, chopped ham and crunchy sweetcorn will appeal to youngsters of all ages.

CORN AND HAM SCRAMBLE

6 eggs

60 ml (4 tbsp) fresh single cream

15 g (½ oz) English butter

198-g (7-oz) can sweetcorn, drained

100 g (4 oz) ham, finely chopped

large pinch of grated nutmeg

salt and freshly ground pepper

4 slices of hot buttered toast to serve

parsley sprigs to garnish

1. Beat the eggs and fresh cream well together. Pour into a frying pan. Add the butter, sweetcorn, ham, nutmeg and seasoning.
2. Scramble over a low heat until just set. Pile equal amounts on to buttered toast and garnish with parsley sprigs.
Serves 4

HOT SUPPER CRUSTIES

4 bread rolls

75 g (3 oz) English butter

rind of ½ orange

5 ml (1 tsp) chopped fresh parsley

freshly ground pepper

100 g (4 oz) boiled bacon, coarsely chopped

1. Cut a thin slice off the tops of the rolls and reserve. Scoop out the centre crumbs leaving a good shell.
2. Beat the butter in a bowl and finely grate in the orange rind. Blend in the parsley and pepper until smooth, then mix in the bacon.
3. Pack the mixture into the rolls and replace the top. Wrap each roll in foil, sealing well. Bake in the oven at 200°C (400°F) mark 6 for 15–20 minutes. Serve hot straight from the foil parcel.
Serves 4

CHEESE AND TOMATO DIP WITH SAUSAGES

40 g (1½ oz) English butter

40 g (1½ oz) flour

300 ml (½ pint) milk

pinch of salt

pinch of cayenne pepper

100 g (4 oz) English Cheddar cheese, grated

60 ml (4 level tbsp) tomato ketchup

500 g (1 lb) pork chipolata sausages, fried and cut in half

1. Melt the butter in a pan, stir in the flour and cook gently for 1 minute, stirring. Remove from the heat and gradually stir in the milk. Bring to the boil and continue to cook, stirring, for 1 minute then remove from heat and add the salt, cayenne pepper, cheese and tomato ketchup. Stir until the cheese has melted.
2. Serve as a dip for hot fried chipolata sausages and pineapple chunks.
Serves 8

BEANY LIVER CASSEROLE

350 g (12 oz) lamb's liver

25 g (1 oz) flour

25 g (1 oz) English butter

1 onion, skinned and chopped

100 g (4 oz) mushrooms, sliced

475-g (17-oz) can red kidney beans

150 ml (¼ pint) beef stock

150 ml (¼ pint) milk

30 ml (2 level tbsp) tomato purée

5 ml (1 level tsp) dried mixed herbs

salt and freshly ground pepper

1. Cut the liver into cubes and coat with flour. Melt the butter in a large saucepan and fry the liver, onion and mushrooms quickly until brown. Add the beans to the liver mixture.
2. Add the remaining ingredients and bring to the boil. Simmer for 20–25 minutes. Serve hot on a bed of rice.
Serves 4

BACON AND CORN PUFFS

125 g (4 oz) flour

pinch of salt

1 egg, separated

150 ml (¼ pint) milk

100 g (4 oz) boiled bacon, finely minced

210-g (7½-oz) can sweetcorn, drained

vegetable oil for deep frying

paprika to garnish

1. Sift the flour and salt into a bowl; make a well in the centre and add the egg yolk.
2. Beat gently, adding the milk gradually, until all the flour is mixed in, then beat hard

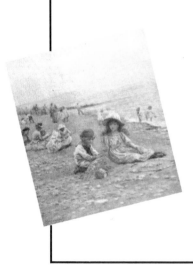

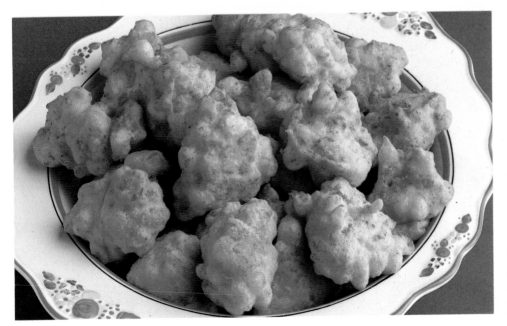

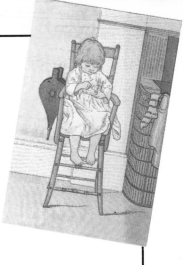

Left:
*BACON AND CORN
PUFFS*
*Flecked with finely chopped
boiled bacon and delicious
sweetcorn, these popular snacks
are made from batter deep-fried
to a golden lightness.*

for about 2 minutes. Leave the batter to stand in a cool place.

3. Just before cooking add the bacon and the sweetcorn to the batter. Stiffly whisk the egg white and fold evenly into the batter.

4. Fry spoonfuls of the mixture in hot deep oil for 3–4 minutes, until crisp and golden.

5. Drain, then dredge lightly with paprika and serve immediately.

Serves 4

CHEESE SCONE TWISTS

450 g (1 lb) self-raising flour

10 ml (2 level tsp) baking powder

pinch of salt

75 g (3 oz) English butter

125 g (4 oz) mature English Cheddar cheese, finely grated

about 300 ml ($\frac{1}{2}$ pint) milk

1. Sift the flour, baking powder and salt together into a bowl, then rub in the butter. Add half the cheese and bind the mixture with milk.

2. Roll out on a floured work surface to 1 cm ($\frac{1}{2}$ inch) thick. Cut rounds with a 7.5-cm (3-inch) cutter and remove the centres using a 3.5-cm ($1\frac{1}{2}$-inch) cutter.

3. Lightly knead trimmings, including the 3.5-cm ($1\frac{1}{2}$-inch) rounds, and roll. Cut out more scone rounds with a hole until all the dough is used.

4. Twist each ring to form a figure of eight and place well apart on buttered baking sheets.

5. Glaze scones with milk and sprinkle over the remaining cheese.

6. Bake in the oven at 220°C (425°F) mark 7 for about 12 minutes, until well risen and golden brown. Serve warm or cold on day of baking.

Makes about 14

CHEESE STRAWS

75 g (3 oz) flour

salt and freshly ground pepper

40 g ($1\frac{1}{2}$ oz) English butter

40 g ($1\frac{1}{2}$ oz) English Cheddar cheese, grated

1 egg, beaten

5 ml (1 level tsp) French mustard

1. Mix the flour and seasonings together and rub in the butter until the mixture resembles fine breadcrumbs. Add the cheese and stir to mix evenly.

2. Combine half the beaten egg with the mustard and stir into the flour mixture to form a soft dough. Turn on to a floured work surface and knead lightly until just smooth.

3. Roll out the dough to a 15-cm (6-inch) square and place on a baking sheet. Brush with the remaining beaten egg. Divide the dough into 7.5 × 1 cm (3 × $\frac{1}{2}$ inch) oblongs and separate out.

4. Bake in the oven at 180°C (350°F) mark 4 for 12–15 minutes until golden. Cool on a wire rack. Store in an airtight container.

Makes about 24

Below:
*CHEESE SCONE TWISTS
Children love these light golden
snacks, tasty and nourishing
with mature Cheddar cheese and
pure English butter. They are
delicious served warm straight
from the oven, or cold on the
day of baking.*

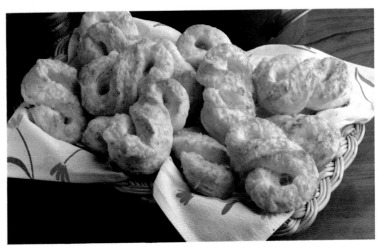

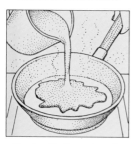

1 Pouring the batter into the hot pan

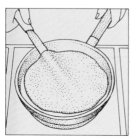

2 Turning the pancake over

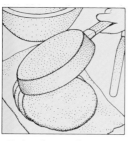

3 Easing the pancake out of the pan

COOK'S TIP

TO SEASON A FRYING PAN. Heat 15 ml (1 tbsp) vegetable oil in the pan. Sprinkle with salt then rub out with kitchen paper. This cleans and conditions the pan in preparation for making pancakes.

Right:
CELERY, ONION AND CHEESE PANCAKES
These crisp delicious pancakes are filled with a tangy celery sauce made with a dash of mustard and are topped with cheese for a tempting finishing touch.

SWEET AND SAVOURY PANCAKES

PANCAKE BATTER

125 g (4 oz) flour
1.25 ml (¼ level tsp) salt
1 egg
300 ml (½ pint) milk
English butter for frying

1. Sift the flour and salt into a bowl, make a well in the centre and add the egg. Beat with a wooden spoon, adding the milk gradually, until incorporated.
2. To make pancakes. Heat a little butter in a 18-cm (7-inch) heavy-based frying pan until very hot, running it round to coat the sides of the pan; pour off any surplus.
3. Ladle or pour in a little batter, rotating the pan at the same time, until enough batter is added to give a thin coating.
4. Cook until the pancake begins to curl around the edges, revealing a golden-brown colour underneath. Ease a palette knife under the centre and flip over.
5. Fry the other side until golden brown, then turn on to a warm plate and cover. Continue cooking pancakes until all the batter is used, adding a small knob of butter to the pan each time.
6. Serve immediately, sprinkled with sugar and lemon juice. Or fill with a sweet or savoury filling.
Makes 8

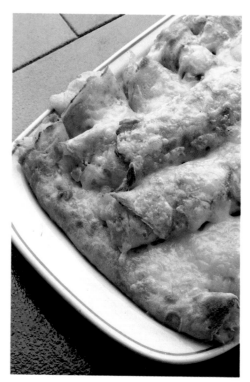

CELERY, ONION AND CHEESE PANCAKES

225 g (8 oz) Lancashire cheese, grated
3–4 sprigs of parsley, finely chopped
1 quantity pancake batter (see left)
175 g (6 oz) celery, cleaned and trimmed
350 g (12 oz) onion, skinned and roughly chopped
50 g (2 oz) English butter
5–10 ml (1–2 level tsp) whole grain mustard
60 ml (4 tbsp) fresh double cream

1. Add 50 g (2 oz) cheese and the parsley to the pancake batter and make eight thin pancakes in the usual way.
2. Sauté the roughly chopped celery and onion in the butter for 7–10 minutes, until soft. Remove from the heat and stir in the mustard, fresh cream and 125 g (4 oz) cheese.
3. Divide the mixture into eight and spread over the pancakes. Roll up and place side by side in a shallow ovenproof dish.
4. Sprinkle with the remaining cheese. Reheat in the oven, uncovered, at 190°C (375°F) mark 5 for 15–20 minutes.
Serves 4

COUNTRY PANCAKES

100 g (4 oz) mushrooms, wiped and chopped
4 large tomatoes, skinned and chopped
25 g (1 oz) English butter
8 pancakes (see left)
300 ml (½ pint) cheese sauce (see page 143)
142 g (5 oz) natural yogurt
25 g (1 oz) Lancashire cheese, crumbled

1. Fry the mushrooms and tomatoes in the butter. Fill the pancakes with this mixture, roll or fold up and arrange in a shallow ovenproof dish.
2. Mix the cheese sauce with the yogurt and pour over the pancakes.
3. Sprinkle with the cheese, brown under a hot grill and serve immediately.
Serves 4

BACON AND MUSTARD PANCAKES

50 g (2 oz) English butter
2 medium onions, skinned and roughly chopped
175 g (6 oz) boiled bacon, finely chopped
225 g (8 oz) apple, peeled and cored
225 g (8 oz) frozen cut beans, cooked
15 ml (1 level tbsp) whole grain mustard
30 ml (2 level tbsp) flour
300 ml (½ pint) milk
125 g (4 oz) English Cheddar cheese

salt and freshly ground pepper

8 pancakes (see opposite)

chopped fresh parsley to garnish

1. Melt 25 g (1 oz) butter in a deep frying pan and fry the onion until softened. Stir in the bacon, apple and beans and sauté for 2–3 minutes. Remove from the heat and stir in the mustard.

2. Melt the remaining butter in a pan, stir in the flour and cook gently for 1 minute, stirring. Remove pan from the heat and gradually stir in the milk. Bring to the boil slowly and continue to cook, stirring, until the sauce thickens. Simmer for a further 2–3 minutes. Add the cheese and seasoning.

3. Fill the pancakes with the bacon filling and roll or fold up. Place side by side in a ovenproof dish and spoon over the cheese sauce.

4. Heat in the oven at 180°C (350°F) mark 4 for 25–30 minutes. Serve garnished with parsley.

Serves 4

CINNAMON APPLE PANCAKES

125 g (4 oz) fresh breadcrumbs

75 g (3 oz) English butter

grated rind and juice of 1 lemon

700 g (1½ lb) cooking apples, peeled and sliced

50 g (2 oz) caster sugar

5 ml (1 level tsp) ground cinnamon

8 pancakes (see opposite)

icing sugar

1. Fry the breadcrumbs in 50 g (2 oz) butter until golden, stirring.

2. Place the remaining butter, lemon rind and juice, apples, sugar and cinnamon in saucepan. Cover and cook to a purée, then add breadcrumbs.

3. Divide the mixture between the pancakes and roll up. Place in an ovenproof dish. Cover with foil and heat in the oven at 180°C (350°F) mark 4 for about 25 minutes. Serve dusted with sifted icing sugar.

Serves 4

NOVELTY CAKES AND BISCUITS
ANIMAL BUTTER BISCUITS

225 g (8 oz) English butter

125 g (4 oz) caster sugar

275 g (10 oz) flour

50 g (2 oz) fine semolina

currants, cocktail sticks, white glacé icing (see page 265) and about 12 small apples to decorate

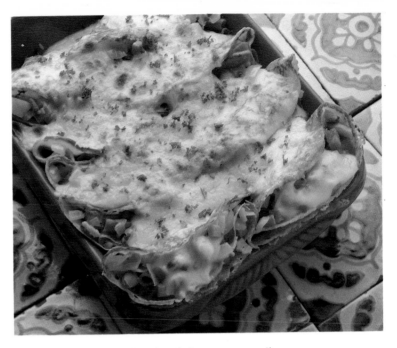

1. Beat the butter well in a bowl, then gradually work in the sugar. Stir in the flour and semolina until well mixed, then knead.

2. Roll out on a lightly floured work surface, half at a time, to a 0.5 cm (¼ inch) thickness. Stamp out animal shapes. If the mixture sticks to the surface, roll out between pieces of non-stick paper.

3. Lift the animals on to baking sheets and press currants into the heads for eyes. Slide cocktail sticks into the bodies of the animals from the base.

4. Bake in the oven at 180°C (350°F) mark 4 for 15–20 minutes; cool on wire racks.

5. Using a fine nozzle, pipe the children's names across the animals with the icing. Make a small hole in the tops of the apples and push in the biscuit sticks.

Makes about 12

Above:
BACON AND MUSTARD PANCAKES
Filled with boiled bacon and topped with a delicious savoury sauce, these substantial pancakes are a quick and tasty family meal.

Below:
ANIMAL BUTTER BISCUITS
Novelty biscuits are fun to eat and are ideal place markers for a children's party. A cocktail stick is slipped into each biscuit before baking. The finished iced biscuits are then pushed into crisp shiny apples for support.

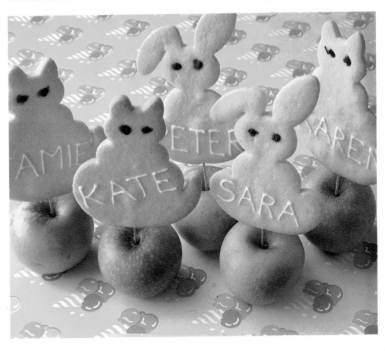

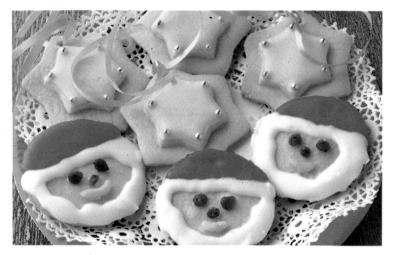

rounds. Make a hole with a skewer about 0.5 cm ($\frac{1}{4}$ inch) from the edge; bake and cool. Use thick red glacé icing to make the hat and white to make the beard. Use marzipan for the nose and mouth and currants for the eyes. Attach these with a blob of white icing. When dry, hang up with ribbon.
Makes about 18

Above:
CHRISTMAS BISCUITS
These delicious biscuits add a colourful note to children's Christmas party fare. The star biscuits twinkle with silver balls and are threaded through with shiny ribbon. The Santas are decorated with red and white glacé icing for a bright and festive effect.

Opposite, top:
KITTEN CAKES
These mouthwatering little kittens' faces are made on a base of white icing with Smarties for eyes, jelly diamonds for ears and angelica strips for the whiskers.

Opposite, below:
EASTER CAKE
Topped with two chirpy marzipan chicks, this luscious chocolate-coated cake is an Easter treat.

Below:
HEDGEHOGS AND LADYBIRDS
Rich chocolate butter frosting and striking red-tinted marzipan are the secret of making these popular 'wild-life' cakes.

CHRISTMAS BISCUITS

125 g (4 oz) English butter, softened

50 g (2 oz) caster sugar

175 g (6 oz) flour

yellow glacé icing (see page 265), silver balls and ribbons to decorate stars

red glacé icing (see page 265), white glacé icing (see page 265), bought marzipan, currants and ribbon to decorate Santa faces

1. Whisk the butter thoroughly in a bowl until really soft, then beat in the sugar a little at a time and finally fold in the flour. Knead lightly until smooth.
2. Roll out the dough on a floured work surface to the thickness of a 10p piece.
3. For the star: using star cutters, cut eight 6.5-cm (2$\frac{1}{2}$-inch) stars and eight 2.5-cm (1-inch) stars. Place a small star on top of a large one and, using a skewer, make a hole in the centre of one of the outer points of each biscuit. Bake in the oven at 150°C (300°F) mark 2 for about 25 minutes; cool. Coat the small stars with yellow glacé icing and place silver balls at smaller star points. Leave to dry before threading ribbon through the holes.
4. For Santa faces: knead and re-roll the dough and stamp out ten 5.5-cm (2$\frac{1}{4}$-inch)

HEDGEHOGS AND LADYBIRDS

50 g (2 oz) English butter

50 g (2 oz) caster sugar

1 egg, beaten

50 g (2 oz) self-raising flour

15 ml (1 tbsp) milk

chocolate butter frosting (see page 265), chocolate buttons, silver or gold balls, and dolly mixtures to decorate hedgehogs

175 g (6 oz) bought marzipan, red colouring, chocolate butter frosting (see page 265), dolly mixtures and Matchmakers to decorate ladybirds

1. Whisk the butter and sugar together thoroughly in a bowl until pale and fluffy, then gradually beat in the egg and finally fold in the flour and milk.
2. Divide the mixture between sixteen well-buttered patty tins with rounded bases. Bake in the oven at 180°C (350°F) mark 4 for about 15 minutes; cool on wire racks.
3. For the hedgehogs: cover half the cold buns with chocolate butter frosting, shaping to form a snout. Decorate with halved chocolate buttons, gold balls for the eyes and dolly mixture jellies for the snout.
4. For the ladybirds: colour the marzipan a deep pink with red colouring, roll out thinly and use to cover remaining buns. Pipe lines and spots on to the ladybirds with butter frosting and use dolly mixtures for the eyes and pieces of Matchmakers for the antennae.
Makes about 16

EASTER CAKE

175 g (6 oz) English butter

100 g (4 oz) caster sugar

2 eggs, beaten

75 g (3 oz) self-raising flour

25 g (1 oz) cocoa powder

175 g (6 oz) icing sugar

45 ml (3 level tbsp) chocolate spread

75 g (3 oz) bought marzipan, red and green colouring and jam to decorate

1. Butter and line the base of two 18-cm (7-inch) sandwich tins.
2. Whisk 100 g (4 oz) of butter and caster sugar together in a bowl until pale and fluffy. Add the eggs a little at a time, beating well after each addition. Fold in the sifted

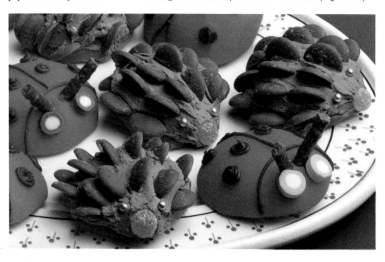

flour and cocoa. Divide the mixture between the tins and level the mixture with a knife.

3. Bake in the oven at 190°C (375°F) mark 5 for about 20 minutes, until well risen and firm to the touch; cool on a wire rack.

4. Whisk the remaining butter, add the icing sugar gradually and beat until smooth. Add the chocolate spread and beat well. Use to fill and top the cake.

5. To make the chicks, use two-thirds of the marzipan to make two large and two small balls. Press the heads to the bodies. Colour half the remaining marzipan and roll out thinly. Cut diamonds for the beaks and small wavy strips for the cocks' combs. Stick on with the jam. Use currants for eyes. Make coloured easter eggs with any remaining marzipan. Place the decorations on the cake.

Serves 6

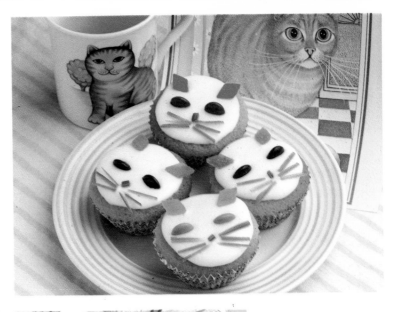

KITTEN CAKES

100 g (4 oz) English butter
100 g (4 oz) caster sugar
2 eggs, beaten
100 g (4 oz) self-raising flour
175 g (6 oz) icing sugar
Smarties, jelly diamonds and angelica to decorate

1. Place twelve paper cases in a 12-hole patty tin.

2. Whisk the butter and caster sugar together in a bowl until pale and fluffy. Add the egg, a little at a time, beating well after each addition. Fold in the flour and divide the mixture between the paper cases.

3. Bake in the oven at 190°C (375°F) mark 5 for about 20 minutes, until golden and risen; cool on a wire rack.

4. Sift the icing sugar into a bowl. Stir in about 15 ml (1 tbsp) water and mix until a smooth icing is formed. Place a little icing on each cake and spread out to cover the tops.

5. To make the kitten faces, press Smarties into the icing for the eyes; halve the jelly diamonds for the ears; cut small pieces of angelica for the nose and whiskers.

Makes 12

TRAIN BIRTHDAY CAKE

225 g (8 oz) English butter
225 g (8 oz) caster sugar
150 g (5 oz) plain chocolate, melted
4 eggs, beaten
225 g (8 oz) self-raising flour
225 g (8 oz) chocolate butter frosting (see page 265)
75 g (3 oz) bought marzipan, coloured with a few drops of brown food-colouring
100 g (4 oz) plain chocolate cake covering
Matchmakers, chocolate mini-rolls, liquorice allsorts, dolly mixtures and candles to decorate

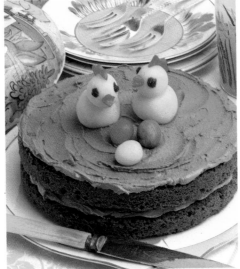

1. Butter and base-line two 20.5-cm (8-inch) round deep cake tins.

2. Whisk the butter and sugar together in a bowl until pale and fluffy. Beat in the cooled melted chocolate.

3. Gradually beat in the eggs and finally fold in the flour. Spoon the mixture into prepared cake tins. Bake in the oven at 180°C (350°F) mark 4 for 35–40 minutes; cool on a rack.

4. To assemble cake, cut a slice 3 cm (1¼ inch) wide off one side and a 7.5-cm (3-inch) round from the centre of each cake. Place cakes upside down on a work surface to make a figure of eight, butting cut sides together.

5. Cover with the butter icing and use brown-coloured marzipan strips and Matchmakers for the rails. Use the mini-roll for the front of the engine and cake 'cut-offs' coated in melted chocolate cake covering for the back of the engine and carriages. Make a tunnel from one centre piece, coat in butter icing and place on the cake. Decorate with sweets and place on Matchmaker signals. Position candles.

Serves 8–10

MAKING A TRAIN
BIRTHDAY CAKE

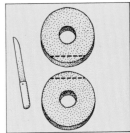

1 Remove a round from the centre of each cake and then cut a slice off the side of each cake. Keep these off-cuts for use in Step 3.

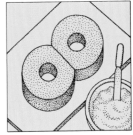

2 Place the cakes on a cake board ready for icing

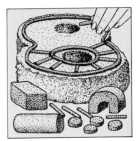

3 Assemble the cake (see the finished cake illustrated in colour on page 266).

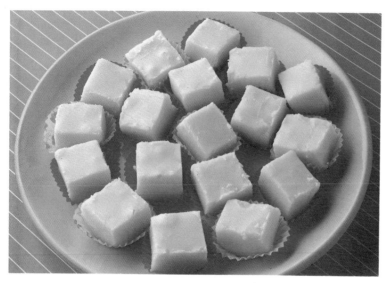

Above:
MILK FUDGE
Made with pure English butter and fresh milk, this mouthwatering fudge is a delicious treat for all the family.

Opposite, top:
BUTTERED POPCORN AND COCONUT ICE BARS
Two traditional treats, firm favourites with generations of children.

Opposite, centre:
CHOCOLATE FUDGE SLICE
Richly flavoured, this luscious slice is wickedly tempting. The recipe is on page 282.

Opposite, below:
PEANUT BUTTER COOKIES
You had better hide these crunchy buttery cookies or they will be snapped up in a moment!

FUDGES AND SWEETS

MILK FUDGE

300 ml (½ pint) milk
800 g (1¾ lb) sugar
100 g (4 oz) English butter
10 ml (2 tsp) vanilla flavouring

1. Pour the milk into a heavy-based saucepan and bring slowly to the boil. Add the sugar and butter. Heat slowly, stirring all the time, until the sugar dissolves and the butter melts. Bring to the boil, cover and boil for 2 minutes.
2. Uncover, and continue to boil steadily, stirring occasionally, for 10–15 minutes, until a little of the mixture, dropped into a cup of cold water, forms a soft ball when rolled between finger and thumb.
3. Remove from the heat. Stir in the vanilla flavouring. Leave to cool for 5 minutes.
4. Beat the fudge until it just begins to lose its gloss and is thick.
5. Transfer to a buttered 18-cm (7-inch) square tin. Mark into squares when cool. Cut up with a sharp knife when firm and set. Store in an airtight container.
Makes about 900 g (2 lb)

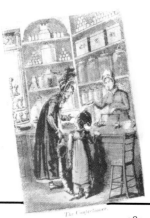

The Confectioner.

BUTTERED POPCORN

30 ml (2 tbsp) oil
75 g (3 oz) popping corn
25 g (1 oz) English butter
30 ml (2 level tbsp) golden syrup

1. Heat the oil in a large, heavy-based saucepan.
2. When the oil is really hot, put in a sparse layer of corn, cover the pan and keep shaking over a high heat. Do not remove the lid until all the popping has stopped.
3. Melt butter and the golden syrup in a saucepan over a gentle heat, add the cooked popcorn and toss in the mixture until it is evenly coated.

COCONUT ICE BARS

450 g (1 lb) sugar
150 ml (¼ pint) milk
150 g (5 oz) desiccated coconut
red food colouring

1. Dissolve the sugar in the milk in a heavy saucepan over a low heat. Bring to the boil and boil gently for about 10 minutes, until a little of the mixture, dropped into a cup of cold water, forms a soft ball when rolled between finger and thumb.
2. Remove from the heat and stir in the coconut. Pour half the mixture quickly into a buttered 20.5×15 cm (8×6 inch) tin. Add a few drops of food colouring to the second half, stir, and pour quickly over the first. Leave until half set, mark into bars and cut or break when cold. Store in an airtight tin.
Makes about 550 g (1¼ lb)

CHOCOLATE FUDGE

450 g (1 lb) sugar
150 ml (¼ pint) milk
150 g (5 oz) English butter
100 g (4 oz) plain chocolate
50 g (2 oz) clear honey

1. Place all the ingredients in a heavy-based saucepan. Stir over a low heat until dissolved. Bring to the boil and boil gently for about 10 minutes until a little of the mixture, dropped into a cup of cold water, forms a soft ball when rolled between finger and thumb. Remove from the heat, stand the pan on a cool surface for 5 minutes, then beat until thick and beginning to grain.
2. Pour into a buttered 20.5×15 cm (8×6 inch) tin, mark into squares and cut when cold. Store in an airtight container.

Variations

Fruit and Nut Fudge: Add 50 g (2 oz) of chopped nuts and 50 g (2 oz) seedless raisins to the mixture before beating.

Marshmallow Fudge: Add 225 g (8 oz) chopped marshmallows to the mixture before beating.

Makes about 700 g (1½ lb)

SWEET-TOOTH SPECIALS

BANANA SPLITS

75 g (3 oz) caster sugar

75 g (3 oz) soft brown sugar

75 g (3 oz) cocoa powder

300 ml (½ pint) milk

5 ml (1 tsp) vanilla flavouring

25 g (1 oz) English butter

4 large bananas

4 scoops of basic dairy ice cream (see page 22)

150 ml (5 fl oz) fresh double cream

25 g (1 oz) walnuts, finely chopped

4 glacé cherries

1. Put the sugars, cocoa, milk, vanilla flavouring and butter into a saucepan. Heat gently, stirring, until the sugar has dissolved. Bring to the boil and boil for 2 minutes without stirring. Cool.

2. Split the bananas lengthwise and sandwich together with ice cream. Whip the fresh cream until stiff.

3. Place the bananas on individual plates and top each with whipped fresh cream. Sprinkle with nuts and put a cherry in the centre of each.

4. Serve immediately. Serve chocolate sauce separately.

Serves 4

PEANUT BUTTER COOKIES

175 g (6 oz) English butter

50 g (2 oz) peanut butter

100 g (4 oz) caster sugar

100 g (4 oz) soft brown sugar

1 egg

275 g (10 oz) flour

1.25 ml (¼ level tsp) salt

1. Mix the butters, sugars and egg together in a bowl, add the flour and salt and mix to firm dough.

2. Make into thirty-six balls. Place on buttered baking trays and flatten with a fork, making a criss-cross pattern.

3. Bake in the oven at 190°C (375°F) mark 5 for 10–12 minutes, until golden. Cool on trays. Store in an airtight container.

Makes 36

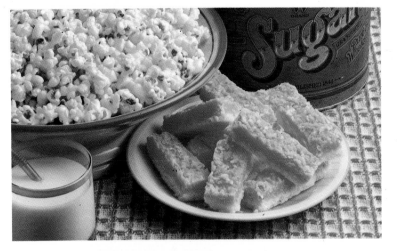

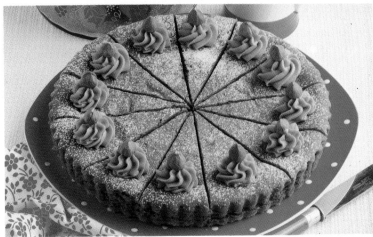

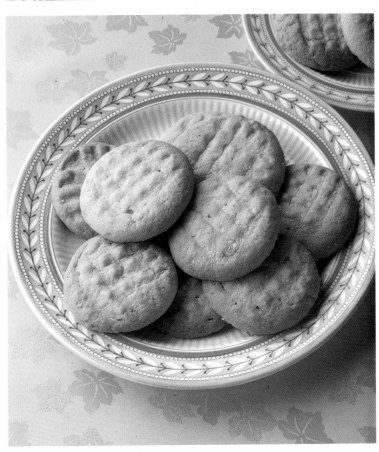

2. Sprinkle the gelatine on 45 ml (3 tbsp) warm water in a bowl, and stir until dissolved. Stir into the chocolate mixture. Whip the fresh cream until softly stiff and fold into the mixture. Spoon the mixture into two 600-ml (1-pint) dampened rabbit moulds.

3. Melt the butter and syrup in a saucepan, stir in the rice crispies, then spread over the chocolate mixture in the moulds. Refrigerate until set. Loosen the edges of the moulds. Dip into hot water and turn out on to a serving plate.

Serves 6–8

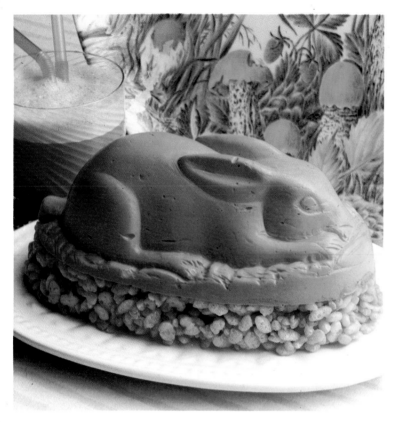

Above:
CHOCOLATE BOBTAILS
Moulds in the shape of a rabbit are essential for these unusual chocolate sweets.

Below:
WALNUT WAFFLES
Give your family a traditional treat and try these crisp, light waffles made extra good with chopped walnuts and a hint of ginger. Let them help themselves to maple syrup or honey as the delectable finishing touch.

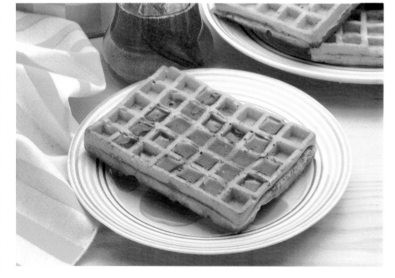

CHOCOLATE BOBTAILS

175 g (6 oz) full fat soft cheese
50 g (2 oz) caster sugar
few drops of vanilla flavouring (optional)
100 g (4 oz) plain chocolate, melted
15 g (½ oz) gelatine
300 ml (10 fl oz) fresh double cream
25 g (1 oz) English butter
30 ml (2 tbsp) golden syrup
65 g (2½ oz) rice crispies

1. Whisk the cheese and sugar together in a bowl until soft, then add the vanilla flavouring. Fold the melted chocolate into the cheese mixture.

CHOCOLATE FUDGE SLICE

175 g (6 oz) English butter
100 g (4 oz) digestive biscuits, crushed
100 g (4 oz) brown sugar
150 g (5 oz) plain flour
25 g (1 oz) cocoa powder
150 ml (¼ pint) milk

1. Melt 50 g (2 oz) butter in a saucepan. Add the biscuit crumbs and mix together. Turn into a 20.5-cm (8-inch) sandwich tin or flan dish and chill.

2. Beat together the remaining butter and sugar until smooth. Add the flour and cocoa. Stir in the milk and spread the mixture over the crumb base.

3. Bake in the oven at 190°C (375°F) mark 5 for 35–40 minutes. Allow to cool before serving. Serve plain with fresh or canned fruit and fresh cream or dredge with icing sugar and decorate with coffee-flavoured butter cream and hazelnuts.

Makes 12 *(illustration on page 281)*

PEPPERMINT FINGERS

50 g (2 oz) English butter
50 g (2 oz) caster sugar
100 g (4 oz) flour
175 g (6 oz) icing sugar
2.5 ml (½ level tsp) peppermint flavouring
175 g (6 oz) plain chocolate

1. Whisk the butter and sugar together until pale and fluffy, then add the flour. Knead to a smooth dough. Press into a small swiss roll tin, prick all over and bake in the oven at 180°C (350°F) mark 4 for 10–15 minutes, until golden brown. Leave until cool.

2. Put the icing sugar into a basin and mix with 15–30 ml (1–2 tbsp) water; add the peppermint flavouring and spread the topping on the shortbread base. Leave until cold.

3. Melt the chocolate in a basin over a pan of hot water and spread over the icing. When cold cut into fingers.

Makes 16–18

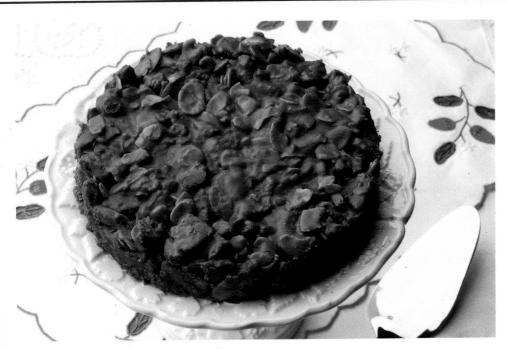

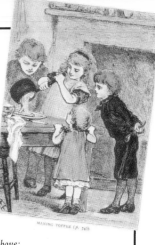

Above:
Making toffee is a cookery session popular with every generation of children.

Cooking is fun for children, as well as gradually giving them an appreciation of good food, but safety in the kitchen from burns, cuts and scalds is of paramount importance.

CHOCOLATE BISCUIT CAKE

100 g (4 oz) plain chocolate
15 ml (1 level tbsp) golden syrup
100 g (4 oz) English butter
30 ml (2 tbsp) fresh double cream
125 g (4 oz) digestive biscuits, broken up
25 g (1 oz) raisins (optional)
25 g (1 oz) glacé cherries, halved
50 g (2 oz) flaked almonds, toasted

1. Butter a loose-bottomed 15–18-cm (6–7-inch) tin or ring.
2. Break the chocolate into pieces and place in a bowl over a pan of hot (not boiling) water. Add the syrup, butter and cream.
3. When the chocolate and butter have melted, remove the pan from the heat and cool slightly.
4. Mix the biscuits, fruit and nuts into the chocolate mixture.
5. Turn the mixture into the prepared tin, lightly level the top, then chill for at least 1 hour before serving.

Serves 8

CRISPY BARS

100 g (4 oz) English butter
100 g (4 oz) marshmallows
100 g (4 oz) caramel toffee
100 g (4 oz) rice crispies

1. Melt the butter, marshmallows and toffee together in a saucepan and boil for 1–2 minutes.
2. Remove from the heat and fold in the rice crispies.
3. Spread into a buttered swiss roll tin and leave to set. Cut into squares.

Makes 12

WALNUT WAFFLES

225 g (8 oz) flour
15 ml (1 level tbsp) baking powder
30 ml (2 level tbsp) caster sugar
5 ml (1 level tsp) salt
5 ml (1 level tsp) ground ginger
3 eggs, separated
300 ml (½ pint) milk
60 ml (4 tbsp) English butter, melted
50 g (2 oz) walnuts, chopped

1. Put the flour, baking powder, sugar, salt and ginger in a mixing bowl. Whisk in the egg yolks, milk and melted butter. Add the walnuts.
2. Just before cooking, stiffly whisk the egg whites and gently fold into the batter.
3. Heat a little oil in a 7.5×10 cm (3×4 inch) waffle iron. Spoon in a little batter and cook for about 1 minute on each side. Keep hot. Repeat until all the batter is used up. Serve hot.

Makes 10

Left:
CHOCOLATE BISCUIT CAKE
Children love this crunchy chocolate cake which is quick to make and scrumptious to eat.

Below:
PEPPERMINT FINGERS
Zesty peppermint icing sandwiched between a shortbread base and a dark chocolate topping, make these a tea-time treat with a difference.

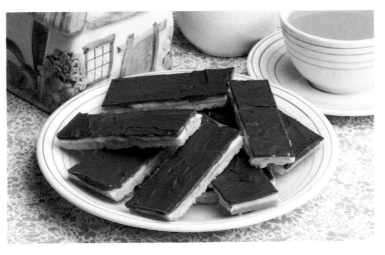

BLACK MAGIC

100 g (4 oz) flour
10 ml (2 level tsp) baking powder
40 g (1½ oz) cocoa powder
150 g (5 oz) sugar
5 ml (1 tsp) vanilla flavouring
150 ml (5 fl oz) fresh single cream
75 g (3 oz) demerara sugar

1. Sift the flour with the baking powder and 30 ml (2 level tbsp) cocoa into a bowl. Stir in the sugar, vanilla flavouring and fresh cream, then beat until smooth. Spread the mixture into a buttered 1.3-litre (2¼-pint) ovenproof dish.
2. Mix the demerara sugar with the remaining cocoa and sprinkle it over the mixture in the dish.
3. Pour 350 ml (12 fl oz) boiling water all over the pudding then bake in the oven at 180°C (350°F) mark 4 for about 50 minutes, until risen and the sponge mixture (which will have come to the top) feels lightly firm to the touch.
4. Turn out and serve with whipped fresh cream or dairy ice cream.

Serves 6

Below, clockwise from top:
CHOCOLATE
MILKSHAKE, BANANA
FLIP AND NUTTY
FRUIT MILKSHAKE
Three delicious thirst-quenchers
whizzed up in a moment with
fresh, cool milk.

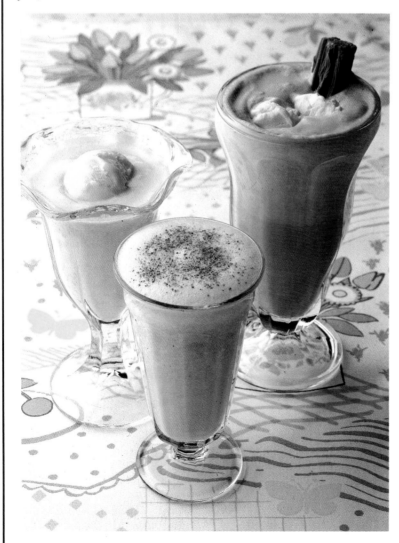

SHAKES AND FLOATS

Honey and Grapefruit Milkshake: Whisk together 568 ml (1 pint) cool fresh milk, 600 ml (1 pint) grapefruit juice, 30 ml (2 tbsp) clear honey and one egg white until thick and frothy. Pour into tall glasses over crushed ice and serve immediately.

Serves 6–8

Chocolate Milkshake: Dissolve 15 ml (3 tsp) drinking chocolate in a little hot water. Cool. Stir in 300 ml (½ pint) cool fresh milk and place 15 ml (1 level tbsp) dairy vanilla ice cream on top. Serve with a chocolate flake bar.

Serves 2

Strawberry Milkshake: Follow the recipe for chocolate milkshake. Use 30 ml (2 level tbsp) strawberry jam instead of the drinking chocolate and omit the chocolate bar.

Serves 2

Nutty Fruit Milkshake: Put 300 ml (½ pint) cool fresh milk, one banana, peeled and sliced and 142 g (5 oz) hazelnut yogurt in a blender and switch on for 1 minute. Pour into chilled glasses, top with 30 ml (2 level tbsp) dairy vanilla ice cream and serve immediately.

Serves 2

Banana Flip: Whisk together 300 ml (½ pint) cool fresh milk, one small banana, peeled and sliced and 15 ml (1 level tbsp) sugar until thick and frothy. Pour into chilled glasses over crushed ice, sprinkle with a little nutmeg and serve immediately.

Serves 4

Choco Mint Shake: Put 568 ml (1 pint) cool fresh milk and 4–8 drops peppermint essence in a blender and switch on for 10 seconds. Add 60 ml (4 level tbsp) dairy chocolate ice cream and blend for a further 30–40 seconds until smooth. Pour into chilled glasses and sprinkle with 50 g (2 oz) grated chocolate. Serve immediately.

Serves 4

Maraschino Float: Put 100 g (4 oz) maraschino cherries with their syrup, 568 ml (1 pint) cool fresh milk and 60 ml (4 level tbsp) dairy vanilla ice cream in a blender and switch on for 25–30 seconds. Pour into chilled glasses, top each with a spoonful of dairy vanilla ice cream, decorate with a cherry and serve immediately.

Serves 4

Pineapple Shake: Put 300 ml (½ pint) cool fresh milk and 142 g (5 oz) pineapple yogurt in a blender and switch on for 30 seconds. Pour into tall chilled glasses. Top with 60 ml (4 level tbsp) dairy vanilla ice cream and serve immediately.

Serves 2